NURSING

GARLAND REFERENCE LIBRARY
OF SOCIAL SCIENCE
(VOL. 66)

NURSING
A Historical Bibliography

Bonnie Bullough
Vern L. Bullough
Barrett Elcano

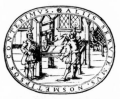

GARLAND PUBLISHING, INC. • NEW YORK & LONDON
1981

Library of Congress Cataloging in Publication Data

Bullough, Bonnie.
   Nursing, a historical bibliography.

   (Garland reference library of social science ;
v. 66)
   Includes index.
   1. Nursing—History—Bibliography. I. Bullough,
Vern L. II. Elcano, Barrett. III. Title.
IV. Series. [DNLM: 1. History of nursing—Bibliog-
raphy. ZWY 11.1 B938n]
Z6675.N7B84 [RT31]   016.61073'09   80-836
ISBN 0-8240-9511-1   AACR2

Printed on acid-free, 250-year-life paper
Manufactured in the United States of America

CONTENTS

INTRODUCTION

This bibliography brings together references pertinent to the history of nursing, something which has never been done before. We were motivated to do this for several reasons: two of the authors are nurses, and the other is a librarian interested in medical and scientific reference materials. We are concerned because most historical and contemporary bibliographies in the medical sciences have ignored nursing. More upsetting to us, many of the bibliographies concentrating on women in history have also ignored nursing, even though nursing has been primarily a women's profession since the time of Florence Nightingale.

We were also concerned with a number of proposed research projects that have come to our attention in recent years. To us, such projects propose to do research on topics that have already been well researched and, in the process, ignore others on which almost nothing has been done. When we queried the authors of the proposed research, we often found that they were totally unaware of what had gone before, and actually thought they were breaking new ground.

A bibliography such as this can also serve as a measuring stick, a method of assessing the nature of research into nursing history. As the number of doctoral dissertations included in this book indicates, there has been a general upgrading of historical research in nursing in the past few years. The bibliography also marks changes in nursing interest. Much of the early historical research which concentrated upon individual nursing leaders was hortatory rather than critical, while the more recent research has turned to the social and economic forces which influence nursing. Although recent research has been more analytical, few quantitative studies have as yet been done. It is also evident from this bibliography that the dominant force in nursing history has been the English-speaking countries, particularly the United States and Great Britain but also Canada, Australia, and South Africa. In recent years Japanese nurses have contributed to nursing research in significant numbers, but nursing literature of any type, as of this writing, is still heavily influenced by those writing in English.

In the process of gathering our materials we have tried to be inclusive rather than exclusive: for example, we have included materials—such as the various brief accounts of Florence Nightingale—which copy from each other without adding additional information or giving any sophisticated analysis. This kind of superficial reporting, however, is part of the history of nursing. As nurses and those who are interested in the history of nursing turn to more sophisticated analysis, the need to be reminded from generation to generation of Florence Nightingale becomes an important historical phenomenon in its own right.

On the other hand, nurses such as Margaret Sanger and Lillian Wald have been comparatively neglected in the official nursing literature. There are, however, a large number of biographical and other studies about these women by writers who were not interested in their nursing background. In these and other cases, we have included only the most well-known studies or a representative sample of the biographies that are available. We have, however, tried to include all material which mentions specifically the nursing aspects of their careers.

This raises the question of what criteria we employed to select the nonnursing materials which have been included. The basis for our selection is the basic bibliography used in writing our own history of nursing; the latest edition is called *The Care of the Sick* (New York: Neale Watson, Prodist Press, 1978). Over the years we have read a vast number of works, collected a number of others for our personal library, and tried to build up a comprehensive bibliography. Obviously, many of these works have only passing references to nursing; these were excluded except where the references were key statements. For those references to ancient and medieval medical writing which we have included scattered statements furnish the basis for most of our knowledge. We estimate that approximately 2500 of the titles in this work have been read by at least one compiler. This leaves an equal number not read but which have been derived from other sources. To assure the accuracy of our citations, we researched more than half of the remaining titles in journals or in libraries. This leaves slightly over 1000 titles that have not been read or examined. We have tried to include only those articles and books which appeared in at least two other bibliographies and seemed neither to derive from each other nor to be derived from a common source. Works in French, German, Spanish, and Italian were personally examined; works in languages other than these, unless there was an English extract, depend upon other references. Some of the English-language titles also depend upon other sources since the journals in which they appeared were not available to us. In general, we tried to be as conservative as possible and eliminated many more titles than we included because we could not verify them from two independent sources.

Only major collections of primary source documents are listed. No attempt was made to inventory the unpublished documents in the archives of nursing schools, hospitals, and nursing organizations. While these sources undoubtedly represent a goldmine of resource materials, they still await scrutiny by the historian and publicity about their existence. Our hope is that any person who wants to find a research topic in the history of nursing can find one through this bibliography. A tremendous amount of research needs to be done. Many of the American states, for example, lack even an informal history while whole areas of the world have been ignored. Moreover, in spite of the emphasis on biographies by early writers on nursing, many important individuals in the recent history of nursing have been neglected.

One of the important uses of a bibliography such as this is to indicate the progress of nursing in the past few decades. This is particularly significant since, in our view, nursing represents the best example of a women's profession trying to establish itself in a world dominated by men. The history of nursing is an ongoing testimony to the inequalities that have existed between the sexes. It is worth noting, however, that men are entering nursing in greater numbers than ever before (including one of the compilers of the bibliography). This work also attempts to demonstrate to those militant feminists who have scorned nursing that much can be learned about the status and position of women in society by studying the profession.

Thanks are due to the various student assistants who helped check citations, arranged our bibliographical cards, and did the preliminary typing: Michell Klees, Donna Krug, Bobbette Cloninger, Jane Dahlroth, Marta Gutierrez, and Delfina Carrillo. The final typing was done by Joy Thornbury. Robert Bullough worked on the index. Special thanks are also due to Lawrence Davidow of Garland Publishing.

A NOTE ON KEEPING CURRENT

One of the difficulties with bibliographies of this sort is that they soon become outdated. We do not think this will be the case for this bibliography: since the 1960s nursing has increasingly come to be included in regularly published bibliographies such as those from the Wellcome Medical Historical Museum and the National Library of Medicine. This bibliography ensures historical coverage of the important relevant literature published through 1978; and it can easily be updated through the indexes and bibliograhies listed in Section 1.

INDEX TO ABBREVIATED TITLES

In general we have followed the abbreviations in the annual *Bibliography of the History of Medicine* issued by the National Library of Medicine and published by the U.S. Department of Health, Education, and Welfare. The abbreviations, journals, and collections used in this bibliography are cited below.

Ann Assoc Coll Surg Eng: Annals of the Association of Colleges of Surgery (England)
Ann Int Med: Annals of Internal Medicine
Ann Medi Hist: Annals of Medical History
Ann Roy Coll Surg: Annals of the Royal College of Surgeons
Ann San Pub Roma: Annali della Sanita Publica
ANPHI Papers: Academy of Nursing of the Philippines (College of Nursing, Univ. of Philippines)
AORNJ: American Association of Operating Room Nurses' Journal
Archi Gesch d Med: Archiv für Geschichte der Medizin (later called *Sudhoffs Archiv für Geschichte der Medizin*)
Arch Intern Med: Archives of Internal Medicine (Chicago)
Ariz Med: Arizona Medicine (Phoenix)
Ariz Pub Hlth News: Arizona Public Health News
Arkansas Gazette Mag: Arkansas Gazette Magazine
Asclepio: Asclepio
Atlan: Atlantic Monthly
Atlanta Med Surg J: Atlanta Medical and Surgical Journal
Aust Nurs J: Australian Nurses' Journal (earlier *Australasian Nurses' Journal*)

Berl Med: Berliner Medizin
Bol Col Prof Enferm PR: Boletín Colegio Professional de Enfermeras PR
Bost Med & Surg J: Boston Medical and Surgical Journal
Bost M Q: Boston Medical Quarterly
Brit J Nurs: British Journal of Nursing
Brit Med J: British Medical Journal
Bruxelles Med: Bruxelles Medical
Bull Am Acad Med or *Bull Acad Med: Bulletin of the American Academy of Medicine*
Bull Am Coll Nurs-Mid: Bulletin of the American College of Nurse Midwives
Bull Am Hosp Assn: Bulletin of the American Hospital Association
Bull Calif State Nurs Assn: Bulletin of the California State Nurses Association
Bull Hist Med: Bulletin of the History of Medicine
Bull Johns Hop Hos: Bulletin of the Johns Hopkins Hospital
Bull Mass Nurses Assn: Bulletin of the Massachusetts Nurses Association
Bull Med Libra Assoc: Bulletin of the Medical Library Association
Bull NY Acad Med: Bulletin of the New York Academy of Medicine
Bull Pan Am Union: Bulletin of the Pan American Union
Bull Texas Nurs Assoc: Bulletin of the Texas Nurses Association

Cah Nurs: Cahiers du Nursing
Calif Nurs: California Nurse
Canad Nurs: Canadian Nurse
Cana J Pub Hlth: Canadian Journal of Public Health
Can J Psy Nurs: Canadian Journal of Psychiatric Nursing
Can Med Assn J: Canadian Medical Association Journal
Caridad Cien Arte: Caridad Ciencia y Arte
Cath Hist Soc Record: Catholic Historical Society Record
Cath Nurs: Catholic Nurse
Cen Afr J Med: Central African Journal of Medicine

Centaurus: Centaurus
Century: Century Magazine
Char and Commons: Charities and the Commons
Charities: Charities, same as *Charities* and the *Commons*
Charities Review: Same as *Charities* and the *Commons.* Ultimately
    the journal was known as *Survey*
Charlotte Med J: Charlotte Medical Journal
Chautauquan: Chautauquan
Chic Med Rec: Chicago Medical Record
Chinese Med J: Chinese Medical Journal
Christ Nurs: Christian Nurse
Ciba Symp: Ciba Symposium
*CICIA Med Nouvelles: Comité International Catholic des Infirmières
    et Assistantes Medico Nouvelles*
Clin Ex: Clinical Excerpts
CNA Bulletin: California Nursing Association Bulletin
Colliers: Colliers Magazine
Colorado Nurse: Colorado Nurse
Columbia Univ Columns: Columbia University Columns
Compr Nurs Q: Comprehensive Nursing Quarterly (Japan)
Conn Med: Connecticut Medicine
Cont Educ Nur: Continuing Education in Nursing, also *Journal of
    Continuing Education in Nursing*
Contemp: Contemporary
Cur Biog: Current Biography
Cur Swed: Current Swedish Periodicals (*Svensk Tidskriftsfoertechning*)

DAB: Dictionary of American Biography
Delineator: Delineator
Del State Med J: Delaware State Medical Journal
Deutsche Hebamme Z: Deutsche Hebammen Zeitschrift (also *Allgemeine
    Deutsche Hebammenzeitung*)
Deutsche Kranken Z: Deutsche Krankenpflege-Zeitschrift
Deutsche Swchwest: Deutsche Schwester Zeitung
Deutsch Gesundh: Deutsche Gesundheitswesen
Deutsch Med Wchnsch: Deutsche Medizinische Wochcnschrift
Dimens Hlth Serv: Dimensions of Health Service
Dis Nerv Syst: Diseases of the Nervous System
Dist Nurs: District Nursing
DNB: Dictionary of National Biography
Domin N Ass News: Dominican Nurses Association Newsletter

Enfermeras: Enfermeras (Colegio Nacional de Enfermeras)
Epheta: Epheta
Epworth: Epworth
Ethos: Ethos

Fam Cord: Family Coordinator
Fam Plan Pop Rep: Family Planning/Population Reporter
Fed Reg: Federal Register
Feldsher Akush: Feldsher i a Kusherka
Filipino J of Nurs: Filipino Journal of Nursing
Fla N: Florida Nurse
FNIB: Fédération Nationale des Infirmières Belges
Forum: Forum

Frontiers: Frontiers
Front Nurs Ser Q Bul: Frontier Nursing Service Quarterly Bulletin

Garde-Malade Canad-Franc: Garde-Malade Canadienne Française
Gaz Clin: Gazzetta Clinica
G Batt Virol Immun: Giorno di Batteriologia e Immunologia
Geo N: Georgia Nursing
George Washington Law Review: George Washington Law Review
Glasgow Med J: Glasgow Medical Journal
Good Housekeeping: Good Housekeeping
Gray's Hosp Rep: Gray's Hospital Reports
Guy's Hosp Rep: Guy's Hospital Reports

Hadassah Newsletter: Hadassah Newsletter
Harpers: Harpers Monthly
Helferin d Arztes: Die Helferin des Arztes
Hellen Adelphe: Hellen Adelphe
High Educ: Higher Education
Hippokrates: Hippokrates
Hist Med: History of Medicine
Hist Recrd: See Catholic Historical Society Record
Hjelp: Hjelpepleieren (Norway)
Hjuk: Hjukurun (Icelandic)
Hlth Lect: Health Lectures
Hlth Serv Rep: Health Services Reports
Hlth Vis: Health Visitor
Hoja Tisiol: Hoja Tisiologica
Hong Kong Nurs J: Hong Kong Nursing Journal
Hosp: Hospitals
Hosp Mgmt: Hospital Management
Hosp Prog: Hospital Progress
Hosp Top: Hospital Topics
Ht & Lung: Heart and Lung: Journal of Critical Care
Human Org: Human Organization
Hygeia: Hygeia

ICN: International Council of Nurses
Ill Med J: Illinois Medical Journal
Illus Monats d'art e Polytech: Illustrirte Monatsschrift des arzt-
    lichen Polytechnik
Image: Image (Sigma Theta Tau National Honor Society of Nursing)
Imprint: Imprint
Indian J His Med: Indian Journal of the History of Medicine
Ind Med J: Indiana Medical Journal
Ind Woman: Indiana Woman (Indiana Weekly)
Infirm Can: Infirmiere Canadienne
Int Asp Nurs Educ: International Aspects of Nursing Education
Int J Hlth Serv: International Journal of Health Services
Int J Nurs Studies: International Journal of Nursing Studies
Int Nurs Bull: International Nursing Bulletin
Int Nurs Rev: International Nursing Review
Ir Nurs J: Irish Nurses Journal
Ir Nurs News: Irish Nursing News

J Adv Nurs: *Journal of Advanced Nursing*
JAMA: *Journal of the American Medical Association*
J Am Assoc Nurs Anes: *Journal of the American Association of Nurse Anesthetists*
J A Med W A: *Journal of the American Medical Women's Association*
Jamaica Nurs: *Jamaican Nurse*
Jap J Nurs Art: *Japanese Journal of Nursing Arts* (*Kango Gijutsu*) (Japan)
Jap J Nurs Ed: *Japanese Journal or Nursing Education* (*Kango Kyoku*) (Japan)
Jap J Nurs Res: *Japanese Journal of Nursing Research* (*Kango Kenkyu*) (Japan)
J Asian Afr Stud: *Journal of Asian and African Studies*
J Bone Jt Surg: *Journal of Bone and Joint Surgery*
J Chris M A: *Journal of the Christian Medical Association* (India)
J Cont Ed Nurs: *Journal of Continuing Education in Nursing*
J Ed: *Journal of Education*
JEN: *Journal of Emergency Nursing*
JGN: *Journal of Gerontological Nursing*
J Hist Med: *Journal of the History of Medicine and Allied Sciences*
J Ind Med Assoc: *Journal of the Indian Medical Association*
J Int Col Surg: *Journal of International College of Surgeons* (now called *International Surgery*)
J M Assn Ala: *Journal of the Medical Association of the State of Alabama*
J Med Ed: *Journal of Medical Education*
J Men Sci: *Journal of Mental Science*
J Mich Med S: *Journal of the Michigan Medical Society*
J Neurosurg Nurs: *Journal of Neurosurgical Nursing*
J Nurs: *Journal of Nursing* (*Hu Li Tsu Chih*) (Chinese)
J Nurs Admin: *Journal of Nursing Administration*
J Nurs Care: *Journal of Nursing Care*
J Nurs Educ: *Journal of Nursing Education*
J Nurs Mid: *Journal of Nurse-Midwifery*
J NY State Nurs Ass: *Journal of the New York State Nurses Association*
J Ob Dis Wom & Chil: *Journal of Obstetrics and the Diseases of Women and Children*
J Ob Gyn Brit: *Journal of Obstetrics and Gynecology of the British Empire*
J Obs Gyn: *Journal of Obstetrics and Gynecology*
JOGN Nursing: *Journal of Obstetric Gynecologic and Neonatal Nursing*
Johns Hop Nursing Alum Mag: *Johns Hopkins Hospital School of Nursing Alumni Magazine*
J Prac Nurs: *Journal of Practical Nursing*
J Psychi Nurs: *Journal of Psychiatric Nursing and Mental Health Services*
J Roy Army Med Cps: *Journal of the Royal Army Medical Corps*
J Roy Brit Nurs: *Journal of the Royal British Nurses' Association*
J Roy Inst Pub Hlth: *Journal of the Royal Institute of Public Health and Hygiene*
J Roy San Institute: *Journal of the Royal Sanitary Institute*
J Sch Hlth: *Journal of School Health*
J Soc His: *Journal of Social History*
J United Reformed Church His Soc: *Journal of the United Reformed Church Historical Society* (London)
J West Aust Nurs: *Journal of the West Australian Nurses*

Kango: Kango/Nursing
Kango G: Kango Gijutsu: Japanese Journal of Nursing Arts
Kango Ken: Kango Kenkyu: Japanese Journal of Nursing Research
Kango Kyo: Kango Kyoku: Japanese Journal of Nursing Education
Kansas Nurse: Kansas Nurse
Keats-Shelly J: Keats-Shelley Journal
Ken N A News: Kentucky Nurses Association Newsletter
Kenya Nurs J: Kenya Nursing Journal
Klin Med: Klinische Medizin
Kor Nurs: Korean Nurse: Taehan Kanho
Krankend: Krankendienst
Krankenpfl: Krankenpflege
Krankensch: Krankenschwester (Vienna)

Labor La J: Labor Law Journal
Ladies Home J: Ladies Home Journal
Lamp: Lamp (New South Wales)
Lancet: Lancet
Lit Dig: Literary Digest
London QR: London Quarterly Review
Long Term C: Long Term Care
*Louisville Mon J M & S: Louisville Monthly Journal of Medicine and
    Surgery*
L R C Societies: League of Red Cross Societies Monthly Bulletin

Maatschap: Maatschappelijke Gezondheidszorg
Mag Traumatol Orthrop: Magyar Traumatologia Orthopaedia
Maine Nurs: Maine Nurse
Manchest Nurs Times: Manchester Nursing Times
Maryl Nurs: Maryland Nurse   `
Mary Med J: Maryland Medical Journal
Mat-Child Nurs J: Maternal-Child Nursing Journal
Matern Child Wel: Maternal and Child Welfare Survey
*Med & Chirurg Fa: Medical and Chirurgical Faculty of Maryland
    Bulletin*
Med Bul U.S. Army: Medical Bulletin of the U.S. Army
Med Care: Medical Care
Med His: Medical History (London)
Med J Aust: Medical Journal of Australia
Med Lib & His J: Medical Library and Historical Journal
Med Mag: Medical Magazine (London)
Med Prog: Medical Progress
Med Rec: Medical Record
Med Rev Mex: Medicina Revista Mexicana
Med Sestra: Meditsinskala Sestra
Med Soc: Medicina Sociale (Turin)
Med Surg Rep: Medical and Surgical Reports
Med Tech Bul: Medical Technicians Bulletin
M.D. Med News Mag: M.D. Medical News Magazine
Mich Alum: Michigan Alumnus (World of Learning)
Mich Med Bul: Michigan University Medical Center Medical Bulletin
Mich Nurs: Michigan Nurse
Mid Hlth Visit: Midwife and Health Visitor (various other titles
    added, such as *and Community Nurse*)
Mid Chron & Nurs Notes: Midwives Chronicle and Nursing Notes

Mid Folklore: Mid South Folklore
Mil Med: Military Medicine
Mil Mem F Q: Milbank Memorial Fund Quarterly
Mil Surg: Military Surgery
Minerva Med: Minerva Medica
Minn Med: Minnesota Medicine
Minn Nurs Accent: Minnesota Nursing Accent
Minn Reg Nurs: Minnesota Registered Nurse
Mis His Rev: Missouri Historical Review
Mis Med: Missouri Medicine
Mis Nurs: Missouri Nurse
Miss Doc: Mississippi Doctor
Mission Rev: Missionary Review (Missionary Review of the World)
Miss RN: Mississippi RN
Mod Hlth Care: Modern Health Care
Mod Hosp: Modern Hospital
Mon Cyc & Med Bul: Monthly Cyclopedia and Medical Bulletin
Monthly Bull Ind Bd of Hlth: Monthly Bulletin of the Indiana Board
    of Health
MS Mag: MS Magazine
Munca Sanit: Municipal Sanitation (Waste Engineering)
Münch Med Wschr: Munchener Medizinische Wochenschrift

Nat Bus: National Business Woman
NAT News: National Association of Theatre Nurses News
NCAB: National Cyclopedia of American Biography
Neb Nurs: Nebraska Nurse
Ned T Geneesk: Nederlandschtijdschrift voor Geneeskunde
New England J Med: New England Journal of Medicine
New Hamp Nurs N: New Hampshire Nursing News
New Rep: New Republic
New Stsm & Nat: New Statesman and Nation
News Lett Florence N Int Nurs Assoc: News Letter Florence Nightin-
    gale International Nurses Association
New York Med J: New York Medical Journal
New Zeal Nurs J: New Zealand Nursing Journal (Kaitiaki)
Niger Nurs: Nigerian Nurse
19th Cent: 19th Century
N J Nurs: New Jersey Nurse
NLN News: National League for Nursing News
N M Nurs: New Mexico Nurse
North Am R: North American Review
Northwest Univ Med School Bull: Northwestern University Medical
    School Bulletin
Nosok: Nosokomeion
N S Med Bull: Nova Scotia Medical Bulletin
Nurs: Nursing/Kango (Japanese)
Nurs Ad Q: Nursing Administration Quarterly
Nursc: Nurscene
Nurs Cl N A: Nursing Clinics of North America
Nurs Dim: Nursing Dimensions
Nurs Ed: Nurse Educator
Nurs Ed Bull: Nursing Education Bulletin
Nurs Forum: Nursing Forum
Nurs Israel: Nurse in Israel/Haachot Be Israel

Nurs J India: Nursing Journal of India (English and Hindi)
Nurs J Pac Cst: Nursing Journal of the Pacific Coast
Nurs J Singapore: Nursing Journal of Singapore/Berita Jukurawat
Nurs Lamp: Nurses Lamp
Nurs Mirror: Nursing Mirror and Midwives Journal (title varies, also
    Nursing Mirror)
Nurs News: Nursing News (Connecticut)
Nurs Out: Nursing Outlook
Nurs Papers: Nursing Papers: Perspectives on Nursing
Nurs Pract: Nurse Practitioner
Nurs Rec: Nursing Record (title varies, also *Nursing Record and
    Hospital World*)
Nurs Res: Nursing Research
Nurs Res Rep: Nursing Research Reports
Nurs Standard: Nursing Standard (Royal College of Nursing)
Nurs Times: Nursing Times
Nurs World: Nursing World
N Y State J M: New York State Journal of Medicine
N Y State Nurs Assn J: New York State Nurses Association Journal
N Y State Nurs Assn R: New York State Nurses Association Report
N Y Times: New York Times
N Y Times Mag: New York Times Magazine

Oberlau Fors: Oberlausitzer Forschung
Obs Gaz: Obstetric Gazette
Obs Gyn: Obstetrics and Gynecology
Occ Health Nurs: Occupational Health Nursing
Oest Hebammen Z: Oesterreichische Hebammen Zeitung
Oest Kranken: Oesterreichische Krankenpflege Zeitschrift
Oest Krankenpflege Z: Oesterreichische Krankenpflege Zeitung
Oest Schwes: Oesterreichische Schwesternzeitung
Ohio Archaeol Hist Q: Ohio Archaeological and Historical Quarterly
Ohio Nurs R: Ohio Nurses Review
Ohio St Med J: Ohio State Medical Journal
Okla Nurs: Oklahoma Nurse
Ontario J Neuro Psychiat: Ontario Journal of Neuro Psychiatry
*Ord Nurs Quebec: Order of Nurses of Quebec News and Notes/Ordre
    des Infirmières and Infirmiers du Quebec--Notes et Nouvelles*
Ore Nurs: Oregon Nurse
Orthopedic Nurs Assn: Orthopedic Nurses Association Journal
Orv Hetil: Orvosi Hetilap (Hungarian)
Orv Szle: Orvosi Szemle
Österr Schwesternztg: Österreichische Schwesternzeitung, formerly
    Krankenschwester
Österr Krankenpflegezeit: Österreichische Krankenpflege Zeitschrift

Pac Cst J Nurs: Pacific Coast Journal of Nursing
Pac Med Surg J: Pacific Medical and Surgical Journal
Peds: Pediatrics
Penn Med J: Pennsylvania Medical Journal
Penn Nurs: Pennsylvania Nurse
Perspect: Perspectives (New Jersey State Nurses' Association)
Perspect Psy Care: Perspectives in Psychiatric Care
Phi Chi Q: Phi Chi Quarterly
Philip J Nurs: Philippines Journal of Nursing

Pict Rev: Pictorial Review
Pieleg Polozna: Pielegniarka I Polozna
Point View: Point of View (United States)
Pop Sci Month: Popular Science Monthly
Prac Nurs Dig: Practical Nurses' Digest
Practitioner: Practitioner (London)
Prair Rose: Prairie Rose (North Dakota State Nurses Association)
Prens Med Ara: Prensa Medica Argentina
Presse Med: Presse Medicale
Prezegl Lek: Prezeglad Lekanski
P Rico Enferm: Puerto Rico y su Enfermera
Proc Am Cong Obs & Gyn: Proceedings of the American Congress on Obstetrics and Gynecology
Proc Am Phil Soc: Proceedings of the American Philosophical Society
Proc Inst Med Chic: Proceedings of the Institute of Medicine of Chicago
Proc Natl Conf Charities and Corrections: Proceedings of the National Conference of Charities and Corrections
Proc Roy Soc Med: Proceedings of the Royal Society of Medicine
Profes Infer: Professioni Infermiertische (Italy)
Prov Med J: Providence Medical Journal
Psychiat: Psychiatry
Psychiat Opin: Psychiatry Opinion
Psychiat Q: Psychiatric Quarterly
Pub Health Mich: Public Health of Michigan
Pub Hlth Nurs: Public Health Nurse
Pub Hlth Nurs Q: Public Health Nursing Quarterly
Pub Hlth Rep: Public Health Reports

Q Bull Front Nurs Serv: Quarterly Bulletin of the Frontier Nursing Service
Q Bull Louisiana Dept Hlth: Quarterly Bulletin of the Louisiana Department of Health
Quart J Chin Nurs: Quarterly Journal of Chinese Nurses
Queensland Nurs J: Queensland Nurses Journal
Queen's Nurs J: Queen's Nurses Journal

Read Dig: Readers Digest
Record, Am Cath Hist Soc: Record, American Catholic Historical Society
Red Cr Courier: Red Cross Courier
Red Cross Bull: Red Cross Bulletin
Red Cr World: Red Cross World
Reg Nurs Or: Registered Nursing Orderly
Res Bull Nat Educ Assoc: Research Bulletin of the National Education Association
Res Nurs Hlth: Research in Nursing and Health
Rev Assist Pub: Revue de l'Assistance Publique à Paris
Rev Brasil Enferm: Revista Brasileira de Enfermagem
Rev Enferm Nov Diemens: Revista Enfermaria Nov Diemens
Rev Fac de Med Bogota and *Rev Fac de Med Colom: Revista la Facultad de Medicina, Colombia*
Rev Infirm: Revue de l'Infirmière
Rev Infirm Ass So: Revue de l'Infirmière de l'Assistance Sociale

*Rev Inform Bull League Red Cro Soc: Review and Information Bulletin
     League of Red Cross Societies*
Rev Int Croix Rge: Revue Internationale de Croix Rouge
Rev Med Chil: Revista Medica de Chile
Rev of Reviews: Review of Reviews
Rev Philanthrop: Revue Philanthropique
RN: RN
RNABC News: Registered Nurses Association of British Columbia News
*RNANS Bulletin: Registered Nurses Association of Nova Scotia
     Bulletin*
RNAO News: Registered Nurses Association of Ontario
Rev Sanid Hig Publica: Revista de Sanidad y Higiene Publica
Rev San Mil Mex: Revista de la Sanidad Militario de México
*Rev Tb Pub Hlth Nurs: Review of Tuberculosis for Public Health
     Nurse*
Rocky Mt Med J: Rocky Mountain Medical Journal

St Barth Hosp J: Saint Bartholomew's Hospital Journal
St Barth Hosp Rep: Saint Bartholomew's Hospital Reports
St Thom Hosp Gazette: St. Thomas Hospital Gazette
Sair-Sjuk: Sairaanhoitaja-Sjukskoterskan
Salub y Assist: Salub y Assistencia
San Tom Nurs J: Santo Tomas Nursing Journal
*Sas Reg Nurs Assoc Bull: Saskatchewan Registered Nurses' Association
     Bulletin*
Sat Eve Post: Saturday Evening Post
Sat Rev: Saturday Review
Sch and Soc: School and Society
Sch Life: School Life
Sch Nurs: School Nurse
Scholas: Scholastic
Sch Phy Bull: School Physicians Bulletin
Schweiz Med Wochens: Schweizerische Medizinische Wochenschrift
Schwes Rev: Schwestern Revue
Sci: Science
Sci Am: Scientific American
SC Nurs: South Carolina Nursing
Slav Rev: Slavic Review
So Afr Nurs J: South Africa Nursing Journal
So Afr Nurs Rec: South African Nursing Record
Socio Med: Sociologiske Meddelelser
Soc Res: Social Research
Soc Serv R: Social Service Review
Soc Stud: Social Studies
Sogo Kan: Sogo Kango (Comprehensive Nursing Quarterly)
SOINS: ·SOINS
Southern Med J: Southern Medical Journal
South Hosp: Southern Hospital
Sovetsk Zdravookhr: Sovetskoe Zdravookhranenie
Span Med Rev Mex: Spanish Medical Review
SPCK: Society for the Propogation of Christian Knowledge
Stat: Statistics
State Hosp Q: State Hospital Quarterly
Stras Med: Strasbourg Médical
Sud Arch Ges Med: Sudhoffs Archiv für Geschichte der Medizin
Sup Nurs: Supervisor Nurse

Sur: Survey
Surg, Gyn & Obs: Surgery, Gynecology and Obstetrics
Sur Graph: Survey Graphic
Sygeplej: Sygeplejersken
Sykeplei: Sykepleien

Tar Heel Nurs: Tar Heel Nurse
Teach Coll Rec: Teachers College Record
Tenn Nurs Assoc Bull: Tennessee Nurses Association Bulletin
Texas Nurs: Texas Nursing
Tex Rep Biol Med: Texas Reports on Biology and Medicine
Thai Nurs Assoc J: Thai Nurses' Association Journal
Tids Jor: Tidskrift for Jormoedre
Tidsk Sver Sjukskot: Tidskrift for Svergiges Sjukskoterskor
Tids Sygepl: Tidskrift for Sygeplejersker
Tijds Bejaar: Tijdschrift voor Bejaarden
Tijds Ziekenver: Tijdschrift voor Ziekenverpleging
Tip Fakulten Mecmuasi: Tip Fakultesi Mecmuasi (Istanbul)
Today's Hlth: Today's Health
Toledo Med Surg J: Toledo Medical and Surgical Journal
Tomorrow's Nurs: Tomorrow's Nurse
Top Clin Nurs: Topics in Clinical Nursing
Trans Am: Transactions of American Medical Association
Trans & Stu Coll Phy Phil: Transactions and Studies of the College
    of Physicians of Philadelphia
Trans Am Gyn Soc: Transactions of the American Gynecological
    Society
Trans Med Soc Virg: Transactions of the Medical Society of Virginia
Trans NY State Med Assoc: Transactions of the New York State
    Medical Association
Tr Nurs: Trained Nurse
Tr Nurs & Hosp Rev: Trained Nurse and Hospital Review
Turk Hemsire Derg: Turk Hemsireler Dergisi
20th Cent: Twentieth Century

UNA Communique: Utah Nurses Association Communique, formerly *Utah*
    Nurse
UNA Nurs J: United Nations Association Nursing Journal
UN Bull: United Nations Bulletin
Univ De Sao Paulo Es De Enferm Rev: Universidade De Sao Paulo Escola
    De Enfermagem Revista
U.S. Bur Educ Bull: U.S. Bureau of Education Bulletin
U.S. Na Med Bull: U.S. Navy Medical Bulletin
Utah Hist Q: Utah History Quarterly

Van Law Rev: Vanderbilt Law Review
VA Nurs Q: Veterans Administration Nursing Quarterly
Via Med--Cad Med: Viata Medicala--Cadre Medii
Vict Ord Nurs Can News: Victorian Order of Nurses for Canada
    Newsletter
Vict Stud: Victorian Studies
Virgin Med Mon: Virginia Medical Monthly
Virg Nurs: Virginia Nurse
VINA Q: Virgin Islands Nurses Association Quarterly
Visit Nurs Q: Visiting Nurses Quarterly

NURSING

1. INDEXES, BIBLIOGRAPHIES, AND ABSTRACTS

INDEXING / ABSTRACTING SERVICES

1. *Medline* (Medlars on-line): 1966- . National Library of Medi-
    cine, Bethesda, MD.

    Designed by the National Library of Medicine, *Medline* provides
    access to citations from over 2,000 medical journals and mono-
    graphs published worldwide. This data base corresponds to the
    printed indexes: *Index Medicus*, *Index to Dental Literature*, and
    International Nursing Index.

2. *Excerpta Medica*: 1974- . Excerpta Medica, Amsterdam, The
    Netherlands.

    Excerpta Medica consists of citations and abstracts from over
    3,500 biomedical journals published throughout the world.
    Coverage is provided on articles dealing with all aspects of
    human medicine and allied disciplines. This base corresponds
    to the more than 40 separate abstract journals and literature
    indexes which make up the printed *Excerpta Medica* services. An
    estimated additional 100,000 records (annually) are included
    that are not listed in the printed counterparts.

3. *Psychological Abstracts*: 1967- . American Psychological
    Association, Washington, DC.

    Psychological Abstracts provides access to articles in over
    900 journals in psychology and related disciplines. Addition-
    ally, over 1,500 books, technical reports, and monographs are
    scanned annually to afford greater coverage of current research.

4. *Sociological Abstracts*: 1963- . Sociological Abstracts, Inc.,
    San Diego, CA.

    Sociological Abstracts provides citations and abstracts to
    articles from over 1,200 journals and serial publications in
    sociology and related behavioral sciences disciplines.

5. *Historical Abstracts*: 1973- . ABC-Clio, Inc., Santa Barbara,
    CA.

    Historical Abstracts indexes and abstracts periodical litera-
    ture covering the history of the world from 1450 to the present
    excluding the United States and Canada. Over 2,000 journals
    published throughout the world are scanned. The base corresponds
    to the printed counterparts *Historical Abstracts Part A*, *Modern
    History Abstracts* (1450-1914); and *Historical Abstracts Part B*,
    Twentieth Century Abstracts (1914 to the present).

6. *America: History and Life*: 1964-   . ABC-Clio, Inc., Santa
    Barbara, CA.

    America: History and Life provides indexing and abstracting
    covering all aspects of United States and Canadian history. The
    base corresponds to the printed counterparts *America: History
    and Life Part A (Article Abstracts and Citations)*, *Part B (Index
    to Book Reviews)*, *Part C (American History Bibliography)*.

7. *ERIC* (Educational Resources Information Center): 1966-
    National Institute of Education, Washington, DC, and ERIC
    Processing and Reference Facility, Bethesda, MD.

    ERIC consists of two major files: *Research in Education*, which
    identifies and abstracts the more significant educational re-
    ports and projects; and *Current Index to Journals in Education*,
    covering more than 700 publications from all areas of education
    (1970-   ).

OTHER BIBLIOGRAPHIC SOURCES

8. Abdellah, F.C. "Letter: National Library of Medicine is Official
    Nursing Archives." *Nurs Res*, 24 (Jan-Feb 1975), 64.

9. *Bibliographies on Nursing*. 10 vols. and supplements. New York:
    National League of Nursing Education, 1952. An annotated list
    of books, pamphlets, articles, audio-visual materials, and
    selected lists of indexes to books, pamphlets, and periodical
    literature. Prepared by a Committee of the League and edited
    by the NLN staff. Volume 2, pp. 21-53, includes a specific
    bibliography on history.

10. Boston University. "Nursing Archive at Boston University."
    Nurs Res, 19 (Jul-Aug 1970), 342. ANA archives are at Boston
    University.

11. *Bulletin of the History of Medicine, The*. Baltimore, MD: Insti-
    tute of Medical History at the Johns Hopkins University and
    the American Association for the History of Medicine. Has an
    annual bibliography of works on American medicine including
    nursing.

12. Callahan, C.L. "A Record of Nursing. Boston University Nursing
    Archive." *Nurs Out*, 20 (Dec 1972), 778-781.

13. Chaff, Sandra L., Ruth Haimbach, Carol Fenichel, and Nina B.
    Wood, eds. *Women in Medicine: A Bibliography of the Litera-
    ture on Women Physicians*. Metuchen, NJ: Scarecrow Press, 1977.
    1,124 pp.

14. Columbia University-Presbyterian Hospital, Department of Nursing.
    Catalogue of the Florence Nightingale Collection. New York:
    Columbia University-Presbyterian Hospital, 1956.

15. *Cumulative Index to Nursing Literature.* Vol. 1, 1956. Seventh
     Day Adventist Hospital Assn., Glendale, P.O. Box 871, Glendale,
     CA 91209. Title later changed to *Cumulative Index to Nursing
     and Allied Health Literature*, now published five times a year
     plus annual accumulation.

16. *Current List of Medical Literature.* Vols. 1-36. Washington,
     DC: National Library of Medicine, 1941-1959. Published weekly
     until June 1950, then monthly; cumulative indexes semi-
     annually. Superseded 1960 by *Index Medicus*. See no. 23.

17. *Current Work in the History of Medicine: An International
     Bibliography.* A quarterly index of articles published by the
     Wellcome Institute for History of Medicine, 183 Euston Road,
     London NW1 2BP. Begun in 1954.

18. Dale, B. "The Archives Room: A Description of the Historical
     Collection at the Toronto Western Hospital." *Canad Nurs*, 57
     (Oct 1961), 974-975.

19. Garrison, F.H., and L.T. Morton. *A Medical Bibliography: A
     Check-List of Texts Illustrating the History of Medicine.*
     London: Grafton & Co., 1943. 2nd ed., New York: Argosy
     Bookstore, 1954.

20. Grandbois, M. "The 'Nursing Literature Index': Its History,
     Present Needs and Future Plans." *Bull Med Libr Assoc*, 52
     (Oct 1964), 676-683.

21. Guerra, Francisco. *American Medical Bibliography 1639-1783: A
     Chronological Catalogue.* New York: Lathrop C. Harper, 1962.
     885 pp.

22. *Index-Catalogue of the Library of the Surgeon-General's Office.*
     See U.S. War Department, no. 41.

23. *Index Medicus: A Monthly Classified Record, The Current Medical
     Literature of the World.* Vols. 1-21. New York: 1879-1899.
     A second series, Vols. 1-18 appeared between 1903 and 1920.
     A third series, Vols. 1-6, 1921-1927. In 1927 the *Quarterly
     Cumulative Index to Current Medical Literature*, 12 vols.,
     1916-1926, was amalgamated with *Index Medicus* to form *Quar-
     terly Cumulative Index Medicus*. This was superseded in 1960
     by a new monthly *Index Medicus* with an annual *Cumulative
     Index Medicus*. The gap 1900-1902 was filled by *Bibliographia
     Medica*, 3 vols., edited by C. Potain and C. Richet.

24. *International Nursing Index.* Vol. 1, 1966, to current vol. 13,
     1978, published quarterly, then in annual volumes by the *Am
     J Nurs* in cooperation with the National Library of Medicine,
     10 Columbus Circle, New York, NY 10019.

25. Miller, Genevieve, ed. *Bibliography of the History of Medicine
     of the United States and Canada, 1939-1960.* Baltimore: Johns
     Hopkins Press, 1964.

26. Morton, Leslie T. *A Medical Bibliography (Garrison and Morton)*.
    3rd ed. Philadelphia: J.B. Lippincott, 1970.

27. Nagatoya, Y. "Bibliography of European and American Nursing
    History." *Jap J Nurs Educ*, 10 (Apr 1969), 68-71.

28. National Library of Medicine. *Bibliography of the History of
    Medicine, 1964 On*. Bethesda, MD: National Library of Medi-
    cine, U.S. Government Printing Office. Annual editions each
    year from 1964 on. Five-year compilations in 1969 and 1974.

29. Nursing History. "At Smithsonian—Hall of Medical Sciences
    Opens." *Pub Hlth Rep* (Washington), 81 (Nov 1966), 72.

30. *Nursing Studies Index*. 4 vols. Vol. 1 1900-1929; vol. 2 1930-
    1949; vol. 3 1950-1956; vol. 4 1957-1959. Philadelphia:
    J.B. Lippincott, 1963-1972. Project under Virginia Henderson.

31. "Official Opening of the Henrietta Stockdale Memorial Library,
    University of the Orange Free State, July 1975." *So Afr
    Nurs J*, 42 (Sep 1975), 30-31.

32. Pings, Vern M. "Nursing Libraries in Historical Perpsectives"
    (Charts). *Am J Nurs*, 65 (Nov 1965), 115-120.

33. Poynter, Frederick Noel Lawrence. *A Catalogue of Incunabula in
    the Wellcome Historical Medical Library*. Compiled by F.N.L.
    Poynter. London: Oxford University Press, 1954.

34. *Quarterly Cumulative Index to Current Medical Literature*.
    12 vols. 1916-1926. See *Index Medicus*, no. 23.

35. *Quarterly Cumulative Index Medicus (1927-1956)*. See *Index
    Medicus*, no. 23.

36. "Reference Sources for Nursing." *Nurs Out*, 24 (May 1976),
    317-322. The ninth revision (including a Canadian supplement)
    of a list of nursing reference works lists items in the fol-
    lowing sections: abstract journals, audiovisuals, bibliog-
    raphies, dictionaries, directories, drug lists and pharma-
    cologies, educational programs, histories, indexes, legal
    guides, library administration and organization, research
    grants, research and statistical data sources, and writers'
    manuals. Author/MS—Descriptors: Nursing, Reference Materials,
    Reference Books, Booklists, Bibliographies, Resource Materials,
    Resource Guides.

37. Schullian, Dorothy M., and Francis E. Sommer. *A Catalogue of
    Incunabula and Manuscripts in the Army Medical Library*. New
    York: Henry Schuman, 1950.

38. Thompson, A.M.C. "The Literature of Nursing." *Bull Med Libr
    Assoc*, 52 (Apr 1964), 427-437.

39. Thompson, Alice M. *A Bibliography of Nursing Literature, 1859-
    1960*. London Library Association for the Royal College of

Nursing and National Council of Nurses of the United Kingdom in association with King Edward's Hospital Fund for London, 1960.

40. *United States: National Library of Medicine Catalog.* 18 vols. Ann Arbor, Washington, New York: 1950-1966. 6 vols. 1950-1954; 6 vols. 1955-1959; 6 vols. 1960-1965. First series under title of *U.S. Armed Forces Medical Library.*

41. United States War Department, Surgeon General's Office. *Index-Catalogue of the Library of the Surgeon-General's Office.* Vol. 1-16; 2nd ser. vol. 1-21; 3rd ser. vol. 1-10; 4th ser. vol. 1-11A-Mn; 5th ser. vol. 1-3 (Washington: U.S. Government Printing Office, 1961). The Surgeon-General's collection started in 1838. J.S. Billings planned and started the *Index Catalogue.* Series 1-4 indexes about 3,000,000 books, journals, articles, and pamphlets. In the fifth series only monographs and theses were included. The name of the library was changed to Armed Forces Medical Library in 1952; in 1956 it became the National Library of Medicine. See no. 22.

42. Wellcome Historical Medical Library. *A Catalogue of Printed Books in the Wellcome Historical Medical Library.* 2 vols. London: Wellcome Historical Medical Library, 1962. Vol. 1 books printed before 1641; vol. 2 books printed from 1641 to 1850.

43. Wellcome Historical Medical Library. *Subject Catalogue of the History of Medicine and Related Sciences. Wellcome Institute for the History of Medicine.* Liechtenstein: KTO Press, 1979 and 1980. 16 vols. in 3 sections: subject section 8 vols.; biographical section 5 vols.; topographical section 3 vols.

44. Wigmore, Ethel. "On Making and Using a Bibliography." *Am J Nurs*, 36 (May 1936), 463-468. Author traces development of bibliographies and outlines sources, procedures, and criteria; extensive, annotated bibliography.

2. HISTORIES OF NURSING

GENERAL

45. Abbott, Maude E. "Lectures on the History of Nursing." *Canad Nurs*, 16 (May 1920), monthly through 19 (Jul 1923). Nine also published separately as *McGill University Publications*, (Montreal), Series VII (Medicine) 25 (1924).

46. Abel-Smith, Brian. *A History of the Nursing Profession*. London: William Heinemann, 1960.

47. Abu-Saad, Huda. *Nursing: A World View*. St. Louis: C.V. Mosby, 1979.

48. Achiba, G. "Nursing as a Field of Study. VI Memo on Nursing History." *Jap J Nurs Educ*, 16 (Sep 1975), 546-553.

49. Ackerknecht, Erwin Heinz. *A Short History of Medicine*. New York: Ronald Press, 1955.

50. Austin, Anne L. *History of Nursing Source Book*. New York: G.P. Putnam's Sons, 1957.

51. Baggallay, Olive. "World Trends in Nursing Over the Last 50 Years." *Nurs Times*, 51 (6 May 1955), 178-181.

52. Balaty, J. "Progress with a Purpose." *Stat*, 41 (Mar 1972), 12 *passim*.

53. Baly, Monica. *History of Nursing*. London: Batsford, 1977.

54. Baumler, Christian. *Über Krankenpflege*. Freiburg, i.B.: J.C.B. Mohr, 1892.

55. Beck, H.G. "The Evolution of Nursing." *Maryland Med J*, 59 (1916), 157-164.

56. Bett, Walter Reginald. *A Short History of Nursing*. London: Faber & Faber, 1960.

57. Bettman, Otto L. *A Pictorial History of Medicine*. Springfield, IL: Charles C. Thomas, 1956.

58. Bradley, M.E. "It's Different Now. Hush. You'll Wake the Patients." *Nurs Times*, 71 (11 Dec 1975), 1982-1983.

59. ———. "It's Different Now. 'Please, Sister.'" *Nurs Times*,
     71 (4 Dec 1975), 1940-1941.

60. ———. "It's Different Now. The Magic of Christmas." *Nurs
     Times*, 71 (25 Dec 1975), 2064-2065.

61. ———. "It's Different Now. Some Sisters are Dragons." *Nurs
     Times*, 71 (18 Dec 1975), 2023-2024.

62. ———. "It's Different Now. Part Your Hair Down the Middle."
     Nurs Times, 71 (20 Nov 1975), 1844-1847.

63. ———. "It's Different Now. Where Are Your Sleeves?" *Nurs
     Times*, 71 (27 Nov 1975), 1900-1901.

64. ———. "It's Different Now. 'Can I Help You?'" *Nurs Times*,
     72 (11 Mar 1976), 365-366.

65. ———. "It's Different Now. Crockery Day." *Nurs Times*, 72
     (8 Apr 1976), 540-541.

66. ———. "It's Different Now. Night Duty Again." *Nurs Times*,
     72 (1 Apr 1976), 494-495.

67. Bridges, Daisy C. "The Growth and Development of a Profession."
     Canad Nurs, 65 (Jun 1969), 32-34.

68. Browne, S. "The Nurse and the Nation: A Survey of Her Position
     in the State Today." *Nurs Times* (5 Nov 1910), 904-931.

69. Brunner, Lillian Sholtis. "Nursing Today." *Nurs World*, 132
     (Jun 1958), 8, illus.

70. Bull, M.R. "Kimberley--A Century of Nursing." *Nurs Mirror*,
     133 (17 Dec 1971), 27-30.

71. Bullough, Vern and Bonnie. *The Care of the Sick: The Emergence
     of Modern Nursing*. New York: Prodist, 1978.

72. ———. *The Emergence of Modern Nursing*. New York: Macmillan,
     1964; 2nd ed., 1969.

73. ———. "Nursing and History." *Nurs Out*, 12 (Oct 1964), 27-29.

74. Burbridge, G.N. "Nursing Care and Nursing Education." Second
     Annual Oration. The New South Wales College of Nursing.
     Aust Nurs J, 52 (Nov 1954), 258-264; (Dec 1954), 284-289.

75. Calder, Jean McKinley. *The Story of Nursing*. London: Methuen &
     Co., 1954; 2nd ed., 1958; 3rd ed., 1960.

76. Candan, M.G. "Nurse, Pioneer of Health." *UN Bull*, (1 Apr 1954),
     270.

77. Carr, E.I. "Evolution of Nursing." *J Mich M Soc* (Grand
     Rapids), 17 (1918), 186-188.

78. Castiglioni, Arturo. *A History of Medicine.* Translated by
    E.B. Krumbhaar. 2nd ed. New York: Alfred A. Knopf, 1947.

79. Chayer, Mary E. *Nursing in Modern Society.* New York: G.P.
    Putnam's Sons, 1947.

80. Christy, T.E. "To Honor Our Past ... To Herald Our Future."
    VA Nurs Q, 45(1) (Spring 1976), 1-15, 17.

81. Clendenning, Logan. *Source Book of Medical History.* New York:
    P.B. Hoeber, 1942.

82. Coleman, V. "Early Nursing." *Nurs Mirror*, 140 (24 Apr 1975),
    72.

83. Cowan, Cordelia. *The Yearbook of Modern Nursing.* New York:
    G.P. Putnam's Sons, 1956 and 1958.

84. Cross, M.B. "Remember Nursing Back When?" *Occup Hlth Nurs*, 17
    (Aug 1969), 21f.

85. Crowley, M.F. "Milestones in the History of Nursing: 1893-
    1969." *Irish Nurs News* (Jan-Feb 1970), 9, 13 *passim.*

86. Dahm, E. "Women as Nurses, A Historical Resume." *Sociol Med*
    (Swe.), 37 (Nov 1960), 353-357.

87. Darbyshire, Miss. "Nursing--Past, Present and Future." *Nurs
    Mirror* (17 Jun 1933), 225.

88. Davison, Wilburt C. "Nursing as the Foundation of Medicine."
    TR Nurs, 111 (Oct 1943), 259-261.

89. Deloughery, Grace. *History and Trends of Professional Nursing.*
    8th ed. St. Louis: C.V. Mosby, 1977; 7th ed. edited by G.J.
    Griffin. See no. 133.

90. De Murillo, G.M. "A Passing Glance at the Profession." *ANEC*,
    5 (Oct 1974), 23-24. (Spa)

91. Densford, Katharine J. "Nursing 1941--For All the People."
    Hosp Mgmt, 51 (1941), 49-50, 52, 54.

92. Dickey, W. "The Evolution of the Modern Trained Nurse." *Am M
    Compend* (Toledo), 18 (1902), 211-216.

93. Dietz, Lena Dixon. *History and Modern Nursing.* Philadelphia:
    F.A. Davis Co., 1963.

94. Dietz, Lena Dixon and Aurelia R. Lehozhy. *History and Modern
    Nursing.* Philadelphia: F.A. Davis Co., 1967.

95. Dillner, Elisabet. *The Stave of Mercy: A Pageant Play of
    Tableaux.* Translated by Ronald de Wolfe. Stockholm: Swedish
    Nurses Assn., 1949.

96.   Dixon, P.W. "A Century of Progress." *Hosp* (London), 55
      (1959), 777-779.

97.   Dock, Lavinia L. *A History of Nursing from the Earliest Times
      to the Present Day, with Special Reference to the Work of
      the Past 30 Years.* New York and London: G.P. Putnam's Sons,
      1912. 340 pp.

98.   Dock, Lavinia L., and Isabel M. Stewart. *A Short History of
      Nursing.* New York: G.P. Putnam's Sons, 1920; 2nd ed., 1925;
      3rd ed., 1931; 4th ed., 1938.

99.   Dodge, Bertha Sanford. *The Story of Nursing.* Boston: Little,
      Brown & Co., 1965.

100. Dolan, Josephine A. *Goodnow's History of Nursing.* 11th ed.
      Philadelphia: W.B. Saunders Co., 1963.

101. ————, ed. *History of Nursing.* 12th ed. Philadelphia:
      W.B. Saunders Co., 1968.

102. ————. *Nursing in Society: A Historical Perspective.* 13th
      ed. Philadelphia: W.B. Saunders Co., 1973; 14th ed., 1978.

103. Domarus, U. "Einiges aus der Geschichte von Krankenhaus und
      Krankenpflege." *Rothe Kreuz*, 32 (1914), 335, 374.

104. Eberle, Irmengarde. *NURSE!* New York: Thomas Y. Crowell,
      1945. 136 pp.

105. Edward, Helen. "Milestones in Nursing, 1854-1914-1939."
      Irish Nurs World, 15 (Sep 1945), 1.

106. Edwarda, Sister M. "Notes on Early Hospital Nursing." *Bull
      Acad Med* #5 (Cleveland), 28(5) (1943), 7, 19.

107. Edwards-Rees, Desrée. *The Story of Nursing.* London: Con-
      stable Young, 1965.

108. D.E. *Recollections of a Nurse.* London and New York: Mac-
      millan & Co., 1889.

109. Ferguson, E.D. "The Evolution of the Trained Nurse." *Am J
      Nurs*, 1 (Mar 1901), 463-468; (Apr 1901), 535-538; (May 1901),
      620-626.

110. "Fifty Years Ago." *Nurs Times*, 71 (2 Jan 1975), 11-13.

111. Fiske, A. "Florence Nightingale, Where is Her Modern Counter-
      part?" *Hygeia*, 14 (May 1936), 394-396.

112. Fitzpatrick, M. Louise. "Nursing." *Signs*, 2 (Summer, 1977),
      818-834.

113. Flaherty, J. "The Present of Today was the Future of Yester-
      day." *RNAO News*, 28 (May-Jun 1972), 11-13.

114.   Fogarty, C.P. "From 1900 to the Present." *New Zeal Nurs J*,
       66 (Feb 1973), 23-25.

115.   Frank, Sister Charles Marie. *Foundations of Nursing*. 2nd
       ed. Philadelphia: W.B. Saunders Co., 1959.

116.   ———. *The Historical Development of Nursing*. Philadelphia:
       W.B. Saunders Co., 1953. 400 pp.

117.   Gabrielson, R.C. "Two Centuries of Advancement: From Un-
       trained Servant to Skilled Practitioner." *J Adv Nurs* (Jul
       1978), 265-267.

118.   ———. "Viewing the Past as Prologue for Changes Today and
       Tomorrow." *SC Nurs*, 25 (Winter 1973), 6 *passim*.

119.   Gage, N.D. "International Relationships: Their Growth in 30
       Years." *Tr Nurs*, 80 (Jun 1978), 724-728.

120.   Gaines, M. Josephine. "Preserving the Structures of the Past."
       Nurs Out, 6 (Feb 1958), 103-104.

121.   Garcia del Cassizo San Millan, M.G. "Precedentes historiscos
       de la profession de enfermera." *Asclepio*, 18-19 (1966),
       407-421.

122.   Garrison, F.H. *Introduction to the History of Medicine*.
       Philadelphia: W.B. Saunders Co., 1929.

123.   Gay, George W. "Nursing as a Vocation." *Aust Nurs J*, 12
       (Jan 1914), 18-24.

124.   Gelinas, Agnes. *Nursing and Nursing Education*. New York:
       Commonwealth, 1946. 72 pp. Summarized in *Hosp Mgmt*, 61
       (June 1946), 70, 72, 74, 76, 78, 80; *Nurs Times*, 42 (17 Aug
       1946), 617-618, (24 Aug 1946), 635-636.

125.   Ghini, Laura. "La Ricerca Applicata alla Professione dell'
       Infermerie." *Annali Di Sociologia*, 10 (1973), 46-55.

126.   Gillette, E. "Times Have Changed for Nurses." *Point View*, 11
       (Jan 1974), 13.

127.   Goodnow, Minnie. 1953. *Nursing History*. 9th ed. Philadel-
       phia: W.B. Saunders Co. 1st ed., 1918; 2nd ed., 1926; 3rd
       ed., 1923, 420 pp; 4th ed., 1928, 472 pp.; 5th ed., 1933,
       517 pp.; 6th ed., 1939, 489 pp.; 7th ed., 1942, 495 pp.;
       8th ed., 1948, 404 pp. Eds. 5 and 6 titled *Outlines of
       Nursing History*.

128.   ———. *Nursing History in Brief*. Philadelphia: W.B. Saun-
       ders Co. 1st ed., 1938, 325 pp.; 2nd ed., 1943, 338 pp.; 3rd
       ed., 1950.

129.   ———. *Nursing History*. Revised by Josephine A. Dolan as
       Goodnow's History of Nursing. Philadelphia: W.B. Saunders
       Co. See Dolan, Josephine A., nos. 100, 101, 102.

130.   Goostray, Stella, et al.   "American Nursing--History and
       Interpretation." *Am J Nurs*, 54 (Jun 1954), 719-721.

131.   Gordon, J.E. "Nursing Through 75 Years." *Nurs Mirror*, pt. 1,
       117 (11 Oct 1963); pt. 2 (18 Oct 1963); pt. 3 (25 Oct 1963);
       pt. 4 (1 Nov 1963).

132.   Greenough, K. "1896-1971: A Story of Evolution." *Nurs Res
       Rep*, 6 (Sep 1971), 2.

133.   Griffin, Gerald Joseph, and Joanne King Griffin. *History and
       Trends of Professional Nursing*. St. Louis: C.V. Mosby Co.,
       1973. A continuation of original work by Jensen (see nos.
       153 and 154).

134.   Grippando, Gloria M. *Nursing Perspectives and Issues*. Albany:
       Delmar, 1977.

135.   Guthrie, Douglas. "Nursing Through the Ages." *Nurs Mirror*,
       97 (17 Jul 1953), 10-12; (24 Jul 1953), 12-14; (31 Jul 1953),
       13-15.

136.   Haeser, Heinrich. *Geschichte Christlicher Kranken-Pflege und
       Pflegerschaften*. Berlin: W. Hertz, 1957; and Bad Reichen-
       hall: Kleinert, 1966.

137.   Hamilton, Anna Emile. *Les gardes malades congréganistes, mer-
       cenaires, professionelles, amateurs*. Paris: Vigot, 1901.

138.   Hampton, Isabel A. et al. *Nursing of the Sick, 1893*. New
       York: McGraw-Hill, 1949. 218 pp.

139.   Harley, G.W. *Native African Medicine*. Cambridge, MA: Har-
       vard University Press, 1941.

140.   Hibbard, A.B. "Diary of a Nurse." *Canad Nurs*, 59 (Dec 1963),
       1158ff.

141.   Hicks, Emily. "The Emergence of a New Profession--Nursing."
       Tr Nurs, 105 (Dec 1940), 435-437, 487, 489, 491; 106 (Jan
       1941), 44-46.

142.   Hirsh, H. "A Brief History of Nursing." *State Hosp Q* (Utica,
       NY), 6 (1920-1921), 225-231.

143.   "History of Nursing." *Int Med Digest* (Jun 1938), 375-380.

144.   "How Much Do You Know About History of Nursing?" *Epheta*, 7
       (Apr-Jun 1968), 30-31.

145.   "Illustrious Past, Challenging Future." *Am J Nurs*, 71 (Sep
       1971), 1773-1777.

146.   "Infirmier." *Encyclopédie ou Dictionnaire des Sciences, des
       Arts et des Metiers*. Edited by Denis Diderot, 17 vols.
       Paris: Briasson et al., 1751-1765; 8, pp. 707-708.

147. Jacobi, A. "The Historical Development of Modern Nursing." *Pop Sc Month*, 23 (1883), 773-787.

148. Jamieson, Elizabeth, and Mary Sewall. *History of Nursing Notebook.* 10th ed. Philadelphia: J.P. Lippincott, 1956.

149. ————, and Mary Sewall. *Trends in Nursing History.* Philadelphia: W.B. Saunders Co., 1940. 2nd ed. 1944; 3rd ed. 1949; 4th ed. 1954.

150. ————, Mary F. Sewall, and Lucile S. Gjertson. *Trends in Nursing History: Their Social, International and Ethical Relationships.* 5th ed. Philadelphia: W.B. Saunders Co., 1959.

151. ————, Mary F. Sewall, and Eleanor R. Suhrie. *Trends in Nursing History.* 6th ed. Philadelphia: W.B. Saunders Co., 1966.

152. Jensen, Deborah MacLurg. *A History of Nursing.* St. Louis: C.V. Mosby Co., 1943.

153. ————. *History and Trends of Professional Nursing.* 2nd ed. St. Louis: C.V. Mosby Co., 1950. 365 pp.; 3rd ed. 1955, 508 pp.; 4th ed. 1959.

154. ————. *History and Trends of Professional Nursing.* St. Louis: C.V. Mosby Co., 1965. Revised by Gerald J. and H. Joanne King Griffin under the title of *Jensen's History and Trends of Professional Nursing.* See no. 133.

155. Johnstone, Mary M. "History of Nursing." *Woman's M J*, 13 (1903), 220-223.

156. Katscher, Liselotte. *Geschichte der Krankenpflege; ein Leitfaden für den Schwesternunterrich.* Berlin: Christlicher Zeitschriften-Verlag, 1969.

157. Kelly, Cordelia. "Those Were the Days." *Am J Nurs*, 54 (1954), 452.

158. Kerr, Margaret, ed. "In the Good Old Days." *Canad Nurs*, 54 (1958), 41, 116, 226, 358, 431, 548, 635, 736, 813, 918, 1028, 1138.

159. Knox, C.A. *The Nursing Years.* Ilfracombe, Gt. Britain: Stockwell, 1967.

160. Laidler, P.W. "The Nurse in General." *So Afr Nurs Rec*, 18 (Mar 1931), 141-145.

161. Lattimore, J.G. "The Transition from Medical Training to Patient Care." *Med Tech Bull* (Sep-Oct 1959), 191-194.

162. Laulen, R. "Nurses of Former Years." *Prese Med*, 61 (18 Mar 1953), 397.

163. McCarrick, H. "Have Times Changed?" *Nurs Times*, 65 (25 Sep 1969), 1248-1249.

164. McCrary, Willard Livingston. *They Caught the Torch*. Milwaukee: Will Ross, Inc., 1939.

165. McKenzie, Dan. *The Infancy of Medicine*. London: Macmillan & Co., 1927.

166. MacLeod, G.K. "Traditions and Trends in Nursing." *Conn Med*, 35 (Sep 1971), 541-542.

167. Mannino, Anthony J. "Bringing Nursing History Up to Date." *Am J Nurs*, 56 (1956), 1004.

168. "The March of Time in Nursing History." *Pac Cst J Nurs*, 36 (1940), 528-533.

169. Markowitz, Gerald E. and David Karl Rosner. "Doctors in Crisis: A Study of the Use of Medical Education Reform to Establish Modern Professional Elitism in Medicine." *Am Q*, 25 (Mar 1973), 83-107.

170. Martin, M.W. "A Postal Gallery of Nursing Art." *Nurs Times*, 68 (2 Nov 1972), 1386-1387.

171. Maxwell, Anna C. "Struggles of the Pioneers." *Am J Nurs*, 21 (Feb 1921), 321-329. See also *Quart J Chin Nurs*, 3 (July 1922), 2-9.

172. Mettler, Cecelia C. *History of Medicine*. Philadelphia: Blakiston, 1947.

173. Monteiro, Lois. "Notes from Another Century." *Nurs Out*, 15 (Feb 1967), 62-63.

174. Morison, Luilla J., and Anna Fegan. *History of Nursing*. Philadelphia: F.A. Davis, 1942.

175. Morten, Honnor. *From a Nurse's Notebook*. London: Scientific Press, 1899.

176. Murphy, Denis G. *They Did Not Pass By; The Story of the Early Pioneers of Nursing*. London: Longmans, Green, 1956.

177. Neidhamer, Sr. Emile, and C. Armington, et al. "Three Score Years in the Upward Spiral of Nursing." *Mo Nurs*, 39 (Oct 1970), 8.

178. Neuberger, Max. *History of Medicine*. Translated by Ernest Playfair. London: Oxford University Press, 1910.

179. Nightingale, Florence. *Die Pflege bei Kranken und Gesunden*. Includes German translation of *Notes on Nursing*. Leipzig: F.A. Brockhaus, 1861. 223 pp.

180. ————. "Notes on Nursing: Military Hospital in India, Hospitals for Military Dependents." *Compr Nurs Q* (Summer 1973), 87-98. (Jap)

181. Nourse, J. "Those Who Came First." *Nurs Mirror*, 134 (26 May 1972), 40-41.

182. "New Century's Greetings." *Nurs Rec & Hosp World*, 26 (5 Jan 1901), 5-8.

183. "The Nursing Profession, Yesterday, Today and Tomorrow." 38th Congress of the National Association of Nurses and State Registered Nurses--Biarritz, May 11-14, 1972, *Rev Infirm*, 22 (Jul-Sep 1972), 675-682. (Fre)

184. "Nurses Through the Centuries." *RN*, 19 (Feb 1956), 46-49.

185. Nutting, M. Adelaide and Lavina L. Dock. *A History of Nursing*. 4 vols. New York: G.P. Putnam's Sons, 1907-1912. First two vols. published in 1907 and carry the history to Florence Nightingale and St. Thomas. Vols. 3 and 4 published in 1912 carry story up to that year. Reprinted Buffalo: Heritage Press, 1974.

186. ————. *Geschichte der Krankenpflege; der Entwicklung der Krankenpflege--Systeme von Urzeiten bis zur Gündung der Ersten Englischen und Amerikanischen Pflegerinnenschulen.* Translated by Sister Agnes Karll. Ubers. Von Berlin: D. Reimer, 1910, 1913.

187. ————. "Malicious Criticism" (editorial). *Am J Nurs*, 13 (Jun-Jul 1913), 660, 742-744. Comment on review of *History of Nursing* appearing in the British periodical, *The Hospital* (8 Mar 1913), ridiculing vols. 3 and 4; copy of letter from M. Adelaide Nutting to editor of *The Hospital* asking for its publication; copy of letter also sent to *Brit J Nurs*.

188. "The Nutting-Stewart Archives." *Nurs Out*, 12 (May 1964), 12.

189. Ott, Frances M. "Nursing in the Early Days." *Tr Nurs & Hosp Rev*, 107 (1941), 103-105.

190. "Outline of Nursing History." *Kango*, 15 (Sep 1971), 24-28. (Jap)

191. "Panorama of Nursing." *Tr Nurs*, 80 (1928), 681, 780.

192. "The Past is Inspiring." *Int Nurs Rev*, 6 (Jul 1959), 7-69.

193. Pavey, Agnes E. *The Story of the Growth of Nursing as an Art, a Vocation and a Profession.* 1st ed., London: Faber & Faber, 1938; 2nd ed., Philadelphia: J.P. Lippincott, 1944; 3rd ed., 1951, 498 pp. 4th ed., 1953, 512 pp.; 5th ed., London: Faber & Faber, 1959.

194. Pelley, Thelma. *Nursing; Its History, Trends, Philosophy,*
      Ethics and Ethos. Philadelphia: W.B. Saunders Co., 1964.

195. Perry, Charlotte Mandeville. "A Brief History of Nursing."
      Tr Nurs, 33 (Aug 1904), 75-79.

196. "Personalities at the Dawn of Modern Nursing." *Jap J Nurs*, 33
      (6 Mar 1969), 83-88. (Jap)

197. Petersen (nfn). "Zur Geschichte der Krankenpflege." *Rothe*
      Kreuz, 12 (1906), 24, 37. (Ger)

198. Pillers, Marjorie E. *The Lamp, A Pageant of Nursing.* Liver-
      Pool: Bennington, 1943.

199. Power, Sir D'Arcy. *A Short History of Surgery.* London: John
      Bale Sons and Danielsson, Ltd., 1933.

200. Pride, Sister. "History of Nursing." *New Zeal Nurs J*, 24
      (Sep 1931), 220, 222, 224; also printed in *S Afr Nurs Rec*,
      19 (Nov 1931), 29-30.

201. Reid, G.L. "Fifty Years of Change: 1913-1963." *Nurs Sci*, 2
      (Jun 1964), 246ff.

202. Rico-Avello, C. "Nurses and Their History." *Caridad Cienc*
      Arte, 8 (Apr-Jun 1971), 30-31. (Spa)

203. Rijcke, L. de. *Geschiendenis van de verplege-Kunde en genees-*
      kunde. Leuven: Aurelia Books, 1973. (Flemish).

204. Robb, Isabel Hampton. "Address of the President Before the
      Third Annual Convention of the Associated Alumnae of Trained
      Nurses in the United States." *Am J Nurs* (Nov 1900), 97-104.

205. Roberts, Mary. "Immortality of Influence." *Am J Nurs*, 58
      (1958), 1523.

206. ————. "New Look at the History of Nursing." *Nurs Out*, 6
      (Feb 1958), 79.

207. Robinson, Victor. *White Caps; The Story of Nursing.* Phila-
      delphia: J.P. Lippincott, 1946. 425 pp.

208. Root, E.H. "The Evolution of Nursing: Woman's Role in the
      Care of the Sick and Wounded in Times Ancient and Modern."
      Nurs World, 3 (1896), 133.

209. Rosen, Richard. *Die Krankenpflege in der arztlichen Praxis.*
      Berlin: H. Kornfeld, 1903. 197 pp.

210. Rowley, Phyllis. "The Progress of Nursing." *Nurs Mirror*, 84
      (5 Oct-26 Oct 1946).

211. Runge, F. *Die Krankenpflege als Feld weiblicher Erwerbstättig-heit gegenüber den religiosen Genossenschaften.* Berlin: 1870.

212. Rupprecht, Paul. [Bernhard Trauyott]. *Die Krankenpflege im Frieden und Kriege.* Leipzig: F.C.W. Vogel, 1894. 443 pp. 4th ed., 1902, 460 pp.; 5th ed., 1905, 464 pp.

213. Russell, E. Kathleen. "Changements in Nursing." [Changes in Patterns of Nursing]. *Canad Nurs,* 54 (1958), 529-535. (Fr)

214. ————. "Fifty Years of Medical Progress: Medicine as a Social Instrument: Nursing." *New England J Med,* 244 (1951), 439-445.

215. ————. "In the Good Old Days." *Canad Nurs,* 53 (1957), 39, 103, 222, 296, 385, 504, 642, 710, 807, 916, 996, 1118.

216. Russell, Sheila MacKay. *The Lamp is Heavy.* London: n.p., 1955.

217. Sanders, R.L. "The Nursing Profession in Retrospect and in Prospect." *Mississippi Dr,* 18 (1940), 203-206.

218. Sandwith, F.M. "Abstract of a Lecture on the Development of Modern Nursing." *Med Mag* (London), 23 (1914), 625-635.

219. Savard, Francoise, and Jean-Marc Gagnon. *Histoire du Nursing.* Montreal: Editions du Renouveau Pedagogique, 1970. (Fr)

220. Scarlett, E.P. "The Nurse of a Century Ago." *Arch Intern Med Chic,* 110 (1962), 272-274.

221. Schorr, T.M. "Editorial: Celebrating the Bicentennial." *Am J Nurs,* 75 (Apr 1975), 585.

222. Schutt, Barbara G. "The Recent Past." *Am J Nurs,* 71 (Sep 1971), 1785-1791.

223. Seidler, Eduard. *Geschichte der Pflege des Kranken Menschen: Leitlinien für den Unterricht in Krankenpflege.* Stuttgart: W. Kohlhammer, 1966.

224. Sellew, Gladys, and C.J. Stet Nuesse. *A History of Nursing.* 1st ed. St. Louis: C.V. Mosby Co., 1946; 2nd ed., 1951.

225. ————, and Sister M. Ethelrede Ebel. *A History of Nursing.* 3rd ed. St. Louis: C.V. Mosby Co., 1955.

226. Seymer, Lucy Ridgely. *A General History of Nursing.* 1st ed. New York: Macmillan & Co., 1933. 317 pp. Revised for American publication by Nina D. Gage. 2nd ed., 1949, 332 pp.; 3rd ed., 1954; 4th ed., 1956.

227.   ———. "A Summary of Nursing History." *League Red Cr Soc
         Mon Bull* (Jun 1934), 113-114; (Jul 1934), 133-134; (Aug
         1934), 161-162; (Sep 1934), 177-178.

228.   ———. "One Hundred Years Ago ..." *Am J Nurs*, 60 (May
         1960), 658-661.

229.   Sheaffer, Susan V. "Nursing--A Bird's Eye View." *Am J Nurs*,
         23 (May 1923), 637-640.

230.   Shryock, Richard H. *The Development of Modern Medicine.* 2nd
         ed. New York: Alfred A. Knopf, 1947.

231.   ———. *The History of Nursing: An Interpretation of the
         Social and Medical Factors Involved.* Philadelphia: W.B.
         Saunders Co., 1959.

232.   ———. "Nursing Emerges as a Profession: The American
         Experience." *Clio Medica*, 3 (1968), 131-147.

233.   Sigerist, Henry E. *The Great Doctors.* New York: W.W. Norton
         & Co., Inc., 1933.

234.   Sleeper, R. "Nursing Care Throughout Fifty Years." *Am J
         Nurs*, 50 (1950), 586-589.

235.   Snyder, Gertrude. "History of Nursing." *Canad Nurs*, 13
         (Aug 1917), 493-494.

236.   Stephenson, Gladys E., and James Liu. "Historical Outlines,
         Showing the Relation of Nursing History to World History."
         Quart J Chin Nurs, 10 (July 1929), 43-58.

237.   Stetson, Halbert G. "Nursing Past and Present." *Tr Nurs*, 30
         (Jan 1903), 1-6.

238.   Stewart, Isabel M., and Agnes Gelinas. *A Century of Nursing.*
         New York: G.P. Putnam's Sons, 1950.

239.   Stewart, Isabel Maitland, and Anne L. Austin. *A History of
         Nursing from Ancient to Modern Times, A World View.* 5th ed.
         New York: G.P. Putnam's Sons, 1962. Earlier editions under
         title of *A Short History of Nursing* by Dock and Isabel M.
         Stewart. See no. 98.

240.   "Stray Memories: Nursing Forty Years Ago." *Nurs Rec & Hosp
         World*, (16 Jun 1928), 724-726.

241.   Tanner, Margaret C. *Trends and Professional Adjustments in
         Nursing.* Philadelphia: W.B. Saunders Co., 1962.

242.   "Then and Now." *Nurs World*, 124 (Jul 1950), 312-313.

243.   Thomas, Margaret. "Modern Nursing in Foreign Lands: A Gift
         from the United States." *Tr Nurs*, 74 (1925), 457-462.

244. Thorup, L. "Forty Years of Nursing." *CNA Bull*, Pt. 1, 60 (Nov 1964); Pt. 2, 60 (Dec 1964), 8.

245. Tucker, K. "Growth of the Social Point of View in Nursing." *Proceedings*, Nat. Conf. Soc. Work (1923), 61-64.

246. Vezin, Heimann. *Ueber Krankenhäuser die Krankenpflege durch christliche Genossen-schaften und über die Winksamkeit*. Munster: Theissing, 1858. 84 pp.

247. Wakeford, C. *The Wounded Soldiers' Friends: The Story of Florence Nightingale, Clara Barton and Others*. London: Headley Brothers, 1917.

248. Walsh, James J. *The History of Nursing*. New York: Kennedy, 1929. 293 pp.

249. Wisconsin State Nurses' Association. *Nursing Through the Ages --A Pictorial History*. Madison: The Association, 1938.

250. Wood, Catherine J. "A Retrospect and a Forecast." International Council of Nurses, *Third International Congress*, Buffalo, NY, Sep 18-21, 1901. Cleveland: J.B. Savage, 1901. Pp. 370-375.

251. Worcester, Alfred. "Modern Nursing." *New England J Med*, 205 (13 Aug 1931), 334-346.

252. ———. *Nurses and Nursing*. Cambridge: Harvard University Press, 1927.

253. Wright, Helen, and Samuel Rapport, eds. *Great Adventures in Nursing*. New York: Harper & Brothers, 1960.

ANCIENT AND PRIMITIVE NURSING

254. Allbutt, Sir Thomas Clifford. *Greek Medicine in Rome*. London: Macmillan & Co., 1921.

255. Aurelianus, Caelius. *On Acute Diseases and on Chronic Diseases*. Translated by I.E. Drabkin. Chicago: University of Chicago Press, 1950.

256. Breasted, James Henry. *The Edwin Smith Surgical Papyrus*. 2 vols. Chicago: University of Chicago Press Oriental Institute Publication, 1930.

257. Brock, Arthur John. *Greek Medicine*. London: J.M. Dent & Sons, Ltd., 1929.

258. Bryan, Cyril. *The Papyrus Ebers*. New York: D. Appleton & Co., 1931.

259.   Cameron, Thomas. "The High Calling of a Nurse." *Nurs Mirror*,
        93 (14 Sep 1951), 450.

260.   ————. "Nurses of the Bible—1. Rebekah's Nurse—Deborah."
        Nurs Mirror, 93 (20 Jul 1951), 282.

261.   Celsus. *De Medicina*. Edited and translated by W.G. Spencer.
        3 vols. London: William Heinemann, 1935-1938.

262.   Cohn-Haft, Louis. *The Public Physicians of Ancient Greece*.
        Northhampton, MA: Smith College, 1956.

263.   Dunbar, Virginia M. "Hippocrates, Father of Nursing, Too?"
        Alum Mag, 64 (Sep 1965), 64-65.

264.   *Ebers Papyrus*. Edited and translated by Bendix Ebbel. London:
        H. Milford for Oxford University Press, 1937.

265.   Edelstein, Emma J., and Ludwig Edelstein. *Asclepius*. 2 vols.
        Baltimore: The Johns Hopkins Press, 1945.

266.   Edelstein, Ludwig. *The Hippocratic Oath*. Baltimore: Johns
        Hopkins Press, 1943.

267.   Feldmann, Gustav. *Jüdische Krankenpflegerinnen*. Cassel:
        Gebr. Gotthelft, 1901, 15 pp.; 2nd ed., 1902, 22 pp.

268.   Galen. *On the Natural Faculties*. Edited and translated by
        Arthur John Brock. London: William Heinemann, 1963.

269.   ————. *On Anatomical Procedures*. Translated by Charles
        Singer. Oxford: Oxford University Press, 1956.

270.   ————. *Hygiene*. Translated by Robert M. Green. Spring-
        field, IL: Charles C. Thomas, 1951.

271.   Ghalioungui, Paul. *Magic and Medical Science in Ancient
        Egypt*. London: Hodder and Stoughton, 1963.

272.   Gorman, Sister Mary Rosaria. *The Nurse in Greek Life. A
        Dissertation Submitted to the Catholic Sisters College of
        the Catholic University of America in Partial Fulfillment of
        the Requirements for the Degree of Doctor of Philosophy*.
        Boston: privately printed, 1917. 51 pp.

273.   *Hippocrates*. Translated and edited by W.H.S. Jones and E.T.
        Withinton. 4 vols. London: William Heinemann, Loeb Clas-
        sical Library, 1938-1948.

274.   Jay, Walter Addison. *The Healing Gods of Ancient Civilization*.
        New Haven: Yale University Press, 1925.

275.   Levine, Edwin B., Myra E. Levine, et al. "Hippocrates,
        Father of Nursing, Too?" *Am J Nurs*, 65 (Dec 1965), 86-88.

276.   Manchester, H.H. "Nursing in Graeco-Roman Times." *Tr Nurs*, 88 (Jan 1932), 33-37.

277.   ———. "Nursing in Ancient Egypt: A Fragmentary Professional Background." *Tr Nurs*, 72 (1924), 329-332.

278.   Mead, Margaret. "Nursing, Primitive and Civilized." *Am J Nurs*, 56 (1956), 1001.

279.   Mooney, James. *The Swimmer Manuscript: Cherokee Sacred Formulas and Medicinal Prescriptions.* Revised and edited by Frans M. Olbrechts. Washington: Smithsonian Institution, Bureau of American Ethnology, *Bull* 99, 1932.

280.   Nichols, R. "The Nurse in a Magic Ridden Society." *Nurs Sci*, 3 (Jun 1965), 178ff.

281.   "The Nurse in Ancient Greece." *Nurs Mirror*, 69 (29 Apr 1939), 179.

282.   Phillips, E.D. *Greek Medicine.* London: Thames and Hudson, 1973.

283.   Pliny. *Natural History.* Translated and edited by H. Rackham, W.H.S. Jones and D.E. Eichholza. 10 vols. London: William Heinemann, 1947-1963.

284.   Robinson, V. "Nurse of Greece." *Bull Hist Med*, 6 (Nov 1938), 1001-1009.

285.   Roff, Miss. "Nursing in Ancient Times." *Pac Cst J Nurs*, 15 (Aug 1919), 477-478.

286.   Rosaria, Sister Mary. *The Nurse in Greek Life.* Boston: Privately printed, 1917. See no. 272.

287.   Scarborough, John. *Roman Medicine.* London: Thames and Hudson, 1969.

288.   Schweisheimer, Waldemar. "Nurses in the Early History of Mankind." *S Afr Nurs J*, 14 (Oct 1938), 18-19, 25.

289.   Sharp, Ella E. "Nursing During the Pre-Christian Era." *Am J Nurs*, 19 (Jun 1919), 675-678.

290.   Sigerist, Henry E. *A History of Medicine.* 2 vols. New York: Oxford University Press, 1951, 1961.

291.   Singer, Charles. *Greek Biology and Medicine.* Oxford: Clarendon Press, 1922.

292.   Soranus. *Gynecology.* Translated and edited by Owsei Temkin. Baltimore: Johns Hopkins Press, 1956.

293.   Thompson, Campbell R. *The Devils and Evil Spirits of Baby-
       lonia.* London: Luzac & Co., 1903.

294.   Thurston, Herbert. "Deaconesses." *Catholic Encyclopedia.*
       16 vols. New York: Appleton, 1908-1914. IV, 651.

295.   Vegetius. *Military Institutions of the Romans.* Translated by
       John Clark. Harrisburg, PA: The Military Service Publishing
       Co., 1944.

296.   Xenophon. *Oeconomicus.* Translated and edited by E.C. Mar-
       chant. London: William Heinemann, 1953.

                              MEDIEVAL NURSING

297.   Arderne, John. *Treatises of Fistula in Ano, Haemorrhoids and
       Cysters.* Middle English ed. Edited by Sir D'Arcy Power.
       London: Kegan Paul, Trench, Trubner & Co., Ltd., 1910.

298.   Barrand, G. "History-Nurses of Middle Ages." *Strasbourg Med,*
       Supl. 99 (15 May 1939), 21-23.

299.   Bonser, Wilfrid. *The Medical Background of Anglo-Saxon
       England.* London: Wellcome Historical Medical Library, 1963.

300.   Bowsky, William M. *The Black Death, A Turning Point in
       History.* New York: Holt, Rinehart, and Winston, 1971.

301.   Bullough, Vern. *The Development of Medicine as a Profession.*
       Basel: S. Karger; New York: Hafner, 1966; New York: Neale
       Watson, 1971.

302.   Chauliac, Guy de. *La Grande Chirurgie.* Edited by E. Nicaise.
       Paris: Felix Alcan, 1890.

303.   ————. *On Wounds and Fractures.* Translated by W.A. Brennan.
       Chicago: Privately printed, 1923.

304.   Clay, Rotha Mary. *The Medieval Hospitals of England.* London:
       Methuen & Co., 1909.

305.   Cockayne, Thomas Oswald. *Leechdoms, Wortcunning, and Star-
       craft of Early England.* 3 vols. London: Longmans Green,
       1864-1866.

306.   Codellas, Pan S. "The Pantocrator, the Imperial Byzantine
       Medical Center of the XIIth Century A.D. in Constantinople."
       Bull Hist Med, 12 (1942), 392-410.

307.   Danvek, K. "A Nurse 700 Years Ago (In the Ados Monastery
       Hospital)." *Zdrav Procovnice,* 13 (1963), 532-533.   (Czech)

308. Fort, George F. *Medical Economy During the Middle Ages.* New York: J.W. Bouton, 1883.

309. Gordon, Benjamin Lee. *Medieval and Renaissance Medicine.* New York: Philosophical Library, 1959.

310. Gordon, J.E. "Nurses and Nursing in Britain. 3. The Medieval Monastic Tradition." *Mid Hlth Visit,* 6 (Aug 1970), 294-301.

311. ————. "Nurses and Nursing in Britain. 2. The Saxon Centuries." *Mid Hlth Visit,* 6 (Jul 1970), 252-257.

312. ————. "Nurses and Nursing in Britain. 7. The Hospital Tradition from the Reformation to the 18th Century." *Mid Hlth Visit,* 6 (Dec 1970), 457-462.

313. Hart, Margaret H. "Some Medieval Nurses in England." *Nurs Times,* 29 (11 Feb 1933), 127; (18 Feb 1933), 150; (25 Feb 1933), 174. See also *Brit J Nurs,* 81 (Mar 1933), 58-60; (Apr 1933), 98-99.

314. Hobson, John Morrison. *Some Early and Later Houses of Pity.* London: George Routledge and Sons, 1926.

315. Hughes, Muriel Joy. *Women Healers in Medieval Life and Literature.* New York: King's Crown Press, 1943.

316. Hume, Edgar Erskine. *Medical Work of the Knights Hospitallers of Saint John of Jerusalem.* Baltimore: Johns Hopkins University Press, 1940.

317. Imbert, Jean. *Les Hôpitaux en Droit Canonique.* Paris: Librairie Philosophique J. Vrin, 1947.

318. King, E.J. *The Knights Hospitallers in the Holy Land.* London: Methuen, 1931. 336 pp.

319. Lanfranc. *Science of Cirurgie.* Edited by Robert Von Fleishhacker. London: Early English Text Society, 1894.

320. McDevitt, B. "Foundations of Nursing in the Middle Ages." *Irish Nurs News* (Mar-Apr 1967), 2-7.

321. MacDonald, Isabel. "Royal Nurses." *Brit J Nurs,* 80 (Sep 1932), 234-235; (Oct 1932), 261-262; (Nov 1932), 298-300, 340, 342-343; 81 (May 1933), 142-144; (Jun 1933), 165-166; (Jul 1933), 196-198; 82 (Sep 1934), 237-238; (Oct 1934), 264-265; 83 (Feb 1935), 40-41; (Jul 1935), 182-183; (Aug 1935), 210-211; 84 (Sep 1936), 235-238; 85 (Jan 1937), 9-10.

322. MacKinney, Loren C. *Early Medieval Medicine.* Baltimore: Johns Hopkins University Press, 1937.

323. Marks, Geoffrey. *The Medieval Plague.* New York: Doubleday, 1971.

324.   Mazakarini, L. "Development of Nursing. Middle Ages Till the
       Time of the Turks with Reference to Viennese City History."
       Osterr Schwesternztg, 24 (May 1971), 135-138. (Ger)

325.   "Medicine and Nursing in the Middle Ages." *Nurs Times*, 33
       (10 April 1937), 356.

326.   "Milestones in the History of Nursing, 1854-1939." *Nurs Times*,
       35 (11 Nov 1939), 13.

327.   Mondeville, Henry de. *Chirurgie*, Edited by E. Nicaise.
       Paris: Felix Alcan, 1893.

328.   *Notes et Souvenirs*. Archives, Religeuses Augustines Hospi-
       taliers de l'Hotel de Paris, n.d. p. 312.

329.   Payne, Joseph Frank. *English Medicine in the Anglo Saxon
       Times*. Oxford: Clarendon Press, 1904.

330.   Riesman, David. *The Story of Medicine in the Middle Ages*.
       New York: P.B. Hoeber, 1935.

331.   Sudhoff, K. "Das kapitel über die Krankenpflege in der
       Beneditinerregel mit althochdeutschen Interlinearglossen in
       einer St. Galler Handschrift des 9 Jahrhunderts." *Archiv
       Gesch d Med*, 14 (1915).

332.   Trotula, Dame. *The Diseases of Women*. Translated by Elizabeth
       Mason-Hohl. Los Angeles: Ward Ritchie Press, 1940.

333.   Welborn, Mary Catherine. "The Long Tradition: A Study in Four-
       teenth Century Medical Deontology." *Medieval and Historio-
       graphical Essays in Honor of James Westfall Thompson*.
       Edited by James L. Cate and E.N. Anderson. Chicago: Uni-
       versity of Chicago Press, 1938.

EARLY MODERN (PRE-NIGHTINGALE) NURSING

334.   Cipolla, Carlo M. *Cristofano and the Plague*. Berkeley: Uni-
       versity of California Press, 1973.

335.   ————. *Public Health and the Medical Profession in the
       Renaissance*. Cambridge: Cambridge University Press, 1976.

336.   Goran, V. "Nursing During the Renaissance and Reformation."
       Tomorrow's Nurse, 4 (Jun-Jul 1963), 20ff.

337.   Hart, Margaret H. "Pre-Reformation Nurses in England." *St.
       Barth Hosp Rep*, 66 (1933), 133-169.

338.   King, Lester S. *The Medical World of the Eighteenth Century*.
       Chicago: University of Chicago Press, 1958.

339. Lallemand, Leon. *Histoire de la Charité.* 4 vols. Paris: Alphonse Picard, 1902-1912.

340. Liddon, H.P. *Life of Edward Bouverie Pusey.* 4 vols. 4th ed. London: Longmans, 1894-1897. See especially vol. 3, chap. 1, "The Early Days of Anglican Sisterhoods."

341. "The Lost Years of Nursing." *Tr Nurs & Hosp Rev,* 124 (Feb 1950), 62-63, 89.

342. McCarthy, Sister de Chantal. *St. Vincent de Paul's Concept of the Care of the Sick Applied to Present Objectives in Nursing Education.* Washington: Catholic University of America, 1938. 40 pp.

343. McMahon, Norbert. *St. John of God: Heavenly Patron of the Sick and Dying, Nurses and Hospitals.* New York: McMullen Books, 1951.

344. Moore, Mary Lou. "Bright Spot in the 18th Century." *Am J Nurs,* 69 (Aug 1969), 1703-1709.

345. Moore, Norman. *The History of St. Bartholomew's Hospital.* 2 vols. London: C. Arthur Pearson, Ltd., 1918.

346. Selvan, Ida Cohen. "Nurses in American History: the Revolution--Part 1." *Am J Nurs,* 75 (Apr 1975), 592-594.

347. Smith, J.M. "A Comparative View of the State of Medicine in the Years 1733 and 1833: An Introductory Lecture." *NY State J M,* 1 (1839), 245.

348. Weiner, D.B. "The French Revolution, Napoleon, and the Nursing Profession." *Bull Hist Med,* 46 (May-Jun 1972), 274-305.

349. ————. "Napoleon and the Professional Nurse: A Missed Opportunity." *Proc Inst Med Chic,* 28 (Nov 1971), 542.

NINETEENTH-CENTURY NURSING

350. Breay, Margaret. "Nursing in the Victorian Era." *Nurs Rec* (19 Jun 1897), 493-502.

351. Christy, Teresa E. "Nurses in American History: The Fateful Decade 1890-1900." *Am J Nurs,* 75 (Jul 1975), 1163-1165.

352. Dickens, Charles. *The Life and Adventures of Martin Chuzzlewit.* New York: The Heritage Press, 1951. (There are many other editions.)

353. Dolan, Josephine. "Nursing Leadership--1895. *Nurs Sci* (Aug-Sep 1963), 224-228.

354.   Edwards, R.   "Health and Medical Care at the Time of the
       American Centennial."   *J Sch Hlth*, 46(2) (Feb 1976), 77-80.

355.   Fox, E.M.   "What the 20th Century Nurse May Learn from the
       19th."   *Brit J Nurs* (26 Nov 1910), 432-434; (3 Dec 1910),
       447-449.

356.   Gordon, J.E.   "The Libel of Sairey Gamp."   *Med News* (28 Jun
       1963), 17, 21.

357.   Halsted, W.S.   "Ligature and Suture Material."   *J Am Med Assoc*,
       60 (13 May 1913), 1123.

358.   Luckes, Eva C.E.   *Hospital Sisters and Their Duties*.   4th ed.
       London: 1912.   234 pp.

359.   McCarrick, H.   "Aristotle's Midwife."   *Nurs Times*, 66 (1970),
       1470-1471.

360.   MacDermot, H.E.   "Nursing in Osler's Student Days."   *Canad
       Nurs*, 46 (Mar 1950), 222-224.

361.   Meigs, A.V.   "The Old Nursing and the New."   *Tr Nurs*, 22
       (1899), 119, 175.

362.   "Nursing in Madras in the 19th Century."   (Extracts from Re-
       ports of General Hospital, Madras, 1895.)   *Indian J Hist Med*,
       2(1) (1957), 43-48.

363.   "Nursing Progress in the 19th Century."   *Nurs Rec*, (Dec 1900),
       512-518.

364.   Ogle, W.   "Nurses; How to Make Them, How to Use Them, How to
       Pay Them."   *Rep Cong San Inst Gr Brit 1879*.   London: 1880,
       I, 100-104.

365.   "On a Summer Day in 1829."   *Nurs Mirror*, 132 (4 Jun 1971),
       30-31.

366.   Plotkin, S.A.   "The Crisis at Guy's."   (Dispute Concerning the
       Hiring of Nurses 1886.)   *Grey's Hosp Gaz*, 75 (1961), 45-50.

367.   "The Role of a Nurse in 1887 ..."   *Nurs Forum*, 10 (1971), 31.

368.   Rosenberg, Charles E.   "Social Class and Medical Care in Nine-
       teenth Century America: The Rise and Fall of the Dispensary."
       J Hist Med, 29 (Jan 1974), 32-54.

369.   Rothstein, William G.   *American Physicians in the 19th Century:
       From Sects to Science*.   Baltimore: Johns Hopkins University
       Press, 1972.

370.   Sandwith, F.M.   "Nursing and Care of the Sick Prior to 1850."
       Hosp (London), 56 (6 Jun 1914), 273-277.

371. Santos, E.H., and E. Stainbrook. "History of Nursing in 19th Century." *J Hist Med*, 4 (1949), 48-74.

372. Seidler, E. "Foundations of Medicine and Nursing in the 19th Century. I." *Deutsch Schwesternzeitung*, 20 (8 Aug 1967), 365-368. (Ger)

373. ————. "Foundations of Medicine and Nursing in the 19th Century. II." *Deutsch Schwesternzeitung*, 20 (10 Sep 1967), 430-432. (Ger)

374. Sherman, Ruth Brewster. "Abbé Gregoire on Nursing." *Am J Nurs*, 3 (Apr 1903), 505.

375. Wood, Catherine. "The Progress of Nursing During the Victorian Era." *Practitioner Lond*, 58 (1897), 709-716.

3. NURSING RESEARCH

376. Carnegie, M. Elizabeth. *Historical Perspectives of Nursing Research.* Boston: Nursing Archive of Boston University, 1976.

377. De Tornyay, R. "Nursing Research--The Road Ahead." *Nurs Res,* 26 (1977), 404-407.

378. Ellis, R. "The Evolution of Research in Nursing in the United States." *Jap J Nurs Res,* 4 (Autumn 1971), 294-300. (Jap)

379. ————. "Research for the Practice of Nursing." *Jap J Nurs Res,* 4 (Autumn 1971), 309-314. (Jap)

380. Ginsberg, Miriam K. *Years of Nursing Research at the Walter Reed Army Institute of Research.* Washington: Walter Reed Army Institute of Research, 1967.

381. Gortner, Susan R. "Research in Nursing: The Federal Interest and Grant Program." *Am J Nurs,* 73 (1973), 1052-1055.

382. McManus, R. Louise. "Nursing Research--Its Evolution." *Am J Nurs,* 61 (Apr 1961), 76-80.

383. Meyer, Burton, and Loretta Heidgerken. *Introduction to Research in Nursing.* Philadelphia: J.B. Lippincott Co., 1962.

384. Notter, L.E. "The Case for Nursing Research." *Nurs Out,* 23 (12) (Dec 1975), 760-763.

385. Pirquet, Clemens. "Should the Nurse Take Part in the Scientific Work of the Medical Profession?" *International Council of Nurses.* Geneva, 1927. pp. 61-62.

386. Simpson, Marjorie. "Research in Nursing--The First Step." *Int Nurs Rev,* 18(3) (1971), 231-247.

387. Whittaker, Elvi Waik, and Virginia L. Oleson. "Why Florence Nightingale?" *Am J Nurs,* 67 (Nov 1967), 2338-2341.

4. NURSING JOURNALS

388. *American Journal of Nursing: The Story of the Journal.* New York: American Journal of Nursing, 1950.

389. Christy, Teresa E. "The First 50 Years." *Am J Nurs,* 71 (Sep 1971), 1778-1784.

390. DeWitt, Katherine, and Helen Munson. "The Journal's First Fifty Years." *Am J Nurs,* 50 (Oct 1950), 590-597.

391. "Excerpts from the Journal (American Journal of Nursing) Fifty Years Ago." *Am J Nurs,* 59 (1959), 1421 *passim;* 60 (1969), 70 *passim.*

392. Fillmore, Anna. "Our First Five Years." *Nurs Out,* 6 (Jan 1958), 14-17.

393. "The First Nursing Journal to be Edited and Controlled by Trained Nurses." *Brit J Nurs,* 104 (Apr 1956), 25.

394. Gordon, J. Elise. "Nursing Mirror Through 75 Years." *Nurs Mirror,* 117 (1963), VI-VIII, XIII, 3041.

395. "Harefooah: Palestine's First Medical Journal." *Am J Nurs,* 20 (1920), 980.

396. "The History of the Journal." *Amer Assoc Industr Nurs J,* 14 (1966), 7-8.

397. Karll, A. "Under the Lazarus Cross. History of Our Society's Periodical." *Krankenpflege,* 27 (Jan 1973), 11-12.

398. Kerr, Margaret E. "Fifty Years Young." *Am J Nurs,* 55 (Mar 1955), 302.

399. *Nurses Journal of the Pacific Coast,* editorial, 20 (Sep 1906), 210.

400. Pfefferkorn, Blanche. "Improvement of the Nurse in Service—an Historical Review." *Annual Report 1928.* New York: National League of Nursing Education, pp. 128-139; *Proceedings of 34th Convention.* New York: The League, 1928. 324 pp.

401. "Resignation of Miss (Lavinia L.) Dock from the Journal Staff," editorial. *Am J Nurs,* 23 (May 1923), 660-661.

402.   Shah, N.A.   "Editorial: Commemoration of the 20th Anniversary
       of the Journal of Nurse Midwifery."   *J Nurs Mid*, 20(2)
       (Summer 1975), 4.

403.   "Thirty-five Years Ago They were Saying--."   *Am J Nurs*, 35
       (Oct 1935), 905-908.

5. HISTORICAL RESEARCH AND THE TEACHING OF THE HISTORY OF NURSING

404. Abbott, Maude E. "History as Force in Nursing Education, How to Teach it." *Canad Nurs*, 27 (Oct 1937), 509-516.

405. Austin, Anne L. "The Historical Method in Nursing." *Nurs Res*, 7(1) (Feb 1958), 4-10.

406. Christy, T.E. "The Methodology of Historical Research: A Brief Introduction." *Nurs Res*, 24(3) (May-Jun 1975), 189-192.

407. ———. "Nursing History Neither Dead nor Dull." *Am Nurs*, 7 (7) (Jul 1975), 10.

408. ———. "Problem Forum: Historical Research; Characteristics of Historical Research and Problems of the Historian." *Nurs Res Conf*, 8 (May 1972), 227-228.

409. Cuthbert, B.L. "Can We Do More In Contributing to History of Nursing?" *Alum Mag* (Baltimore), 65 (Sep 1966), 67-68.

410. Depierri, K.P. "One Way of Unearthing the Past." *Am J Nurs*, 68 (Mar 1968), 521-524.

411. Desch, Sister Mary Digna. *An Analytical Study of Content and Achievement in the History of Nursing Course*. Washington: Catholic University of America, 1936. 55 pp.

412. Dock, Lavinia L. "History of Nursing." *Am J Nurs*, 11 (Feb 11), 379-381. (Ger)

413. ———. "When We Wrote a History." *Johns Hop Nurs Alum Mag*, 49 (1950), 59-60.

414. Dolan, Josephine A. "Using Postage Stamps to Teach History of Nursing." *Nurs Out*, 9 (Mar 1961), 164-165.

415. Dunbar, Virginia M. "The Instructor of History of Nursing." *Nurs Out*, 10 (May 1962), 307-310.

416. Fauerbach, Gale. "More Vital Instruction in the History of Nursing." *Tr Nurs*, 76 (May 1926), 541-542.

417. Flack, Holly. "A History-of-Nursing Society." *Am J Nurs*, 27 (Jul 1927), 553-555.

418.   Goostray, Stella. "Nationwide Hunt for Nursing's Historical Treasures." *Nurs Out*, 13 (Jan 1965), 26-29.

419.   Hahn, Ruth E. "A History of Nursing Scrapbook." *Am J Nurs*, 27 (Apr 1927), 279-280.

420.   "History of Nursing." *Tr Nurs & Hosp Rev*, 87 (Sep 1931), 324-325.

421.   "History of Nursing Comes Alive." *Christian Nurs*, 216 (Dec 1967), 15ff.

422.   Howard, W. "Ladies and Hospital Nursing." *Contemp Rev*, 34 (1879), 490-503.

423.   Kalisch, Beatrice J., and Philip A. Kalisch. "Is History of Nursing Alive and Well?" *Nurs Out*, 24(6) (Jun 1976), 362-366.

424.   Koyama, R. "Nursing Study at the High School Nursing Courses, Teaching Methods in History of Nursing and Their Evaluation." *Jap J Nurs Educ*, 15(8) (Aug 1974), 520-525. (Jap)

425.   Kubo, S. "Nursing Seminar. History and Ethics of Nursing." *Kango*, 18 (May 1974), 20-33. (Jap)

426.   Leahy, M. "History of Nursing Can Be Fascinating." *Nurs Out*, 54 (1954), 464.

427.   "The March of Time in Nursing History." *Pac Cst J Nurs*, 36 (Sep 1940), 528-532.

428.   Meij de Leur, A Prande van der. "History-Why and How." *Tijdschr Ziekenverpl*, 24 (Feb 1972), 117-119. (Dut)

429.   Monteiro, L.A. "Forum on Historical Research Response in Anger--An Unsent Letter to the Editor: Investigation of a Letter Written by Florence Nightingale." *Ninth Nurs Res Conf Proceedings* (ANA Publications) (21-23 Mar 1973), 283-293.

430.   ———. "Research into Things Past: Tracking Down One of Miss Nightingale's Correspondents." *Nurs Res*, 21 (Nov-Dec 1972), 526-529.

431.   Morison, Luella J., and Anna C. Fegan. *Continued Study Unit in History of Nursing*. Philadelphia: F.A. Davis, 1941. 72 pp.

432.   Nagatoya, Y. "Establishment of Nursing History as a Study." *Jap J Nurs Educ*, 12 (May 1971), 53-57. (Jap)

433.   National League for Nursing. Committee on Early Nursing Source Materials. *Source Materials in Nursing Education*. No. 1. New York: The League, 1952. 57 pp.

434. ————. *Source Materials in Nursing Education.* No. 2. New
      York: The League, 1954. 56 pp.

435. National League of Nursing Education. Committee on Early
      Nursing Source Materials. *A Century of Nursing.* New York:
      G.P. Putnam's Sons, 1950. 172 pp.

436. Newton, Mildred E. "The Case for Historical Research." *Nurs
      Res*, 14 (Winter 1965), 20-26.

437. Notter, L.E. "The Case for Historical Research in Nursing."
      Nurs Res, 21 (Nov-Dec 1972), 483.

438. Pakkala, K. "Museum Activities are Lifetime Ambition."
      Sairaanhoitaja, 54(9) (1978), 18-19. (Fin)

439. Roberts, Mary M. "New Look at History of Nursing." *Nurs Out*,
      6 (1958), 79.

440. Ryan, Patricia, and R. Fawson. "Project in History of
      Nursing." *Canad Nurs*, 51 (1955), 873.

441. Shopa, M.A. "Letter: Historical Materials in Nursing." *Nurs
      Res*, 24(4) (Jul-Aug 1975), 308.

442. Smith, Dorothy M., Madeline Hines, and Eleanor Tourtillot.
      "Instruction in History of Nursing in a Collegiate School,
      A Diploma School, and An Associate Degree Program." *Nurs
      Out*, 8 (Nov 1960), 631-635.

443. "Society of Teresians: An Outline for Study in Nursing His-
      tory." *Am J Nurs*, 7 (Dec 1906), 199-200.

444. Stewart, Isabel Maitland. "A Bird's-eye View of Nursing
      History." *Am J Nurs*, 17 (Jul 1917), 958-966. Also in *NLNE
      Annual Report, 1917 and Proceedings of 23rd Convention.*
      New York: NLNE, 1918.

445. "Visualizing Nursing in Pageantry." *Tr Nurs & Hosp Rev*, 104
      (1940), 530-531.

446. Walker, Lena Dixon. "History of Nursing Maps." *Am J Nurs*, 28
      (Jan 1928), 23-25.

447. Yamane, N. "In Search of Unknown Nursing Literature (5).
      Nursing Literature in 1890's and early 1900." *Jap J Nurs
      Educ*, 16(10) (Oct 1975), 634-639. (Jap)

448. ————. "In Search of Unknown Nursing Literature (6). The
      Nursing Literature in Early 1900 and the Publication by the
      Japan Red Cross." *Jap J Nurs Educ*, 16(11) (Nov 1975), 682-
      687. (Jap)

6. NURSES' UNIFORMS

449. Carbary, L.J. "Nursing School Pins Are Priceless Possessions." *RN*, 34 (Dec 1971), 27-31.

450. Central Health Services Council Standing Nursing Advisory Committee. *Report of a Subcommittee on the Design of Nurses' Uniforms*. London: HMSO, 1959.

451. "The History of Queen's Uniform and Badges." *District Nursing* (May 1961), 36.

452. Kerling, N.J.M. "The First Blue Uniform (of the Matron, Sisters and Officers of St. Bartholomew's Hospital in the 16th Century)." *St Bart Hosp J*, 67 (1963), 47.

453. Knowles, Lois N. "The Collar That Became a Cap." *Am J Nurs* (Sep 1958), 1246-1248.

454. Lapointe, G. "Yesteryear Uniforms in Reminiscences Over the Years." *Infirm Can*, 14 (Aug 1972), 34-37. (Fr)

455. Michaels, Roberta. "What's New in Uniforms." *RN* (Mar 1958), 52-59.

456. Nelson, Jean. "Ladies Who Had Style." *Nurs Mirror*, 141 (20 Nov 1975), 79.

457. Newcastle Regional Hospital Board. *Report on Design of Nursing Uniforms*. Newcastle Regional Hospital Board, England, 1954.

458. "The Nurse and Her Outfit in Hospital, on District, in Private and Midwifery, Work in Government Service and Abroad." *Nurs Times* (13 Nov 1909), 920-933.

459. "The Nurse and Her Uniform." *Nurs Times* (7 Oct 1955), 1111-1112.

460. "Nurse's Uniform, New American Ideas." *Nurs Times* (7 Oct 1955), 1128-1130.

461. "The Nurse's Uniform, Editorial." *Nurs Mirror* (20 Dec 1957), 868.

462. Rees, S.A.H. "Staff Uniforms." *Hosp & Hlth Mgmt* (Jan 1964), 58-60.

463.   Robson, P.L.   "Nurses' Uniforms (1) Standards and Patterns."
       Nurs Mirror (17 Nov 1960), 541-542.

464.   Smith, Marion E.   "Uniforms." *Nurs Rec* (5 Sep 1896), 183-185.

465.   Sticker, A.   "The Nurse's Headdress--Head Covers of Religious
       Orders and Deaconesses." *Agnes Karll Schwest*, 23 (Dec 1969),
       574-576.   (Ger)

466.   Stratford, D.O.   "Women in Uniform: IV. A Brief Account of
       Nursing in the Crimea Giving Details of Uniform Worn." *So
       Afr Nurs J* (1961), 26-27.

467.   Tanno, I.   "Role of Uniforms in History." *Jap J Pub Hlth Nurs*,
       31(9) (Sep 1975), 566-570.   (Jap)

468.   "The Territorial Force Nursing Service--Uniform." *Brit J Nurs*
       (27 May 1911), 415.

469.   "The Tides of Style--In Professional Garb From 1891 to 1941."
       Tr Nurs & Hosp Rev, 106 (1941), 206-211, 235, 237, 239.

470.   Villermay, D. De.   "Pro or Con Uniforms." *Rev Infirm*, 24
       (Jun 1974), 513-520.   (Fr)

471.   Watkin, B.   "Cap and Apron (Nursing Uniforms)." *Med News*
       (17 Sep 1965).

472.   Watkin, Brian V.   "The Story of Nurses' Uniforms." *Nurs Times*
       (11 Oct 1963), 1279-1283.

473.   "Why a Cap? The Evolution of the Nurse's Cap in Some Schools
       Established Before 1895." *Am J Nurs*, 40 (1940), 384-387.

474.   *Why a Cap? A Short History of Nursing Caps from Some Schools
       Organized Prior to 1891.* Philadelphia: J.B. Lippincott,
       1940.

475.   Yates, Eileen.   "The Apron Story." *Nurs Mirror* (10 Jun 1966),
       12-13.

7.   BIOGRAPHIES AND AUTOBIOGRAPHIES

Standard biographical dictionaries such as *Who's Who* are not listed here nor included in the Bibliography.

GENERAL

476.   *Alumnae Biographical Register, 1894-1953.* New York: Dept. of Nursing, Columbia University and Alumnae Association, Presbyterian Hospital, 1953.

477.   *American Journal of Nursing.* Biographical material in obituaries, occasional biographical sketches, photographs, et al. More detailed biographies are listed separately in this section.

478.   *American Women.* 3 vols. Los Angeles: American Publication, Inc., 1935-1940. Women are listed by their profession.

479.   "Autographs of Beloved Nurses." *Tr Nurs & Hosp Rev*, 104 (1940), 26-27.

480.   *British Journal of Nursing.* Obituaries, biographies, et al.

481.   *Canadian Nurse.* Biographical material in obituaries and in periodic biographical sketches. More detailed biographies are listed separately in this section.

482.   Derieux, Mary. *One Hundred Great Lives.* New York: Greystone, 1948. pp. 191-198.

483.   DeWitt, William A. *Illustrated Minute Biographies.* New York: Grosset, 1949. p. 118.

484.   "Eminent Teachers." *Am J Nurs*, 29 (1929), monthly except for October.

485.   *Filipino Nurse.* Periodic sketches of nursing leaders. Articles on the more prominent leaders are listed separately in this section.

486.   Fitzhugh, Harrie Lloyd (le Porte), and P.K. Fitzhugh. *Concise Biographical Dictionary of Famous Men and Women.* Rev. ed. New York: Grosset, 1949. pp. 502-504.

487. "Friends of Nursing." *Am J Nurs*, 32 (1932), monthly.

488. "Historical Collections." *Am J Nurs*, 30 (May 1930), 551-556.
      Memorabilia of various nurses at Johns Hopkins Hospital
      School of Nursing collected by Adelaide Nutting. Much on
      Florence Nightingale. See also *Brit J Nurs*, 78 (Jun 1930),
      154-155.

489. Hume, R.F. *Great Women of Medicine*. New York: Random House,
      1964.

490. "Interesting People." *Canad Nurs*, 40 (1944). Biographical
      notes and photographs of nurses. First appeared in October
      1944. Renamed "Nursing Profiles" in 1948.

491. National League of Nursing Education. *Biographic Sketches,
      1937-1940*. New York: The League, 1940. Biographical
      sketches and photographs of 40 nursing leaders.

492. ————. *Early Leaders of American Nursing*. New York: The
      League, 1922. Biographical sketches and photographs of 24
      nurses.

493. ————. *Nursing and Nurses, Old and New*. New York: National
      League of Nursing Education, 1929.

494. Newcomb, Ellsworth. *Brave Nurse: True Stories of Heroism*.
      New York: Appleton, Century, 1945.

495. *Nursing Mirror and Midwives Journal*. Periodic sketches of
      nursing leaders as well as obituaries of prominent nurses.

496. *Pacific Coast Journal of Nursing*. Section entitled "Who's Who
      in the Western Nursing World" appeared sporadically.

497. Pennock, Meta Rutter. *Makers of Nursing History: Portraits
      and Pen Sketches of Fifty-Nine Prominent Women*. New York:
      Lakeside Pub. Co., 1928. 128 pp.

498. ————. *Makers of Nursing History: Portraits and Pen Sketches
      of One Hundred and Nine Prominent Women*. New York: Lakeside
      Pub. Co., 1940. 142 pp.

499. *Philippine Journal of Nursing*. Regular biographical sketches
      of nurses.

500. *Queen's Nurses Magazine*. Regular department giving brief
      obituaries of members of Queen's Institute of District
      Nursing.

501. Ross, Will. *They Caught the Torch*. Milwaukee: Ross, 1939.
      Color drawings and biographical notes on nurses.

502. Safier, Gwendolyn. *Contemporary American Leaders in Nursing:
      An Oral History*. New York: McGraw-Hill Book Co., 1977.

503.   ————. "I Sensed the Challenges: Leaders Among Contemporary
        U.S. Nurses." *The Oral History Review* (1975).

504.   Sewell, W. Stuart, ed. *Brief Biographies of Famous Men and
        Women.* New York: Permabook, 1949. pp. 143-144.

505.   "Some Leaders Along the Way." *Tr Nurs & Hosp Rev*, 100 (Apr
        1938), 410.

506.   "Some Specialists." *Am J Nurs*, 30 (1930); 31 (1931), *passim.*

507.   Stephenson, Gladys E. *Some Pioneers in the Medical and Nurs-
        ing World.* Shanghai: Nurses' Assn. of China, 1924. 52 pp.

508.   Thomas, Adah H. *Pathfinders—A History of Progress of Colored
        Graduate Nurses.* New York: McKay, 1929. Biographies of
        some black nurses.

509.   "Who's Who in the Nursing Profession." *Filipino Nurse*, 4
        (1930).

510.   "Who's Who in the Nursing World." *Am J Nurs*, 21-28 (1921-
        1928), an on-going series.

511.   "Who's Who in the Who's Who or Don't Be So Modest Ladies."
        Nurs Out, 8 (1960), 15.

512.   Yost, Edna. *American Women of Nursing.* Philadelphia: J.B.
        Lippincott, 1955.

INDIVIDUAL

        Individuals who are not nurses, but who had some
        influence on nursing, such as Jane Addams, are in-
        cluded, although not in any exhaustive way.

ABELGAS, IRENE M.

513.   "Who is Who: Irene M. Abelgas." *Filipino Nurs*, 10 (Jul 1935),
        16.

ADDAMS, JANE

514.   "Looking Back—Jane Addams and Lillian Wald." *Nurs Out*, 8
        (Sep 1960), 492.

515.   Thomson, Elnora E. "Jane Addams—A Tribute." *Pac Cst J Nurs*,
        31 (Jul 1935), 36.

AIKENS, CHARLOTTE A.

516.   "Charlotte A. Aikens." *Tr Nurs & Hosp Rev*, 123 (Dec 1949), 279.

AINSLIE, RUTH (MCCONNELL)

517.   Mendez, C. "My Most Unforgettable Characters." *Read Digest*,
        104 (Apr 1974), 145-149.

AITKENHEAD, MARY AUGUSTINE (MOTHER BISHOP)

518.   "Mary Aitkenhead (1787-1858)." *Nurs Mirror*, 108 (Oct 1958),
        7; and *Nurs Times*, 55 (23 Jan 1959), 120.

ALCOTT, LOUISA MAY

519.   Cheney, Edna D., ed. *Life, Letters and Journal (Louisa May
        Alcott)*. Boston: Roberts Brothers, 1889.

520.   Gulliver, Lucile. *Louisa May Alcott: A Bibliography*. Boston:
        Little, Brown & Co., 1932.

521.   Hosmer, Gladys E.H. "Louisa May Alcott: War Nurse." *Tr Nurs*,
        89 (Aug 1932), 145-151; and *Nurs Mirror*, 56 (26 Nov 1932),
        150-151.

522.   Meigs, Cornelia Lynde. *The Story of the Author of Little
        Women: Invincible Louisa*. Boston: Little, Brown & Co., 1933,
        1961.

523.   Stern, Madeline Bettina. *Louisa May Alcott*. Norman: Univer-
        sity of Oklahoma Press, 1950.

524.   Worthington, Marjorie Muir. *Miss Alcott of Concord: A Bio-
        graphy*. Garden City, NY: Doubleday, 1958.

ALETRINO, MRS. E.J. (VAN STOCKUM)

525.   "Nurses of Note: Mrs. (E.J.) Aletrino née Van Stockum." *Brit
        J Nurs*, 39 (26 Oct 1907), 330.

ALEXANDER, B.G.

526.   "Death of Miss B.G. Alexander--Irreparable Loss to Nursing."
        So Afr Nurs J, 15 (Aug 1949), 38-40. See also *Int Nurs Bull*,
        5 (Suppl) (Autumn-Winter 1949) and earlier biographical
        sketch, *Nurs Times*, 40 (Jan 1944), 3.

527.   "New President of South African Trained Nurses' Association--
        B.G. Alexander." *So Afr Nurs Rec*, 17 (Mar 1930), 146-147.

ALEXANDRA, PRINCESS OF CONNAUGHT

528.   Alexandra, Princess of Connaught. *A Nurse's Story by Alexandra*.
        London: Bumpus, 1955. 159 pp.

ALKIN, ELIZABETH

529.   Gordon, J.E. "Distinguished British Nurses of the Past. 1:
       Elizabeth Alkin--Nurse and Secret Agent, 1616-1655." *Midwife
       Hlth Visit Com Nurs*, 11(3) (Mar 1975), 77-81.

530.   ————. "17th Century Florence Nightingale." *Country Life*,
       150 (28 Oct 1971), 155-157.

531.   MacDonald, Isabel. *Elizabeth Alkin, A Florence Nightingale of
       the Commonwealth*. Keighley: Wadsworth & Co., 1935. 23 pp.

ALLEN, JAN C.

532.   Hansen, Anne L. "Miss (Jane C.) Allen's Resignation." *Pub
       Hlth Nurs*, 20 (Aug 1928), 397. For note on her appointment,
       see *Am J Nurs*, 26 (Jul 1926), 556.

ALLINE, ANNA LOWELL

533.   *Early Leaders of American Nursing (Calendar 1923)*. New York:
       National League of Nursing Education, 1922.

AMURO, C.

534.   "Confrontational." *Newsweek*, 68 (1 Aug 1966), 26.

535.   "They are All Dead." *Newsweek*, 68 (25 July 1965), 18-20.

536.   Wainwright, L. "Who the Gentle Victims Were." *Life*, 61
       (29 Jul 1966), 19-26.

ANDERSON, ELIZABETH

537.   "Pioneer of Women Practitioners. Elizabeth Garrett Anderson,
       M.D." *Aust Nurs J*, 16 (Mar 1918), 90-95. She was also a
       nurse.

ANDERSON, LOUISA GARRETT

538.   *Elizabeth Garrett Anderson, 1836-1917*. London: Faber & Faber,
       1939. 338 pp. Deals with her relationship to nursing.

ANNESTASIA, SISTER

539.   Cosby, V. "Sister Annestasia." *Ladies Home J*, 67 (Oct 1950),
       269-270.   \

ANTHONY, SUSAN B.

540.   Fenwick, Ethel Gordon. "Apotheosis of Susan B. Anthony."
       Brit J Nurs, 37 (18 Aug 1906), 136-137.

541.   "Miss Susan B. Anthony, editorial." *Am J Nurs*, 6 (Apr 1906),
       424-425; (May 1906), 506; (Dec 1906), 97-98. Deals with her
       relationship to nursing.

APPLEBEE, RHODA

542.   *No Greater Calling: The Story of a Nursing Sister.* St. Ives,
       Cornwall, Eng.: United Writers Pubs., 1974. 270 pp.

ARCHARD, THERESA

543.   *G.I. Nightingale: The Story of an American Army Nurse.* New
       York: W.W. Norton, 1945.

ARENDT, SISTER HENRIETTE

544.   Kent, Beatrice. "Sister Henriette Arendt." *Brit J Nurs*, 52
       (6 Jun 1914), 507-509; see also 52 (27 Jun 1914), 568.

ARMIGER, SISTER BERNADETTE

545.   "Two Sister Nurses Claimed by Cholera." *Nurs Out*, 12 (Sep
       1964), 54, 56.

ARNSTEIN, MARGARET G.

546.   "M.G. Arnstein." *Nurs Times* (9 Oct 1972), 34.

ARTHUR, PRINCESS OF CONNAUGHT

547.   "New President of the Royal British Nurses' Association."
       Brit J Nurs, 72 (Jan 1924), 11-12.

548.   "The Princess Arthur of Connaught, S.R.N., President of Royal
       British Nurses' Association." *Brit J Nurs*, 87 (May 1939),
       117; see also 78 (Jun 1930), 13.

AVERY, L.M.

549.   "Secretary-General of the Australian Nursing Federation."
       Aust Nurs J, 49 (Mar 1951), 46.

BACON, MRS. FRANCIS

550.   "Official Reports. Death of Mrs. Francis Bacon." *Am J Nurs*, 6
       (Mar 1906), 403.

BAGGALLAY, OLIVE

551.   "News from the Nursing World." *Nurs Mirror*, 59 (25 Aug 1934),
       395.

BAILEY, A.

552. "The Passing to the Great Beyond of a Gallant Nurse and a
Lover of Africans. Tribute to Mother Mary Martin." *Niger
Nurs*, 7(2) (Apr-Jun 1975), 28-29.

BAILEY, HARRIET

553. Obituary. *New York Times* (24 May 1953), 88.

BAILEY, MARGARET E.

554. "Top Nurse in Uniform." *Ebony*, 21 (Sep 1966), 50ff.

BALL, MARY

555. Earl, Laurence. *She Loved a Wicked City: The Story of Mary
Ball*. New York: Dutton, 1962. 240 pp. Also published as
One Foreign Devil. London: Hodder, 1962. 140 pp.

BANNON, DOROTHY E.

556. "Dorothy E. Bannon." *Nurs Mirror*, 70 (10 Feb 1940), 445-446.

BARNETT, RICHARD WHIELDON

557. "Richard Whieldon Barnett, Kt" editorial. *Brit J Nurs*, 78
(Nov 1930), 281-283. His role in influencing nursing
legislation.

BARTLETT, CLAUDE

558. "Mental Nurse Becomes Chairman of T.U.C." *Nurs Mirror*, 108
(18 Sep 1959), 1301.

BARTON, CLARA

559. Bailey, Helen Miller. *40 American Biographies*. New York:
Harcourt, Brace & World, 1964. pp. 125-129.

560. Baker, Harry J. *Biographical Sagas of Will Power*. New York:
Vantage Press, 1970. pp. 160-161.

561. "Clara Barton." *Am J Nurs*, 16 (Feb 1916), 385-386; see also
Brit J Nurs, 47 (20 Apr 1921), 314; and *Pac Cst J Nurs*, 12
(May 1916), 260-261.

562. "Clara Barton: A Biographical Sketch." *Grade Teach*, 71 (Mar
1954), 38ff.

563. Barton, William E. *The Life of Clara Barton*. 2 vols. Boston:
Houghton Mifflin Co., 1922.

564. Barton, William Eleazar. *Life of Clara Barton, Founder of the American Red Cross.* 2 vols. New York: AMS Press, 1969.

565. Berman, J.K. "Florentia and the Clarabellas--A Tribute to Nurses." (Nightingale, Barton, C., and Maas, C.) *J Ind Med Assoc*, 67 (Aug 1974), 717-719.

566. Bird, Caroline. *Enterprising Women.* New York: W.W. Norton and Co., 1976. pp. 98-100.

567. Carmen, Carl Lamson, ed. *Cavalcade of America.* New York: Crown, 1956. pp. 311-313 (por.).

568. Christian Science Sentinel. *Mary Baker Eddy Mentioned Them.* Boston: Christian Science Publ., 1961. pp. 25-26.

569. DeWitt, William A. *Illustrated Minute Biographies.* New York: Grosset, 1949. p. 20 (por.).

570. D'Humy, Fernand Emile. *Women Who Influenced the World.* New York: Library Publications, 1955. pp. 227-277.

571. Epler, Percy Harold. *Life of Clara Barton.* New York: Macmillan Co., 1915. 438 pp.

572. Hall, Kenneth. *They Stand Tall.* New York: Warner Press, 1953. pp. 43-53.

573. Heath, Monroe. *Great Americans at a Glance.* Vol. 4. Menlo Park, CA: Pacific Coast Publs., 1957. p. 15.

574. Humphrey, Grace. *Women in American History.* Freeport, NY: Books for Libraries Press, 1968. pp. 189-206.

575. McGrady, Mike. *Jungle Doctors.* Philadelphia: J.B. Lippincott, 1962. pp. 103-106.

576. McKown, Robin. *Heroic Nurses.* New York: G.P. Putnam's Sons, 1966. pp. 101-102.

577. Morris, Richard Brandon, ed. *Encyclopedia of American History.* New York: Harper and Row, 1953. 634 pp.

578. Muir, Charles Stothard. *Women, The Makers of History.* New York: Vantage Press, 1956. 172 pp.

579. Pace, Dixie Ann. "Clara Barton." In *Valiant Women.* New York: Vantage Press, 1972. pp. 67-73 il.

580. Pan American Columbus Society. *Clara Barton, Protector of the Cuban Reconcentrados.* The Society, 1954. 18 pp. il.

581. Paris, L. "Angel of the Battlefield." *Scholastic*, 69 (4 Jan 1957), 15.

582. Park, Roswell. "Clara Barton." *Am J Nurs*, 6 (Nov 1905), 92.

583. Ramsay, A.G. "She Walked with Kings." *Ind Woman*, 35 (Jun 1956), 4-6.

584. Ross, Ishbel. *Angel of the Battlefield: The Life of Clara Barton*. New York: Harper and Row, 1956. 305 pp.

585. Samuels, G. "Legacy of Clara Barton." *NY Times Mag* (26 Feb 1961), p. 30ff.

586. Sewell, W. Stuart, ed. "Clara Barton." In *Brief Biographies of Famous Men and Women*. New York: Permabooks, 1949. pp. 144-145.

587. Stoddard, Hope. "Clara Barton." In *Famous American Women*. New York: Thomas Y. Crowell, 1970. pp. 59-70.

588. Wefer, M. "Miss Barton's in Charge." *Scholastic* (2 Dec 1946), 17-18.

589. Williams, Blanche Colton. *Clara Barton*. Philadelphia: J.B. Lippincott, 1941. 468 pp.

590. Young, Charles Sumner. *Clara Barton. A Centenary Tribute*. Boston: Richard C. Badger Gorham Press, 1922. 444 pp.

BATTERHAM, MARY ROSE

591. "Nursing. First R.N." *Southern Hosp*, 6 (Jan 1938), 11.

BEARD, MARY

592. Gregg, Alan. "Mary Beard--Humanist." *Am J Nurs*, 47 (Feb 1947), 103-104; see also biographical sketch in *Pub Hlth Nurs*, 39 (Jan 1947), 2.

593. Obituary. *NY Times* (5 Dec 1946), 31.

594. Obituary. *Pub Hlth Nurs*, 39 (19 Jan 1947), 2.

595. Obituary. *Time*, 48 (16 Dec 1946), 80.

BEULAH, LOIS

596. "Miss Lois Beulah, S.R.N., D.N., S.C.M., M.D." *Nurs Mirror*, 94 (5 Oct 1951), 17.

BECK, FREDA

597. Gridley, Marion E., ed. *Indians of Today*. n.p.: ICFP, Inc., 1971. 4.

BEEBY, NELL

598.   "Biography." *NCAB*, 45 (1962), 345-346.

599.   "Death of Miss N.V. Beeby, RN. Loss to Nursing World." *So Afr Nurs J*, 24 (Jul 1957), 29.

600.   Fillmore, Anna M. "Nell V. Beeby, 1896-1957." *Nurs Out*, 5 (Jun 1957), 340-343.

601.   "H M Salutes Nell V. Beeby, Executive Editor AJN Co." *Hosp Mgmt*, 86 (Jun 1957), 36.

602.   "In Memoriam." *Canad Nurs*, 53 (Jul 1957), 628.

603.   "Miss Beeby Receives the Nutting Award." *Am J Nurs*, 57 (Apr 1957), 469.

604.   "Nell V. Beeby, 1896-1957." *Am J Nurs*, 57 (Jun 1957), 730.

605.   Obituary. *NY Times* (18 May 1957), 19.

606.   Roberts, Mary M. "The Journal Editors." *Am J Nurs*, 49 (Jun 1949), 330-331; see also *Canad Nurs*, 46 (Sep 1949), 680-681; and *Pub Hlth Nurs*, 41 (Jun 1944), 366.

BELL, ESTHER HOPE

607.   Simpson, Cora E. "Our New Secretary." *Quart J Chin Nurs*, 7 (Jan 1926), 29; see also *Brit J Nurs*, 74 (Aug 1926), 77.

608.   "Miss Jane Bell, O.B.E." *Aust Nurs J*, 45 (Feb 1947), 36-37.

BENNETT, B.A.

609.   "Distinguished Portrait Gallery--5. Mrs. B.A. Bennett, O.B.E., S.R.N., D.N." *Nurs Mirror*, 93 (13 Jul 1951), 261.

BEST, ELLA

610.   "Addition to Staff." *Am J Nurs*, 30 (Aug 1930), 1077.

611.   McIver, Pearl. "A Job Well Done" (ed). *Am J Nurs*, 58 (Jul 1958), 965.

BETHKE, ANNIE

612.   Haskin, Dorothy (Clark). *Medical Missionaries You Would Like to Know*. Grand Rapids, MI: Zandervan, 1957. pp. 5-13.

BICKERDYKE, MARY ANN

613.   Baker, Nina Brown. *Cyclone in Calico*. Boston: Little, Brown & Co., 1952. 278 pp.

614.   ———. "Cyclone in Calico" (abr). *Read Digest*, 61 (Dec
        1952), 141-162.

615.   Bird, Caroline. *Enterprising Women*. New York: W.W. Norton,
        1976. pp. 92-93.

616.   Cunningham, Dru. "Mother Bickerdyke--A Nursing Tradition."
        Am Leg Mag, 102 (May 1966), 22.

617.   Davis, M.B. *The Woman Who Battles for the Boys in Blue--Mother
        Bickerdyke*. San Francisco: Pacific Press Publishing House,
        1886.

618.   DeLeeuw, Adele. *Civil War Nurse: Mary Ann Bickerdyke*. New
        York: Julian Messner, 1973. 158 pp.

619.   Dunlop, R. "Nurse Who Outranked the General." *Today's Health*,
        48 (May 1970), 56ff.

620.   Erlandson, E.V. "The Story of Mother Bickerdyke." *Am J Nurs*,
        20 (May 1920), 628-631.

621.   Kellogg, Florence Shaw. *Mother Bickerdyke as I Knew Her*.
        Chicago: United Publishing Co., 1907.

622.   McKown, Robin. "Mother Bickerdyke." *Heroic Nurses*. New
        York: G.P. Putnam's Sons, 1966. pp. 77-100.

BLACK, MILDRED (WOLFE)

623.   *Reminiscences of a Country Doctor's Wife*. New York: Exposi-
        tion Press, 1975. 80 pp.

BLACKWELL, ELIZABETH

624.   Fleming, Thomas P. "Dr. Elizabeth Blackwell on Florence
        Nightingale (Comments from or Collection of Autographed
        Letters by Elizabeth Blackwell." *Columbia Univ Columns*, 6
        (1956), 37-43.

625.   Hays, Elinor Rice. *Those Extraordinary Blackwells*. New York:
        Harcourt, Brace and World, 1967.

626.   Ross, Ishbel. *Child of Destiny: The Life Story of the First
        Woman Doctor*. New York: Harper & Bros., 1949; London:
        Gollancz, 1950. See also Tabor, Margaret E., no. 945
        (E. Fry).

627.   Wohlfarth, P. "Die erste Arztin im englischparachigen Rau."
        Berl Med, 15 (1964), 651-652.

BLACKWOOD, HERMIONE

628.   "Nurses of Note: Lady Hermione Blackwood." *Brit J Nurs*, 40
        (30 May 1908), 429.

BLANCHFIELD, FLORENCE A.

629. Aynes, Edith A. "Colonel Florence A. Blanchfield." *Nurs Out*,
      7 (Feb 1959), 78-91.

630. Obituary. *Cur Biog*, 32 (June 1971), 44.

631. Obituary. *Cur Biog Yrbk*. (1971, 1972), p. 460.

632. Obituary. *NY Times* (13 May 1971), 48.

633. "R.N.: A Salute for Col. (Florence A.) Blanchfield." *RN*, 10
      (Sep 1947), 31, 86.

BOARDMAN, MABEL THORP

634. "A Famous Woman and Her Home." *Nurse*, 2 (Jun 1915), 446-450.

BOLTON, FRANCES PAYNE

635. Loth, David. *A Long Way Forward: The Biography of Congress-
      woman Frances P. Bolton*. New York: Longmans, 1957. 302 pp.

BONZER, SALLY (CUMMINGS)

636. Thurelsen, R. "Registered Nurse." *Sat Eve Post*, 220 (3 Apr
      1948), 34-35.

BORCHERDS, M.G.

637. "Retirement of Miss M.G. Borcherds and Miss J. McLarry."
      So Afr Nurs J, 19 (Feb 1953), 46-47.

BOTHMA, J.H.

638. "First Woman to Become a Doctor Must First Be a Nurse." *So
      Afr Nurs J*, 39 (Mar 1972), 10-12.

BOTTARD, MILE

639. Wortabet, Edla R. "Maman Bottard." *Brit J Nurs*, 38 (5 Jan
      1907), 9-10; see also *Nurs Rec*, 27 (17 Aug 1901), 126.

BOWE, E.J.

640. "Honorary Nursing Sister to the Queen." *Aust Nurs J*, 55 (Jul
      1957), 159.

BOWMAN, J. BEATRICE

641. "Who's Who in the Nursing World." *Am J Nurs*, 24 (Nov 1924),
      1122.

642. National League of Nursing Education. *Biographic Sketches, 1937-1940.* New York: The League, 1940.

BOYD, BELLE

643. *Belle Boyd in Camp and Prison.* New York: Blelock & Co., 1865; revised by Curtis Carroll Davis. South Brunswick, NJ: T. Yoseloff, 1968.

BOYLE, RENA E.

644. "Boyle to Head New Research Branch." *Nurs Res*, 8 (Summer 1959), 180-181.

BRANDSTROM, ELSA

645. "A Memorial to Elsa Brandstrom." *Z Krankenpflege*, 10 (Dec 1956), 525-529. (Ger)

BREAY, MARGARET

646. "Margaret Breay, S.R.N., S.C.M." *Brit J Nurs*, 88 (Jan 1940), 2-3.

BRECKINRIDGE, MARY

647. "A Pioneer's Dream Fulfilled." *Brit J Nurs*, 100 (Sep 1952), 83-85.

648. Breckinridge, Mary. *Wide Neighborhoods.* New York: Harper and Row, 1952. 366 pp.

649. Browne, Helen E. "A Tribute to Mary Breckenridge." *Nurs Out*, 14 (May 1966), 54-55.

650. Gardner, Caroline. "Frontier Nurse Chieftain." *Arkansas Gazette Mag* (27 Oct 1935).

651. McKown, Robin. "Mary Breckinridge." In *Heroic Nurses.* New York: G.P. Putnam's Sons, 1966. pp. 69-88.

652. "Mary Breckinridge." *Am J Nurs*, 30 (Mar 1930), 311-312.

653. "Mary Breckenridge." National League of Nursing Education. *Biographic Sketches, 1937-1940.* New York: The League, 1940.

654. Obituary. *NY Times* (17 May 1965), 35.

655. Poole, Ernest. *Nurses on Horseback.* New York: Macmillan, 1933.

656. Wilkie, K.E., and E.R. Moseley. *Frontier Nurse: Mary Breckinridge.* New York: Julian Messner, 1969.

BRIDGE, SISTER JOYCE

657.   "Sister Joyce Bridge." *Aust Nurs J*, 45 (Oct 1947), 241.

BRIDGES, DAISY CAROLINE

658.   "Distinguished Portrait Gallery--2. Miss Daisy Bridges, R.R.C.,
       S.R.N." *Nurs Mirror*, 93 (May 1951), 116-118.

659.   "Internationalists in the Making." *Am J Nurs*, 37 (Dec 1937),
       1367-1368.

660.   "The New Executive Secretary of the ICN." *Int Nurs Bull*, 4
       (Spring 1948), 2; see also *Aust Nurs J*, 46 (May 1948), 109-
       110; *Filipino Nurs*, 17 (Jan 1948), 128; *S Afr Nurs*, 14 (Apr
       1948), 19; *Canad Nurs*, 44 (Apr 1948), 294; *Brit J Nurs*, 96
       (May 1948), 68.

BRIDGES, ELIZABETH RUTH

661.   Bridges, Daisy C. "Miss E. Ruth Bridges." *Int Nurs Bull*, 6
       (Winter 1950), 6.

662.   "Miss E.R. Bridges" (obituary). *New Zeal Nurs J*, 43 (Dec
       1950), 229.

BRINK, FRANCES V.

663.   Adda, Eldredge. "Frances V. Brink." National League of
       Nursing Education. *Biographic Sketches 1937-1940*. New
       York: The League, 1940.

664.   Brinton, John H. *Personal Memoirs*. New York: Neale Publish-
       ing Co., 1914.

BRINTON, MARY (WILLIAMS)

665.   Brinton, Mary (Williams). *My Cap and My Cape: An Autobiog-
       raphy*. New York: Dorrance, 1950. 262 pp.

BRODERICK, MADELINE

666.   "Distinguished Service Awards of the American School Health
       Association for 1969." *J Sch Hlth*, 39 (Nov 1969), 600-601.

BROE, ELLEN JOHANNE

667.   "Florence Nightingale International Foundation: Appointment of
       Director." *Int Nurs Bull*, 6 (Winter 1950), 3; see also *Brit
       J Nurs*, 98 (Oct-Nov 1950), 120; (Dec 1950), 129; *New Zeal
       Nurs J*, 44 (Feb 1951), 19; *Nurs J India*, 42 (Feb 1951), 75;
       So Afr Nurs J, 17 (Jan 1951), 25.

BROWN, ELIZABETH S.

668.   "Retirement of Dominion Secretary." *New Zeal Nurs J*, 50
        (Feb 1957), 3-4.

BROWN, MARIA DEAN

669.   Brown, Harriet Connor. *Grandmother Brown's Hundred Years,*
        1827-1927. Boston: Little, Brown & Co., 1929.

BROWNE, SIDNEY

670.   "Dame Sidney Browne." *Nurs Mirror*, 30 (6 Mar 1920), 415.

BRYCE, ABBIE HUNT

671.   "Who's Who in the Nursing World." *Am J Nurs*, 22 (Jul 1922),
        816.

BULLEN, JANE

672.   *Galloping Nurse (Her) Story, as Told to Genevieve Murphy.*
        London: Paul, 1970. 136 pp.

BULLOCK, LINDA (NICHOLARDES)

673.   Elliott, L. "All We Had to Give Was Ourselves." *Redbook*, 127
        (May 1966), 58ff.

BUNGE, HELEN

674.   Hilbert, Hortense. "Five Years of Leadership." *Nurs Res*, 6
        (Oct 1957), 51.

BURGESS, ELIZABETH CHAMBERLAIN

675.   "Elizabeth C. Burgess, R.N., M.A." *Am J Nurs*, 34 (Dec 1934),
        183-184.

676.   Gage, Nina D. "Elizabeth Chamberlain Burgess." *National*
        League of Nursing Education: Biographic Sketches 1937-1940.
        New York: The League, 1940.

677.   Obituary. *NY Times* (23 Jul 1949), 11; see also *Sch & Soc*, 70
        (30 Jul 1949), 77-78.

678.   Stewart, Isabel Maitland. "Elizabeth Chamberlain Burgess."
        Am J Nurs, 58 (Aug 1958), 1101.

679.   "Who's Who in the Nursing World (Elizabeth C. Burgess)."
        Am J Nurs, 28 (Jul 1928), 714.

BURGESS, MAY AYRES

680.   Obituary. *NY Times* (16 Jul 1953), 21.

681.   Obituary. *Wilson Lib Bull*, 28 (Sep 1953), 30.

BURNS, ALVERTA

682.   Hosokawa, B. "Angel of the Hills." *Sat Eve Post*, 228 (26 May
        1956), 44ff.

BURROW, BRUNETTIE

683.   Burrow, Brunettie. *Angels in White*. San Antonio: Naylor,
        1959. 132 pp.

683.1   ————. *I Lay Down My Cap*. San Antonio: Naylor, 1961. 96 pp.

BUTLER, IDA F.

684.   Adams, Eleanor. "End of a Pioneer Era." *Red Cr Courier*, 28
        (Apr 1949), 22-23.

685.   "Nursing Service Has a New Director." *Red Cr Courier*, 16
        (Dec 1936), 22.

686.   Obituary. *NY Times* (12 Mar 1944), 18.

687.   Stimson, Julia C. "Ida F. Butler." National League of Nursing
        Education. *Biographic Sketches, 1937-1940*. New York: The
        League, 1940.

BYRNE, AGNES ISABELLE

688.   Obituary. *NY Times* (22 Nov 1950), 25.

CALLEN, MAUDE

689.   "Nurse's Midwife." *Life*, 31 (3 Dec 1951), 135-145.

CARMEN, MABEL

690.   "Flexible Autocrat." *Time*, 57 (2 Apr 1951), 57-58.

CARR, ADA M.

691.   Rand, Winifred. "Ada M. Carr." *National League of Nursing
        Education: Biographic Sketches, 1937-1940*. New York: The
        League, 1940.

CARSON-RAE, A.

692. "Nurses of Note. A. Carson-Rae." *Brit J Nurs*, 44 (30 Apr
      1910), 349.

CARTWRIGHT, F.F.

693. "President's Address. Miss Nightingale's Dearest Friend."
      Proceedings Roy Soc Med, 69(3) (Mar 1976), 1169–1175.

CARTWRIGHT, SISTER SOPHIA ELLEN

694. "Nurses of Note. Sister Sophia Ellen Cartwright." *Brit J
      Nurs*, 73 (Apr 1925), 73.

CASEY, CLARE M.

695. Obituary. *NY Times* (19 Apr 1959), 86.

CASSELMAN, MARGARET

696. North Caroline Poetry Society. *A Time for Poetry*. Winston-
      Salem: J.F. Blair, 1966. pp. 127–129.

CATCHINGS, MILDRED

697. "Distinguished Service Awards for 1975." *J Sch Hlth*, 46
      (Jan 1976), 44.

CAVELL, EDITH

698. Adam, George Jefferys. *Treason and Tragedy*. London: Cape,
      1929. 253 pp.

699. Aymer, Brandt, and Edward Sagarin. *Pictorial History of the
      World's Great Trials from Socrates to Eichmann*. New York:
      Crown, 1967. pp. 225–227.

700. Berkeley, Reginald. *Dawn. A Biographical Novel of Edith
      Cavell*. New York: Sears, 1928. 246 pp.

701. Bowie, Walter Russell. *Woman of Light*. New York: Harper and
      Row, 1963. pp. 128–139.

702. Bullwinkel, V. "Edith Cavell Memorial Service." *UNA Nurs J*,
      65 (May 1967), 139.

703. Cabot, Ella Lyman. "The Message of Edith Cavell." *J Ed*, 83
      (6 Jan 1916), 5–6.

704. Canning, John, ed. *100 Great Modern Lives*. New York: Haw-
      thorne, 1965. pp. 285–291.

705.   Clark-Kennedy, Archibald Edmund. *Edith Cavell: Pioneer and
       Patriot*. London: Faber and Faber, 1965. 248 pp.

706.   *Correspondence with the United States Ambassador Respecting
       the Execution of Miss Cavell at Brussels*. Text of letters
       between officials of British, Belgian, German, and American
       Authorities Presented to Both Houses of Parliament, Oct.
       1915. London: HMSO, 1915.

707.   "A Crime Against Humanity." *Brit J Nurs*, 55 (23 Oct 1915),
       328-330.

708.   "Edith Cavell." *Aust Nurs J*, 34 (Oct 1936), 205; see also
       Brit J Nurs, 78 (Dec 1930), 312; *Hosp* (24 May 1919), 177-
       178; *Pac Cst J Nurs*, 17 (Jan 1921), 11-13.

709.   "Edith Cavell as a Pupil Knew Her." *Tr Nurs & Hosp Rev*, 63
       (Aug 1919), 72-77.

710.   "Edith Cavell's Body Taken to England." *Am J Nurs*, 19 (May
       1919), 678.

711.   "Edith Cavell's Last Letter to Her Nurses in Brussels." *Aust
       J Nurs*, 94 (12 Oct 1951), 31.

712.   *Execution of Miss Cavell at Brussels*. London: HMSO, 1915.
       15 pp.

713.   Fellowes-Gordon, Ian. *Heroes of the Twentieth Century*. New
       York: Hawthorne, 1960. pp. 24-37.

714.   Felstead, S. Theodore. *Edith Cavell: The Crime That Shook
       the World*. London: G. Newnes, 1940. 211 pp.

715.   Fitzgerald, Alice. *The Edith Cavell Nurse from Massachusetts*.
       Boston: Butterfield, 1917.

716.   Franklin, Charles. "Edith Cavell." In *Great Spies*. New
       York: Hart, 1967. pp. 42-43.

717.   Fredericks, P.G. "She Was More Than a Patriot." *NY Times Mag*,
       (5 Dec 1965), 110.

718.   Gibson, Hugh. *A Journal From Our Legation in Belgium*.
       Garden City, NY: Doubleday, 1917. 360 pp.

719.   Goodnow, Minnie. "Edith Cavell." *Tr Nurs*, 35 (Sep 1930),
       346-347.

719.1 Got, Ambroise, ed. *The Case of Miss Cavell*. London: Hodder
       and Stoughton, 1920. (From unpublished documents.)

720.   Grey, Elizabeth. "The Essential Meaning of Edith Cavell's
       Life." *Nurs Mirror*, 109 (9 Oct 1959), 15-16.

721.   Hallowes, Ruth M. "Distinguished British Nurses--Edith Cavell."
       Nurs Mirror, 100 (8 Oct 1954), 117.

722.   Harrison, E. "Memories of a Childhood Friendship." *Nurs
       Mirror*, 141 (9 Oct 1975), 51-52.

723.   Harvey, I. "Edith Cavell--How Much Did She Care?" *Nurs Times*,
       70 (10 Oct 1974), 1585-1587.

724.   Hellyer, R. "My Matron (Edith Louisa Cavell)." *Nurs Mirror*,
       141 (9 Oct 1975), 50-51.

725.   Hill, William Thomson. *The Martyrdom of Nurse Cavell*. London:
       Hutchinson, 1915. 55 pp.

726.   Hoehling, A.A. *A Whisper of Eternity: The Mystery of Edith
       Cavell*. New York: Thomas Yoseloff, 1957.

727.   ------. "The Story of Edith Cavell." *Am J Nurs*, 57 (Oct
       1957), 1320-1322.

728.   "Homecoming of Edith Cavell." *Brit J Nurs*, 62 (17 May 1919),
       326; 62 (24 May 1919), 345-346.

729.   "How Miss (Edith) Cavell Was Shot." *Nurs Times*, 11 (4 Dec
       1915), 1495.

730.   "In Memory of Edith Cavell." *Nurs Times*, 35 (7 Oct 1939),
       1229.

731.   Judson, H. *Edith Cavell*. New York: Macmillan Co., 1941.

732.   Kambara, H. "Achievement of Edith Louisa Cavell and the
       Description of her Home." *Jap J Nurs Educ*, 14 (Aug 1973),
       513-518.

733.   Kent, Beatrice. "Transfiguration of a Prison Cell and Some-
       thing Else." *Brit J Nurs*, 73 (Apr 1925), 86-87.

734.   Kyle, R.A. "Edith Louisa Cavell." *J Am Med Assoc*, 228
       (3 Jun 1974), 1255.

735.   "A Last Message from Edith Cavell." *Am J Nurs*, 17 (Mar 1917),
       472-473; see also *Brit J Nurs*, 58 (7 Apr 1917), 238.

736.   Leeds, Herbert. *Edith Cavell; The Story of Her Life*. London:
       Jarrold, 1915. 92 pp.

737.   McKown, Robin. "Edith Cavell." *Heroic Nurses*. New York:
       G.P. Putnam's Sons, 1966. pp. 145-167.

738.   "Martyrdom of Nurse Edith Cavell." *Nurs Times*, 11 (30 Oct
       1915), 1327-1329.

739.   "Memories of a British Nursing Heroine." *Nurs Mirror*, 90
       (8 Oct 1949), 31-32.

740.   "Miss [Edith] Cavell's Fate" (ed). *Brit Med J*, 2 (Oct 1915),
       651.

741.   Moore, Aileen H. "Nurse Cavell." *Tr Nurs*, 93 (Nov 1934),
       459-461.

742.   Muir, Charles S. *Women, the Makers of History*. New York:
       Vantage Press, 1956. pp. 148-152.

743.   Mussallem, H.K. "Mount Edith Cavell: Canada's Tribute to a
       Gallant Nurse." *Canad Nurs*, 68 (Feb 1972), 231/6; same
       article in *Infirm Can*, 14 (May 1972), 18-21. (Fr)

744.   Needer, Ned. *Bold Leaders of World War I*. Boston: Little,
       Brown & Co., 1974. pp. 39-57.

745.   "A Note from the Past" (On Edith Cavell). *Nurs Notes & Mid
       Chron*, 47 (Dec 1934), 181-182.

746.   "Nurse Cavell--Dawn, Oct 12." *Aust Nurs J*, 46 (7 Oct 1950),
       1039.

747.   Olga, Sister. "Edith Cavell." *Nurs Mirror*, 74 (11 Oct 1941),
       15.

748.   "Prussian Law in Belgium and Nurse Edith Cavell." *Brit J
       Nurs*, 59 (20 Oct 1917), 256-257.

749.   Ryder, Rowland. *Edith Cavell*. London: Hamish Hamilton,
       1975. 278 pp.

750.   Scovil, Elizabeth Robinson. "An Heroic Nurse (Edith Cavell)."
       Am J Nurs, 16 (Nov 1915), 118-121.

751.   Smith-Dampies, John Lucius. "Edith Cavell." *East Anglican
       Worthies*. London: Blackwell, 1949. pp. 42ff.

752.   Sticker, A. "Institute Edith Cavell--Marie Depage; In
       Memoriam." *Infirmière*, 43 (Oct 1965), 8. (Fr)

753.   Stuart, Christina. "A New Look At an Old Legend." *Nurs
       Times*, 54 (10 Oct 1958), 1195-1196.

754.   Swanson, M. "Edith Cavell and Nursing Today." *Q Bull North-
       west Uni Med Sch* (Summer 1962), 167-171.

755.   Takami, A. "Edith Cavell." *Jap J Nurs* (Sep 1971), 52-55;
       (Oct 1971), 46-49; (Nov 1971), 72-76; (Dec 1971), 48-54.

756.   Thomas à Kempis. *Of the Imitation of Christ. The Edith Cavell
       Edition*. London: Oxford University Press, 1920. 229 pp.

757.   "To a British Nurse." *Nurs Mirror*, 10 (14 Oct 1955), 117.

758.   "Topical Notes--Statue of Edith Cavell." *Aust Nurs J*, 47
       (13 Oct 1951), 1004.

759.   van Til, Jacqueline. "Most Unforgettable Character I've Met."
         Readers Digest, 76 (Feb 1961), 111-115.

760.   ————. *With Edith Cavell in Belgium.* New York: H.W. Bridges,
         1922. 156 pp.

761.   Number deleted.

CELLIER, ELIZABETH

762.   Gordon, J.E. "Distinguished British Nurses of the Past, 3.
         Mrs. Elizabeth Cellier." *Mid Hlth Visit*, 11 (May 1975),
         139-142.

CELMINS, MARTHA

763.   "Martha Celmins." *Int Nurs Rev*, 11 (Apr 1937), 147-149.

764.   Haydon, M. Olive. "A Great Midwife." *Brit J Nurs* (18 May
         1907), 379-380; 39 (20 Jul 1907), 59-60.

CHAPTAL, LEONIE

765.   Blair-Fish, Hilary M. "Mademoiselle (Leonie) Chaptal, 1873-
         1937." *Nurs Times*, 34 (1 Oct 1938), 1001-1002.

766.   Peltier, M. "Mademoiselle (Leonie) Chaptal." *Int Nurs Rev*,
         11 (July 1937), 303-305; see also *Am J Nurs*, 37 (May 1937),
         567-569; *Brit J Nurs*, 85 (Apr 1937), 96-97; *Canad Nurs*, 33
         (May 1937), 233; *Brit J Nurs*, 86 (Jun 1938), 144.

CHARLEY, IRENE H.

767.   Hills-Yound, E. "In Grateful Memory of Irene H. Charley."
         News Lett Florence N Int Nurs Assoc, 11 (1973), 4.

CHOW, MEI-YU

768.   "Welcome for a Famous Woman General." *Nat Bus Woman*, 39
         (Feb 1960), 10.

CHRISTIAN, PRINCESS

769.   "Royal British Nurses' Association Supplement. Her Royal
         Highness, The Princess Christian." *Brit J Nurs*, 70 (16 Jun
         1923), 376-378.

CHUNG, ELSIE MOWFUNG

770.   "Elsie Mowfung Chung." *Quart J Chin Nurs*, 11 (Jan 1930), 2-3.

CHURCH, ELLEN

771.   Furlong, W.B. "Firstest with the Hostess." *NY Times* (15 May
        1960), 73-74.

CLAUDIA, SISTER MARY

771.1   Obituary. *NY Times* (16 Nov 1965), 47.

CLAYTON, S. LILLIAN

772.   Goodrich, Annie Warburton. "S. Lillian Clayton." *Am J Nurs*,
        30 (Jul 1930), 871-875.

773.   "In Memoriam--S. Lillian Clayton, 1874-1930." *Am J Nurs*, 30
        (Jun 1930), 678-688.

774.   Mackey, Harry A. "An Appreciation of Miss (S. Lillian)
        Clayton." *Am J Nurs*, 5 (Jul 1930), 343-344.

775.   Roberts, Mary M. "S. Lillian Clayton, 1876-1930." *Am J Nurs*,
        54 (Nov 1954), 1360-1363.

776.   Saltzman, Lillian. "Little Lady in White." *RN*, 20 (May
        1957), 56-59, 110.

777.   Tucker, Katherine. "S. Lillian Clayton" (editorial). *Pub
        Hlth Nurs*, 22 (Jun 1930), 1279-1280.

CLEMENT, MARTHA JANE

778.   Obituary. *NY Times* (11 Oct 1959), 86.

CLOUGH, MARTHA

779.   Roxburgh, R. "Miss Clough, Miss Nightingale and the Highland
        Brigade." *Victorian Stud*, 15 (Sep 1971), 75-79.

780.   Roxburgh, R. "Miss Nightingale and Miss Clough: Letters from
        the Crimea." *Victorian Stud*, 13 (Sep 1969), 71-79.

CNOCKHAERT, MARTHA

781.   Taylor, E. "Cult of the Secret Agent." *Horizon*, 17 (Spring
        1975), 61.

COCKAYNE, ELIZABETH

782.   "Britain's Chief Nurse" (editorial). *Nurs Times*, 54 (23 May
        1958), 585-586.

783.   "Distinguished Portrait Gallery--8. Miss E. Cockayne, S.R.N.,
        S.C.M." *Nurs Mirror*, 93 (14 Sep 1951), 442.

784.   "New Year Honours (Elizabeth Cockayne, Roberta Whyte and Others)." *Nurs Times*, 51 (7 Jan 1955), 3.

COLEMAN, LOUISE M.

785.   "Women Who Occupy High Office in American Hospital Association." *Bull Am Hosp Assoc*, 2 (Jan 1928), 16-17.

COLLINS, ANNA

786.   Hurd, H.G. "Two Ladies and a Lake." *Ind Woman*, 33 (Apr 1954), 128-129.

CONYERS, EVELYN AUGUSTA

787.   "Evelyn Augusta Conyers." *Aust Nurs J*, 42 (Nov 1944), 139.

COOKE, GENEVIEVE

788.   McCarthy, Theresa Earles, and S. Gotea Dozier. "Genevieve Cooke." *Pac Cst J Nurs*, 24 (Mar 1928), 146-147.

789.   "Our Professional Editors." *Brit J Nurs*, 36 (27 Jan 1906), 72; see also *Brit J Nurs*, 76 (Apr 1928), 100-101.

790.   "Who's Who in the Nursing World (Genevieve Cooke)." *Am J Nurs*, 23 (Jul 1923), 852.

CORDINER, M.H.

791.   "Distinguished Portrait Gallery--19. Miss M.H. Cordiner." *Nurs Mirror*, 94 (25 Jan 1952), 368.

CORTES, MARCIANA B.

792.   Nicanor, Precioso M. *Profile of Notable Filipinos in the U.S.A.* New York: Pre-Mer Pub. Co., 1963, I, 65-69.

COTE, GABRIELLE D.

793.   "*Canadian Nurse* Names Editor for French Edition." *Am J Nurs*, 59 (May 1959), 612.

COWDRY, VISCOUNTESS (ANNIE)

794.   "News from the Nursing World (Annie, Viscountess Cowdry)." *Nurs Mirror*, 55 (23 Apr 1932), 57.

CRAIG, MARGETTA

795.   "Personal Notes and News." *Nurs J of India*, 49 (Aug 1958), 244-245.

CRAIN, CLARA (MOORE)

796.   *We Shall Rise.* New York: Pageant, 1955. 68 pp.

CRANDALL, ELLA PHILLIPS

797.   "Miss (Ella Phillips) Crandall's Resignation (as NOPHN Execu-
        tive Secretary)." *Pub Hlth Nurs*, 12 (Jul 1920), 553-555.

798.   "National Organization for Public Health Nursing: Ella Phil-
        lips Crandall (News)." *Pub Hlth Nurs*, 30 (Dec 1938), 726-
        727.

799.   "Who's Who in the Nursing World (Ella Phillips Crandall)."
        Am J Nurs, 23 (Nov 1922), 129.

CRAVEN, MRS. DACRE (FLORENCE LEES)

800.   Hallowes, Ruth M. "Distinguished British Nurses, Mrs. Dacre
        Craven." *Nurs Mirror*, 102 (23 Dec 1955), 3-4.

CRAVEN, MARJORIE E.

801.   "Nursing Echoes, Marjorie E. Craven." *Brit J Nurs*, 101 (Dec
        1953), 145.

CRISTINA, PRINCESS

802.   Trono, L. del. "La principessa Christina Trivulzio di Belgio-
        joso e l' assistenza infermieristica femminite." *Med Soc*
        (Torino), 12 (1962), 314-317; see also *Minerva Med*, 53
        (1962), 1249-1254.

CROMWELL, GERTRUDE E.

803.   DeWesse, A.O. "Presentation of the Howe Award to Gertrude E.
        Cromwell, R.N." *J Sch Hlth*, 24 (Nov 1954), 249-255.

804.   "President 1950-1951: Gertrude E. Cromwell." *J Sch Hlth*, 21
        (Feb 1951), 84.

CROSSLAND, MARY

805.   Seymer, Lucy R. "Mary Crossland, A Pioneer Teacher." *Nurs
        Times*, 58 (2 Feb 1962), 141-143.

806.   ———. "Mary Crossland, Further Notes." *Nurs Times*, 58
        (9 Feb 1962), 176-178.

CRUICKSHANK, JOANNA MARGARET

807.   "Dame Joanna Cruickshank, D.B.E., R.R.C., A Great Pioneer Dies."
        Nurs Mirror, 107 (29 Aug 1958), 632.

808.   "In Mrs. Rome's Place." *Nurs Times*, 34 (17 Sep 1938), 935.

CULLINGWORTH, CHARLES

809.   Collingwood, Frances. "Pioneer in Midwifery Legislation--
       Charles Cullingworth, 1841-1908." *Nurs Mirror*, 107 (16 May
       1958), 503.

CUMMING, KATE

810.   *A Journal of Hospital Life in the Confederate Army of Tennessee
       from the Battle of Shiloh to the End of the War.* Louisville,
       KY: Morton, 1866.

CUMMINGS, MARIETTA BRADY

811.   "A Bellevue (Hospital, New York, N.Y.) Pioneer." *Nurs J Pac
       Cst*, 4 (Jun 1908), 249-250.

DAKIN, FLORENCE

812.   Murdoch, Jessie M. "Florence Dakin, R.N." *Am J Nurs*, 34
       (Jun 1934), 575-576.

DALLAS, RITA

813.   Dallas, R., and M. Cheshire. "My 8 Years as the Kennedys'
       Private Nurse." *Ladies' Home J*, 88 (Feb 1971), 77ff.

814.   ———, and Jeanira Ratcliffe. *The Kennedy Case*. New York:
       G.P. Putnam's Sons 1973. 352 pp.

DAMER, ANNIE

815.   "Annie Damer" (editorial). *Am J Nurs*, 15 (Sep 1915), 1077.

816.   Fisher, Lucy B. "Miss Annie Damer, President of (Nurses')
       Associated Alumnae (of the United States). *Nurs J Pac Cst*,
       3 (Apr 1907), 150-154.

817.   "Nurses of Note. Miss Annie Damer." *Brit J Nurs*, 47 (8 Jul
       1911), 24.

DARBYSHIRE, RUTH

818.   "Ruth Darbyshire." *Nurs Mirror*, 70 (23 Mar 1940), 599-600.

DARCHE, LOUISE

819.   Dock, Lavinia L. *Louise Darche. A Reformer in Nursing and in
       the Civil Service.* New York: Privately printed, n.d.
       16 pp.

820.   "Louise Darche." *Early Leaders of American Nursing*. New
       York: National League of Nursing Education, 1921.

DAUSER, SUE

821.   "Sue Dauser." *Pac Cst J Nurs*, 35 (Mar 1939), 150.

DAVIES, MABLE

822.   Obituary. *NY Times* (21 Dec 1960), 31.

DAVIS, DOROTHY

823.   "Five Who Sued." *Sat Rev*, 47 (16 May 1964), 71.

DAVIS, ELIZABETH

824.   Williams, J. *The Autobiography of Elizabeth Davis, a Balaclava
       Nurse*. London: Hurst & Blackett, 1957.

DAVIS, MARY E.P.

825.   "Mary E.P. Davis." *Early Leaders of American Nursing*. New
       York: National League of Nursing Education, 1922.

826.   "Mary E.P. Davis" (editorial). *Am J Nurs*, 24 (Jul 1924),
       811-812.

DAY, HELEN CALDWELL

827.   Day, Helen Caldwell. *Color, Ebony*. New York: Sheed and Ward,
       1951. 182 pp.

828.   ————. *Not Without Tears*. New York: Sheed and Ward, 1954.
       270 pp.

829.   Romig, Walter. "Helen Caldwell Day." *Book of Catholic
       Authors*. Detroit: Romig, 1957. pp. 69-73.

DAY, RUTH

830.   Hurd, H.G. "Two Ladies and a Lake." *Ind Woman*, 33 (Apr 1954),
       128-129.

DEANS, AGNES GARDINER SHEARER

831.   "Who's Who in the Nursing World (Agnes Gardiner Shearer
       Deans)." *Am J Nurs*, 24 (Jun 1924), 736; see also *Am J Nurs*,
       26 (Aug 1926), 624.

DELANO, JANE A.

832. "Appointment of Jane A. Delano as Supt. of Army Nurse Corps."
      Am J Nurs, 9 (Sep 1909), 875.

833. Boardman, Mabel. "Relation of Jane A. Delano to the American
      Red Cross, the Army, and the Nursing Profession." *Proceed-
      ings, 29th Convention, American Nurses Association.* New
      York: 1934. 439–443.

834. Clarke, Mary A. *Memories of Jane A. Delano.* New York: Lake-
      side, 1934. 63 pp. Published serially originally in *Tr
      Nurs*, 90 (May–Jun 1934).

835. Erdmann, Anna H. "Miss Delano Through the Eyes of a Life-Long
      Friend, Sylveen Nye." *Tr Nurs*, 106 (Apr 1941), 280–281.

836. Foley, Edna L. "The Red Cross. Jane A. Delano, R.N., Last
      Honors." *Am J Nurs*, 19 (Jun 1919), 688–700.

837. Gladwin, M.E. *The Red Cross and Jane Arminda Delano.*
      Philadelphia: W.B. Saunders, 1931.

838. "Jane A. Delano." *Early Leaders of American Nursing.* New
      York: National League of Nursing Education, 1921.

839. "Jane A. Delano." *Pac Cst J Nurs*, 26 (May 1930), 291–292; 27
      (Mar 1931), 172–173; 28 (Mar 1932), 163; 29 (Mar 1933),
      141–142; 32 (Mar 1936), 146–148.

840. "Jane A. Delano." *Red Cr Courier*, 10 (16 Mar 1931), 71–74.

841. "Miss Delano Resigns from the (U.S.) Army Nurse Corps." *Am J
      Nurs*, 12 (Apr 1912), 548–549; see also *Brit J Nurs*, 48
      (20 Apr 1912), 314.

842. "Miss Jane A. Delano Dies in France." *Red Cr Courier*, 3
      (12 May 1919).

DELEHANTY, MARY E. BROWN

843. Obituary. *NY Times* (21 Jun 1966), 43.

DEMING, DOROTHY

844. Ross, Grace. "Dorothy Deming." *National League of Nursing
      Education: Biographic Sketches, 1937–1940.* New York: The
      League, 1940.

845. Wales, Marguerite A. "Dorothy Deming." *Am J Nurs*, 36 (Apr
      1936), 325–327.

846. Ward, Martha E., and D.A. Marquardt. "Dorothy Deming." In
      Authors of Books for Young People. Metuchen, NJ: Scarecrow
      Press, 1964. p. 61.

DENNINSON, CLARE

847.   Obituary. *NY Times* (16 Feb 1954), 25.

DENNY, LINA

848.   "Denny, Lina: Doctor of Humanities." *RN*, 15 (Aug 1952), 46-47.

DENSFORD, KATHARINE (DREVES)

849.   Geister, Janet M. "We Present Katharine Densford." *Tr Nurs*,
        113 (Oct 1944), 275-279.

850.   "Katharine Densford Dreves Dies." *Am J Nurs*, 78 (Nov 1978),
        1823, 1826, 1841.

851.   "Katharine June Densford." *Current Biog Yearbook* (1947),
        pp. 166-168.

DePELCHIN, KEZIA PAYNE

852.   Matthews, Harold J. *Candle by Night*. Boston: Humphries,
        1942. 272 pp.

DEUTSCH, NAOMI

853.   "Public Health Nurses' Page Naomi Deutsch." *Pac Cst J Nurs*,
        32 (Jan 1936), 34-35.

DEWITT, KATHARINE

854.   DeLee, Joseph B. "Katharine DeWitt-Student Nurse, and Private
        Duty Nurse." *Am J Nurs*, 32 (Sep 1932), 963-966.

855.   "Katharine DeWitt." *Am J Nurs*, 32 (Dec 1932), 1233-1237; see
        also *Pac Cst J Nurs*, 23 (Dec 1932), 729.

856.   "National Tribute to Miss DeWitt, A." *Am J Nurs*, 32 (Nov
        1932), 1147.

DIOMEDOUS, MARINA

857.   "Outstanding Figures in Nursing, Recently Departed: Marina
        Diomedous." *Krankenschwester*, 18 (Oct 1965), 145-146. (Ger)

DIX, DOROTHEA LYNDE

858.   Blair, Donald. "Dorothea Dix." *Nurs Mirror*, 100 (18 Feb
        1955), 3-4.

859.   Borhuda. "Be Glad You're You and Not a Teammate of Dorothea
        Dix." *RN*, 21 (Oct 1958), 61-63.

860.   Bothma, J.H.   "Dorothea Lynde Dix: Reformer and Nurse Without Equal."   *SA Nurs J*, 39 (Jun 1972), 29-30 *passim*.

861.   "Dorothea Lynde Dix" (editorial).   *Am J Nurs*, 49 (Dec 1949), 743.

862.   "Dorothea Lynde Dix."   *J Educ*, 53 (Mar 28 1901), 202.

863.   Marshall, Helen E.   *Dorothea Dix: The Forgotten Samaritan*. Chapel Hill: University of North Carolina Press, 1937. 298 pp.

864.   Tiffany, F.   *Life of Dorothea Lynde Dix*. Boston: Houghton Mifflin, 1937.

864.1 Wilson, Dorothy C.   *Stranger and Traveler*. Boston: Little, Brown & Co., 1975.

DOCK, LAVINIA LLOYD

865.   Christy, Teresa E.   "Portrait of a Leader: Lavinia L. Dock." *Nurs Out*, 17 (Jun 1969), 72-75.

866.   Dunbar, V.   "A Glimpse of Lavinia Dock in Her 90th Year." *Alumn Mag*, 68 (Sep 1969), 66.

867.   "Lavinia Lloyd Dock" (editorial).   *Nurs Out*, 4 (May 1956), 298-299.

868.   "Lavinia Dock."   National League of Nursing Education, *Early Leaders of American Nursing (Calendar 1922)*. New York: The League, 1921.

869.   Monteiro, L.A.   "Lavinia L. Dock (1947) on Nurses and the Cold War."   *Nurs Forum*, 17 (1978), 46-54.

870.   Obituary.   *NY Times* (18 Apr 1956), 31; see also *Wilson Lib Pub*, 30 (Jun 1956), 740.

871.   "Obituary. Death of Lavinia Dock."   *So Afr Nurs J*, 22 (Jul 1956), 17.

872.   "Obituaries. Lavinia Lloyd Dock."   *Am J Nurs*, 56 (Jun 1956), 712.

873.   "Passing of Lavinia Lloyd Dock."   *Brit J Nurs*, 104 (Apr 1956), 27.

874.   Roberts, Mary M.   "Lavinia Lloyd Dock--Nurse, Feminist, Internationalist."   *Am J Nurs*, 56 (Feb 1956), 176-179.

875.   "Self Portrait of Lavinia Dock."   *Nurs Out*, 25 (Jan 1977), 23-26.

876.   Taylor, Effie J.   "Lavinia Lloyd Dock; In Memoriam."   *Int Nurs Rev*, 3 (Oct 1956), 65-66.

877.   "Who's Who in the Nursing World (Lavinia L. Dock)." *Am J
        Nurs*, 22 (Feb 1922), 349.

DOLAN, MARGARET (BAGGETT)

878.   "Nurse and Public Health Official." *Am J Pub Hlth*, 64 (May
        1974), 578.

DOLIN, MARY M.

879.   Ward, Martha E., and D.A. Marquardt. "Mary M. Dolin." *Authors
        Authors of Books for Young People*. Metuchen, NJ: Scarecrow
        Press, 1967. p. 84.

DOMITILLA, SISTER MARY

880.   English, Irene. "Sister Mary Domitilla." *National League of
        Nursing Education: Biographic Sketches, 1937-1940*. New York:
        The League, 1940.

DORA, SISTER (DOROTHY WYNDLOW PATTISON)

881.   Hallowes, Ruth M. "Distinguished British Nurses." *Nurs
        Mirror*, 102 (13 Jan 1956), 1001.

882.   Mabie, Hamilton W., and Kate Stephens, eds. "Sister Dora."
        Heroines Every Child Should Know. New York: Grosset & Dun-
        lap, 1908. 281 pp.

883.   "Nursing Echoes (Sister Dora)." *Brit J Nurs*, 100 (Feb 1952),
        15; see also 78 (1930).

884.   "The Nursing Outlook. Centenary of Sister Dora." *Nurs Mirror*,
        54 (23 Jan 1932), 332; see also 54 (16 Jan 1932); 56 (21 Jan
        1933), 318.

885.   Wigg, Harold. "Sister Dora." *Nurs Times*, 25 (9 Feb 1929),
        153.

d'YOUVILLE, MARGARET

885.1   Mitchell, E. *Margaret d'Youville, Foundress of the Grey Nuns*.
        Montreal: Palm Publishers, 1965.

DOWLING, MARY T.

886.   Obituary. *NY Times* (14 Feb 1947), 22.

DOWNING, EVELYN HUNT

887.   Obituary. *NY Times* (8 Mar 1950), 25.

DOYLE, GLADYS SULLIVAN

888.   McCarthy, Theresa Earles.   "Gladys Sullivan Doyle, R.N., A
        Modern Santa Filomena."   *Pac Cst J Nurs*, 29 (Aug 1933),
        488, 508.

DROWN, LUCY LINCOLN

889.   "A Pioneer Passes."   *Am J Nurs*, 34 (Sep 1934), 841-842.

890.   "Who's Who in the Nursing World (Lucy Lincoln Drown)."   *Am J
        Nurs*, 22 (Nov 1921), 92.

DUERK, ARLENE

891.   "Biography."   *Cur Biog* (Sep 1973), 11-12; see also *Cur Biog
        Yrbk 1973* (1974), 109-111.

892.   Slater, C.   "Navy's Only Woman Admiral Predicts Ship Command
        for a Woman."   *Biog News*, 1 (Mar 1974), 271.

DUNANT, HENRY

893.   Boissier, Leopold.   "Au Temps de Florence Nightingale de Henry
        Dunant."   *Bruxelles Med*, 37 (Nov 1957), 1141-1149.   (Fr)

894.   "Florence Nightingale and Henri Dunant."   *Red Cr World*, 40
        (1960), 21-22.

DUNNING, CHARLOTTE M.

895.   Obituary.   *NY Times* (1 Nov 1949), 27.

DWYER, MARITA

896.   Bauer, D.   "Night in the Life of a Lady Cop."   *Today's Hlth*,
        53 (Sep 1975), 40ff.

EDMONDS, EMMA

897.   Dannett, Sylvia G. (Liebovitz).   *She Rode with the Generals;
        The True and Incredible Story of Sarah Emma Scelye, Alias
        Franklin Thompson*.   New York: Nelson, 1960.   326 pp.

898.   Hoyt, H.R.   "Emma Edmonds, Nurse and Spy of the Civil War."
        Three Thousand Years of Espionage.   Edited by K.D. Singer.
        Englewood Cliffs, NJ: Prentice-Hall, 1948.   pp. 122-133.

899.   ————.   "Union Spy in Men's Breeches."   *Double Dealers*.
        Edited by Alexander Klein.   Philadelphia: J.B. Lippincott,
        1958.   pp. 328-334.

900.   Kinchen, Oscar A. *Women Who Spied for the Blue and Gray*. New
        York: Dorrance, 1973. pp. 14-24.

901.   Singer, Kurt Deutsch. *Spies and Traitors*. New York: Allen,
        1953. pp. 100-110.

EDWARDS, M.M.

902.   "Distinguished Portrait Gallery--20. Miss M.M. Edwards."
        Nurs Mirror, 94 (29 Feb 1952), 488.

EGBERT, JEAN

903.   "An International Appointment." *Am J Nurs*, 32 (Feb 1932), 125.

ELDREDGE, ADDA

904.   "Adda Eldredge" (news). *Am J Nurs*, 55 (Dec 1955), 1456, 1458.

905.   "Who's Who in the Nursing World (Adda Eldredge)." *Am J Nurs*,
        21 (July 1921), 735.

ELLIS, KATHLEEN WILHELMINA

906.   "Nursing Profiles--Kathleen Wilhelmina Ellis." *Canad Nurs*, 51
        (Aug 1955), 636-637.

EMORY, F.H.

907.   "C. Kotlarsky, A Pioneer in Nursing Education." *Canad Nurs*,
        67 (Nov 1971), 33-35.

FARMBOROUGH, FLORENCE

908.   Lester, F. "Nurse at the Russian Front (Miss Florence Farm-
        borough)." *Nurs Mirror*, 139(16) (17 Oct 1974), 47.

FEDDE, ELISABETH

909.   Rolfsrud, Erling Nicolai. *Borrowed Sister: The Story of
        Elisabeth Fedde*. Minneapolis: Augsburg Publishing House,
        1953. 118 pp.

FENWICK, ETHEL GORDON (MANSON)

910.   Biography. *DNB 1941-1950* (1959). pp. 246-247.

911.   Breay, Margaret. "Complimentary Dinner to Mrs. Bedford Fen-
        wick." *Brit J Nurs*, 49 (21 Dec 1912), 492-497; see also 64
        (15 May 1920), 286-288; 65 (6 Nov 1920), 255.

912. ———. "Mrs. Fenwick's Jubilee." *Brit J Nurs*, 85 (Nov 1937), 286.

913. Hallowes, Ruth M. "Distinguished British Nurses: Ethel Gordon Fenwick." *Nurs Mirror*, 101 (13 May 1955), 2-3.

914. Hardy, Gladys M. "The Late Mrs. Bedford Fenwick." *Brit J Nurs*, 95 (Mar 1947), 25-26; see also 95 (Apr 1947), 37-43; 95 (May 1947), 53; (Jun 1947), 61-62. For other obituaries see *Canad Nurs*, 43 (May 1947), 378; *Nurs Mirror*, 84 (22 Mar 1947), 430; *So Afr Nurs J*, 13 (May 1947), 21; *Int Nurs Bull*, 3 (Sep 1947), 5.

915. Hector, Winifred Emily. "Personal Memories of Mrs. Bedford Fenwick." *Nurs Times*, 69 (24 May 1973), 681-682.

916. ———. *The Work of Mrs. Bedford Fenwick and the Rise of Professional Nursing.* London: Royal College of Nursing, 1973.

FISH, JANET

917. Obituary. *NY Times* (10 Aug 1970), 29.

FISHER, ALICE

918. Cope, Zachary. *Six Disciples of Florence Nightingale.* London: Pitman Medical, 1961. pp. 57-74.

FITZGERALD, ALICE L.

919. "Alice Fitzgerald Given an Important Position" (editorial). *Am J Nurs*, 20 (Dec 1919), 181-182; see also *Brit J Nurs*, 64 (20 Mar 1972), 172; *Pac Cst J Nurs*, 15 (Jan 1920), 11-12.

920. "Miss (Alice) Fitzgerald." *Filipino Nurs*, 3 (Oct 1928), 40.

921. Noble, Iris. *Nurse Around the World: Alice Fitzgerald.* New York: Julian Messner, 1964. 191 pp.

922. Obituary. *NY Times* (11 Nov 1962), 88.

FITZMAURICE, SISTER ANTHONY MARIE

923. Obituary. *NY Times* (18 Nov 1970), 50.

FLIEDNER, FRIEDERIKE

924. Saunders, L. Metta. "Friederike Fliedner." *Brit J Nurs*, 36 (26 May 1906), 415-416; 36 (2 Jun 1906), 436-437; 36 (9 Jun 1906), 453-454; 36 (16 Jun 1906), 494-495; 36 (30 Jun 1906), 515-517; 36 (7 Jul 1906), 26-27.

FLIEDNER, PASTOR

925. "Life of Pastor Fliedner of Kaiserwerth." *Kurzer Abriss seines Lebens*. Kaiserwerth, 1859. Translated by Catherine Winkworth. London: Longmans, 1867.

FOLEY, EDNA L.

926. Fox, Elizabeth Gordon. "Miss Edna L. Foley." *Pub Hlth Nurs*, 35 (Sep 1943), 522.

927. "Who's Who in the Nursing World (Edna L. Foley)." *Am J Nurs*, 23 (Apr 1923), 560.

FORREST, CHRISTINA F.

928. Breay, Margaret. "The Passing of a Signatory to the Royal Charter." *Brit J Nurs*, 74 (May 1926), 97-98.

FORSYTH, A.E.

929. Obituary. *NY Times* (28 Feb 1950), 29.

FOX, ELIZABETH GORDON

930. Deming, Dorothy. "Elizabeth Gordon Fox." *National League of Nursing Education: Biographic Sketches, 1937-1940*. New York: The League, 1940.

931. Obituary. *NY Times* (15 Nov 1958), 23.

932. "Who's Who in the Nursing World (Elizabeth Gordon Fox)." *Am J Nurs*, 23 (Jan 1923), 308.

FRANCE, BEULAH SANFORD

933. Obituary. *NY Times* (19 Jan 1972), 40.

FRANCIS, SUSAN C.

934. Goostray, Stella. "Susan C. Francis." *National League of Nursing Education: Biographic Sketches, 1937-1940*. New York: The League, 1940.

FRICKE, IRMA

935. "Distinguished Service Awards." *J Sch Hlth*, 35 (Dec 1965), 441-442.

FRY, ELIZABETH

936.   Cobb, Ruth. "Home of Elizabeth Fry Now the Norwich (England)
       Municipal Maternity Hospital." *Nurs Mirror*, 85 (20 Sep
       1947), 470.

937.   Douglas, Eileen. *Elizabeth Fry*. London: Salvation Army Book
       Dept., 1913. 115 pp.

938.   Holmes, Marion. *Elizabeth Fry. A Cameo Life Sketch*. 2nd ed.
       London: Womens Freedom League, n.d. 23 pp.

939.   Jacobs, Henry Barton. "Elizabeth Fry, Pastor Fliedner and
       Florence Nightingale." *Ann Med Hist*, 3 (Spring 1921), 17-25.

940.   *Memoirs of the Life of Elizabeth Fry*. Edited by Katherine Fry
       and R.E. Crosswell. London: J. Hatchard, 1848.

941.   *Memoirs of the Life of Elizabeth Fry: Life and Labors of the
       Eminent Philanthropist, Preacher, and Prison Reformer*. New
       York: E. Walker's Sons, 1884.

942.   Pitman, Mrs. E.R. *Elizabeth Fry*. Boston: Little, Brown & Co.,
       1901. 269 pp.

943.   Richards, Laura E. *Elizabeth Fry, The Angel of the Prisons*.
       New York: Appleton, 1916. 206 pp.

944.   Scott, Eleanor. *Heroic Women*. London: Nelson, 1939. 310 pp.
       One of five women profiled.

945.   Tabor, Margaret E. *Pioneer Women. Elizabeth Fry, Elizabeth
       Blackwell, Florence Nightingale, Mary Slessor*. London:
       Sheldon, 1925. 126 pp; Boston: Little, Brown & Co., 1936.

946.   Whitney, Janet. *Elizabeth Fry, Quaker Heroine*. Boston:
       Little, Brown & Co., 1937. 337 pp.

GAGE, NINA DIADAMIA

947.   Obituary. *NY Times* (19 Oct 1946), 21; see also *Sch & Soc*, 64
       (26 Oct 1946), 293-294.

GALARD, GENEVIEVE DE

948.   "Angel of Dienbienphu." *Inst Int Educ N Bull*, 31 (Oct 1955),
       35.

949.   "Angel's Return." *Time*, 63 (31 May 1954), 23.

950.   "ANA Pays Tribute to French Nurse." *Am J Nurs*, 54 (1954), 999.

951.   Biography. *Brit Bk Yr* (1955), 349-350; see also *Collier's Yr Bk* (1955), 475; *Cur Biog*, 15 (Oct 1954), 23-26; same biography (1954), 294-296.

952.   McKown, Robin. "Genevieve de Galard." *Heroic Nurses.* New York: G.P. Putnam's Sons, 1966. pp. 267-290.

953.   "Mlle Merit Awards." *Mlle*, 40 (Jan 1955), 62.

954.   "Return of the Angel of Dienbienphu." *Newsweek*, 43 (31 May 1954), 38.

955.   Taylor, E. "Heroic Nurses of Dienbienphu." *Reporter*, 11 (20 Jul 1954), 26-30.

956.   Vargas, Basurto, F.R. "Address in Honor of Genevieve de Galard, the Angel of Dienbienphu." *Rev San Mil Mex*, 9 (Oct-Dec 1956), 10-12.

GALLAGHER, JEAN (KELLY)

957.   Winchester, J. "Air Force Nurse." *Scholastic*, 69 (1 Nov 1956), 6.

GALT, E.

958.   Obituary. *NY Times* (25 May 1961), 37.

GARDELIUS, PAT

959.   Asbell, B. "Trial of Patricia Gardelius." *Redbook*, 126 (Dec 1956), 46ff.

960.   Dunne, J.G. "Embattled Nurse of Jackrabbit Flats." *Sat Eve Post*, 238 (20 Nov 1965), 42-44.

GARDNER, MARY SEWALL

961.   Kent, Beatrice. "A Very Welcome Visitor." *Brit J Nurs*, 63 (26 Jul 1919), 68, 70.

962.   Nelson, Sophie C. "Mary Sewall Gardner." *Nurs Out* (Dec 1953), 668-670.

963.   "Who's Who in the Nursing World (Mary S. Gardner)." *Am J Nurs*, 26 (May 1926), 390.

GARONE, M.

964.   "Mike the Cop Studies to be Mike the Nurse." *Life*, 70 (14 May 1971), 47ff.

GEISTER, JANET

965.   Obituary. *NY Times* (10 Dec 1964), 58.

966.   "This I Believe About My Half-Century in Nursing." *Nurs Out*,
       12 (Mar 1964), 58, 61.

GEYMONAT, ENCLIDA

967.   Lee, Elizabeth Meredith. *She Wears Orchids and Other Latin
       American Stories*. New York: Friendship Press, 1951. pp.
       116-123.

GIBSON, WINNIE

968.   Gove, G.F. "Specialists in Personnel." *Ind Woman*, 30 (Feb
       1951), 55.

GIFFARD, MARIE FRANCIS

969.   Dimitry, Theodore J. "The First North American Nurse." *Tr
       Nurs*, 91 (Nov 1933), 409-411, 461.

GILES, IDA F.

970.   "Ida F. Giles--A Pioneer." *Am J Nurs*, 28 (Jul 1928), 692.

GILL, ANNIE WARREN

971.   "A Great Loss to the Profession." *Nurs Times*, 26 (8 Mar 1930),
       281.

GILLESPIE, HELEN S.

972.   "Brigadier Dame Helen S. Gillespie." *Nurs Mirror*, 99 (30 Jul
       1954), 1.

GIVEN, LEILA IONE

973.   Obituary. *NY Times* (14 Feb 1959), 21.

GLADWIN, MARY ELIZABETH

974.   Crane, Celia. "Mary Elizabeth Gladwin." *National League of
       Nursing Education: Biographic Sketches, 1937-1940*. New
       York: The League, 1940.

975.   "Mary Elizabeth Gladwin." *Tr Nurs*, 103 (Dec 1939), 526-527.

GOLDMAN, EMMA

976.   *Living My Life.* New York: Dover Publications, Inc., 1970.
        Many other editions.

GOODALL, FRANCES G.

977.   Bruce, J. "Quite Definitely No Amateur." *Ind Woman*, 33
        (Mar 1954), 90.

978.   "Distinguished Portrait Gallery--4. Miss Frances Goodall,
        O.B.E., S.R.N." *Nurs Mirror*, 93 (22 Jun 1951), 206.

979.   "Frances Goodall, C.B.E., S.R.N." *Nurs Mirror*, 105 (3 May
        1957), 624.

980.   "Whitley Council (Staff Side) New Chairman" (editorial). *Nurs
        Times*, 52 (5 Oct 1956), 977-978.

GOODMAN, MARGARET

981.   *Experiences of an English Sister of Mercy.* London: Smith
        Elder, 1821.

GOODRICH, ANNIE WARBURTON

982.   "Annie Warburton Goodrich." *Am J Nurs*, 55 (Feb 1955), 158,
        160.

983.   "Annie W. Goodrich--Crusader." *Am J Nurs*, 34 (Jul 1934),
        669-680.

984.   *Annie W. Goodrich at Bellevue, February 16, 1907 to Septem-
        ber 1, 1910. Her Contributions to Nursing Education and the
        Professional Development of Nursing.* New York: Bellevue
        Hospital Training School for Nurses, n.d.

985.   "Annie W. Goodrich--Representing Tomorrow's Nurse." *Am J Nurs*,
        46 (Apr 1946), 215-218.

986.   "Annie Warburton Goodrich--80 Years." *Am J Pub Hlth*, 36 (Apr
        1946), 428.

987.   Barrett, Adelaide E. "On Discovering a Personality." *Am J
        Nurs*, 46 (May 1946), 339-340.

988.   Biography. *NCAB*, 42 (1958), 326-327.

989.   "Dean of Nurse Educators Dies (News)." *Nurs Out*, 3 (Feb 1955),
        107-110.

990.   Embree, Edwin R. "Miss (Annie W.) Goodrich Chosen as Dean of
        the Yale School of Nursing (New Haven, Conn.)." *Tr Nurs*,
        70 (May 1923), 401; see also *Am J Nurs*, 23 (Jun 1923), 762-

763; 23 (Jul 1923), 824; *Brit J Nurs*, 70 (19 May 1923), 807-808; *Red Cr Courier*, 2 (9 Jun 1923), 2.

991. Henderson, Virginia. "Annie Warburton Goodrich." *Am J Nurs*, 55 (Dec 1955), 1488-1492.

992. "Honors to Whom Honor is Due." *Sch & Soc*, 63 (16 Mar 1946), 183.

993. Koch, Harriett Berger. *Militant Angel*. New York: Macmillan Co., 1951.

994. "The Late Miss Annie Goodrich, Dean Emeritus." *Nurs Times*, 51 (14 Jan 1955), 29.

995. "Miss Annie Warburton Goodrich." *Int Nurs Rev*, 2 (Apr 1955), 16.

996. "New President of the International Council of Nurses." *Brit J Nurs*, 46 (24 Aug 1912), 157-158.

997. Obituary. *NY Times* (1 Jan 1955), 15.

998. Roberts, Mary M. "Annie Warburton Goodrich, 1866-1954" (editorial). *Am J Nurs*, 55 (Feb 1955), 63.

999. Werminghaus, Esther A. *Annie W. Goodrich: Her Journey to Yale*. New York: Macmillan Co., 1950. 104 pp.

1000. "Who's Who in the Nursing World (Annie W. Goodrich)." *Am J Nurs*, 23 (Dec 1922), 2-10.

GOOSTRAY, STELLA

1001. Bliss, Mary E.G. "Stella Goostray." *National League of Nursing Education: Biographic Sketches, 1937-1940*. New York: The League, 1940.

1002. "Ladies with Lamps" (editorial). *New England J Med*, 253 (1 Dec 1955), 989-990.

1003. Nelson, Sophie. "Public Health Statesman." *Am J Nurs*, 60 (Sep 1960), 1268-1269.

1004. Roberts, Mary M. "Stella Goostray--Distinguished Administrator, Professional Leader, and Good Neighbor." *Am J Nurs*, 58 (1958), 352.

GORDON, J.E.

1005. "Nurses and Nursing in Britain." *Mid Hlth Visit*, 9 (Jan 1973), 17-22.

GRANT, AMELIA H.

1006.   "Amelia Grant." *Pac Cst J Nurs*, 32 (Feb 1936), 81.

1007.   Obituary. *NY Times* (15 Aug 1967), 39.

1008.   Wales, Marguerite A. "Amelia Grant." *National League of Nursing Education: Biographic Sketches, 1937-1940.* New York: The League, 1940.

GRANT, L. DUFF

1009.   "Distinguished Portrait Gallery--16. Miss L. Duff Grant, R.R.C." *Nurs Mirror*, 94 (7 Dec 1951), 221.

GRAY, CAROLYN E.

1010.   Gillett, Harriet. "Carolyn E. Gray." *National League of Nursing Education: Biographic Sketches, 1937-1940.* New York: The League, 1940.

1011.   "Who's Who in the Nursing World (Carolyn Elizabeth Gray)." *Am J Nurs*, 23 (Sep 1923), 1022.

GREENOUGH, KATHERINE

1012.   Obituary. *Am J Nurs*, 75 (Oct 1975), 1872.

GREGG, ELINOR D.

1013.   *Indians and the Nurse.* Norman, OK: University of Oklahoma Press, 1965. 173 pp.

1014.   Nelson, Sophie C. "Elinor D. Gregg." *National League of Nursing Education: Biographic Sketches, 1937-1940.* New York: The League, 1940.

GREGORY, ALICE SOPHIA

1015.   Hallowes, Ruth M. "Distinguished British Nurses." *Nurs Mirror*, 101 (1 Apr 1955), 5-6.

1016.   Morland, Egbert. *Alice and the Stork--The Life of Alice Gregory, 1867-1944.* London: Hodder and Stoddard, 1951. 88 pp.

GRENFELL, WILFRED

1017.   "(Wilfred) Grenfell of Labrador." *Brit J Nurs*, 88 (Oct 1940), 171.

1018.   Grenfell, Wilfred. *Forty Years for Labrador.* Boston: Houghton Mifflin, Co., 1932. 372 pp.

GRETTER, LYSTRA E.

1019. Knox, Sally. "She Wrote the Nightingale Pledge." *Tr Nurs*, 108 (Jun 1942), 430-432.

1020. "Lystra E. Gretter." *Am J Nurs*, 51 (May 1951), 352.

1021. Munson, Helen W. "Lystra E. Gretter." *Am J Nurs*, 49 (Jun 1949), 344-348.

1022. National League of Nursing Education: Early Leaders of American Nursing (Calendar 1923) (Lystra E. Gretter). New York: The League, 1922.

GREY, H.D.

1023. "Honour for President of A.N.F. (H.D. Grey)." *Aust Nurs J*, 46 (Aug 1948), 172.

GROSS, SAMUEL D.

1024. *Autobiography of Samuel D. Gross.* Philadelphia: G. Barrie, 1887.

GULLAN, MARION AGNES

1025. "Miss Marion Agnes Gullan." *Nurs Times*, 54 (11 Jul 1958), 820.

GUTHRIE, THERESA (KRAKER)

1026. Obituary. *NY Times* (11 Nov 1959), 35.

GUZMAN, GENERA S.M. de

1027. Montellano, Patrocinio J. "Genera S.M. de Guzman." *Filipino Nurs*, 17 (Oct 1948), 323-335.

HAGIWARA, TAKE

1028. "Take Hagiwara." *Int Nurs Rev*, 10 (Aug 1936), 237-238.

HALKETT, LADY ANNE

1029. "Distinguished British Nurses of the Past, Lady Anne Halkett." *Mid Hlth Visit*, 11(4) (Apr 1975), 114-117.

HALL, CARRIE M.

1030. "Carrie M. Hall." *Am J Nurs*, 37 (Jun 1937), 686-687.

1031. "Carrie May Hall, Who's Who in the Nursing World." *Am J Nurs*, 25 (Jul 1925), 582.

1032.   Johnson, Sally. "Carrie M. Hall." *National League of
        Nursing Education: Biographic Sketches 1937-1940.*   New
        York: The League, 1940.

1033.   "Leader in Nursing Education (Carrie May Hall)." *Nurs Times*,
        25 (31 Aug 1929), 1005.

1034.   "Miss Hall Represents the Harmon Association (For the Advance-
        ment of Nursing)." *Tr Nurs*, 98 (May 1937), 501-502.

HALL, MAUDE HELEN

1035.   "Maude Helen Hall." *Canad Nurs*, 36 (Sep 1940), 626; 43 (Jun
        1947), 452-453; 44 (Dec 1948), 1003.

HAMILTON, ANNA

1036.   "Changes at the Bordeaux School." *Am J Nurs*, 34 (Oct 1934),
        990.

1037.   Goodnow, Minnie. "A Distinguished Visitor." *Tr Nurs*, 62
        (Mar 1919), 157-158.

1038.   "In Memoriam. Dr. Anna Hamilton, Standard Bearer." *Brit J
        Nurs*, 83 (19 Dec 1935), 319; 84 (Jan 1936), 23.

1039.   Obituary. *Tr Nurs*, 96 (Feb 1936), 152; see also *Am J Nurs*,
        35 (Dec 1935), 1208-1209.

1040.   "A Nursing Pioneer in France." *Brit J Nurs*, 54 (2 Jan 1915),
        3-4.

1041.   Selizer, M. "Dr. Anna Hamilton and the Florence Nightingale
        School of Nursing, Bordeaux." *Int Nurs Rev*, 5 (May 1930),
        181-184.

1042.   Winckler, Marguerite. "Anna Hamilton." *Int Nurs Rev*, 10
        (Feb 1936), 6.

HANCOCK, CORNELIA

1043.   *South After Gettysburg; Letters of Cornelia Hancock from the
        Army of the Potomac, 1863-1865.* Edited by Henrietta
        Stratton Jaquette. New York: Crowell, 1956; reprinted
        Freeport, NY: Books for Libraries Press, 1971. 287 pp.

HANSEN, ANNE LYON

1044.   "In Memoriam (Anne Lyon Hansen)." *Pub Hlth Nurs*, 30 (May
        1938), 308.

HARMER, BERTHA

1045.   "Scholar and Teacher." *Canad Nurs*, 30 (Sep 1934), 415.

HASLAM, PHYLLIS

1046.   Pickles, Wilfred. *Ne'er Forget the People*. London: W.
        Laurie, 1953. pp. 43–49.

HAUPT, ALMA C.

1047.   Obituary. *Am J Nurs*, 56 (May 1956), 564; see also *NY Times*
        (17 Mar 1956), 19.

1048.   "Nursing Leader Dies." *Nurs Out*, 4 (Apr 1956), 235.

1049.   "Well Known Public Health Nurse Retires." *Nurs Out*, 1 (Jun
        1953), 365.

HAUSSKNECHT, EMMA

1050.   "Missionary From Lambarene." *Time*, 63 (24 Jan 1954), 82.

HAVEY, I. MALINDE

1051.   "I. Malinde Havey." *Red Cr Courier*, 18 (Oct 1938), 9–10; see
        also *Pub Hlth Nurs*, 301 (Oct 1938), 602–605.

1052.   "The Forgotten Family Remembered." *Red Cr Courier*, 16 (Feb
        1937), 7–10.

HAWKINS, SALLIE

1053.   Minney, D. "Nebraska Nurse Looks Ahead." *Ind Woman*, 35
        (Jun 1956), 118.

HAWKINSON, NELLIE XENIA

1054.   Carrington, Margaret. "Nellie X. Hawkinson." *National League
        of Nursing Education: Biographic Sketches, 1937-1940*. New
        York: The League, 1940.

HAY, HELEN SCOTT

1055.   "Distinction to Miss Helen Scott Hay." *Pac Cst J Nurs*, 10
        (Jul 1914), 291.

1056.   "Helen Scott Hay" (obituary). *Am J Nurs*, 33 (Jan 1933), 67–
        68; see also *Pac Cst J Nurs*, 29 (Jan 1933), 25–26; *Red Cr
        Courier*, 12 (Feb 1933), 241–244; *Tr Nurs*, 90 (Jan 1933), 41.

1057.   "New Chief Nurse of American Red Cross Commission for Europe."
        Red Cr Bull, 4 (Mar 1920), 8.

HAYES, MARGARET

1058.   *Captive of the Simbas*. New York: Harper and Row, 1966. 191
        pp.; also published as *Missing--Believed Killed*. London:
        Hodder & Stoughton, 1966. 192 pp.

HEELY, PATRICIA I.

1059.   Obituary. *NY Times* (7 Feb 1961), 33.

HEILMAN, CHARLOTTE M.

1060.   Obituary. *NY Times* (8 Dec 1956), 19.

HELENA, EMPRESS

1061.   "The Empress Helena: Fragments of Nursing History." *J Br
        Nurs*, 2 (Dec 1950), 155-156.

HELM, ELEANOR M.

1062.   Obituary. *NY Times* (3 May 1960), 39.

HENLEY, SISTER

1063.   "Maternity Sister." *Nurs Mirror*, 104 (7 Dec 1956).

HENRIETTA, SISTER (STOCKDALE)

1064.   Haynes, C.M. "Sister Henrietta." *Afr Nurs J*, 8 (Mar 1943),
        79.

1065.   Loch, Elizabeth, and Christina Stockdale. *Sister Henrietta*.
        London: Longmans Green, 1914. 157 pp.

1066.   "Memorial to Sister Henrietta." *So Afr Nurs J*, 20 (Jan 1954),
        245.

1067.   "Passing Bell. Sister Henrietta of Kimberley." *Brit J Nurs*,
        47 (14 Oct 1911), 311.

1068.   "Sister Henrietta--South Africa's Pioneer Nurse." *So Afr
        Nurs J*, 17 (Feb 1951), 18-19.

HERBERT, SIDNEY

1069.   Stanmore, Arthur H-G. *Sidney Herbert, Lord Herbert of Lea: A
        Memoir*. London: Hazell, Watson & Viney, 1906.

HERRERA, BEATRIZ RESTREPO

1070.   Wiesner, Vanegas L. "Founder of the National Association of
         Nurses." *ANEC*, 5(13) (Oct 1974), 13-14. (Spa)

HERSEY, MABEL FRANCES

1071.   Allder, Elsie. "Mabel Frances Hersey." *Canad Nurs*, 40 (Feb
         1944), 101-103.

HERTZLER, ARTHUR E.

1072.   *The Horse and Buggy Doctor*. New York: Hoeber, 1938.

HESSELBALD, MOTHER MARIA ELIZABETH

1073.   Tjader, Marguerite. *Mother Elizabeth: The Resurgence of the
         Order of Saint Birgitta*. London: Herder & Herder, 1972.
         231 pp.

HIBBARD, MARY EUGENIE

1074.   "M. Eugenie Hibbard Retires." *Am J Nurs*, 27 (Aug 1927), 660.

HICKEY, MARY A.

1075.   "Mary A. Hickey." *National League of Nursing Education:
         Biographical Sketches, 1937-1940*. New York: The League,
         1940.

1076.   Obituary. *NY Times* (16 Feb 1954), 25.

1077.   "Who's Who in the Nursing World." *Am J Nurs*, 34 (Dec 1934),
         1209.

HIGBEE, LENAH STUTLIFFE

1078.   Hasson, Esther V. "The New Navy Nurse Corps Superintendent."
         Am J Nurs, 11 (May 1911), 474; see also *Pac Cst J Nurs*, 19
         (Jan 1923), 11-12; *Am J Nurs*, 23 (Jan 1923), 293 for
         retirement.

HILBERT, HORTENSE

1079.   "National Organization for Public Health Nursing: Miss Hil-
         bert Comes to the N.O.P.H.N." *Pub Hlth Nurs*, 34 (Jan 1942),
         51.

HILL, ELIZABETH

1080.   "This Issue's Personality-Elizabeth Hill." *Philippine J Nurs*,
         24 (Jul-Sep 1955), 99, 131.

HILL, JANE (CORUTHERS)

1081.   Kooiman, Helen. Silhouettes: *Women Behind Great Men.* Waco,
        TX: Word Books, 1972. pp. 161-168.

HILLIARD, AMY MAY

1082.   "Amy M. Hilliard Receives Nightingale Medal." *Am J Nurs,* 22
        (Jun 1922), 731.

HILLYERS, GLADYS V.

1083.   "A Loss to the Profession." *Nurs Times,* 44 (29 May 1948),
        381-382.

HODGINS, AGATHA COBOURG

1084.   "Agatha Cobourg Hodgins." *J Am Assoc Nurs Anes,* 14 (May
        1946), 32-35; see also *Tr Nurs,* 114 (Jun 1945), 435.

HOGAN, A.

1085.   "A Tribute to the Pioneers. Hogan A." *J Nurs Mid,* 20(2)
        (Summer 1975), 6-11.

HOLGATE, E.

1086.   McLean, Hester. "Hers Was a Great Era." *New Zeal Nurs J,* 65
        (Sep 1972), 21.

HOLOKAVA, ANNA

1087.   "A Modern Joan of Arc." *Pac Cst J Nurs,* 15 (Nov 1919), 653-
        655.

HOPE, MARY E.

1088.   "Lamp on the Snow." *Nurs Times,* 52 (6 Jan-22 Jun 1956),
        serial installments weekly.

HORDER, LORD

1089.   "A Great Physician." *Nurs Times,* 51 (19 Aug 1955), 909.

HORWOOD, H.C.

1090.   Obituary. *So Afr Nurs J,* 22 (Jan 1956), 28-29.

HOSOKAWA, B.

1091.   "Angel of the Hills." *Sat Eve Post*, 228 (26 May 1956), 44-45.

HOWARD, JOHN

1092.   Baumgartner, Leona. *John Howard: Hospital and Prison Reformer.* Baltimore: Johns Hopkins Press, 1939.

1092.1 Southwood, M. *John Howard: Prison Reformer.* London: Independent Press, Ltd., 1958.

HOWELL, MARION GERTRUDE

1093.   Goodrich, Annie Warburton. "Marion Howell." *National League of Nursing Education: Biographic Sketches, 1937-1940.* New York: The League, 1940.

1094.   "In Memoriam. Ruth Weaver Hubbard. 1897-1955." *Nurs Out*, 4 (Jan 1956), 34.

1095.   Obituary. *Am J Nurs*, 56 (Feb 1956), 218-219.

HUDSON, ELIZABETH

1096.   Obituary. *Keats-Shelley J*, 23 (1947), 7.

HUGHES, AMY

1097.   "Miss Amy Hughes." *Aust Nurs J*, 8 (Jun 1910), 183-184.

1098.   "Nurse of Note. Miss Amy Hughes." *Brit J Nurs*, 37 (4 Aug 1906), 86.

HUGHES, LORA WOOD

1099.   *No Time for Tears.* New York: Houghton, Mifflin, 1946.   305 pp.

HULME, ANNIE E.

1100.   "Miss Annie Hulme." *Brit J Nurs*, 52 (Feb 1914), 112.

HUNT, DAME AGNES

1101.   Hallowes, Ruth M. "Distinguished British Nurses." *Nurs Mirror*, 10 (Jul 1955), 6-7, 14.

1102.   "Hunt, Dame Agnes--Biography." *DNB 1941-1950.* (1959), 416-417.

1103.   Hunt, Agnes. *This is My Life.* Autobiography. New York:
        G.P. Putnam's Sons, 1942.

1104.   Watson-Jones, Reginold. "Agnes Hunt, 1862-1948; An Apprecia-
        tion." *J Bone Jt Surg,* 30B (Nov 1948), 709-713; issue
        dedicated to her memory.

HUNTER, TRENNA

1105.   "Trenna Hunter, President." *Canad Nurs,* 52 (Oct 1956), 799-
        800.

HUXLEY, MARGARET

1106.   "An Appreciation of the Late Miss Margaret Huxley, R.G.N.,
        M.A." *Brit J Nurs,* 88 (Feb 1940), 27-28.

1107.   "Miss Margaret Huxley." *Brit J Nurs,* 50 (31 May 1913), 429.

INADA, UYKI

1108.   "New President of the Imperial Nursing Association of Japan."
        Brit J Nurs, 85 (Apr 1937), 88.

ISAACS, GERTRUDE

1109.   "Receives World's First Ph.D. in Nursing Science." *Today's
        Hlth,* 41 (Nov 1963), 84.

JAMES, ANNIE

1110.   Davey, Cyril. *Fifty Lives for God.* Valley Forge, PA: Judson
        Press, 1973. pp. 79-81.

JAMMÉ, ANNA C.

1111.   "Anna C. Jammé" (news). *Am J Nurs,* 36 (Aug 1936), 856-857.

1112.   Obituary. *Pac Cst J Nurs,* 35 (Aug 1939), 459-461; see also
        35 (Sep 1939), 533-536; *Tr Nurs,* 103 (Aug 1939), 147-148.

1113.   Wayland, Mary Marvin. "Anna C. Jammé." *National League of
        Nursing Education: Biographic Sketches, 1937-1940.* New
        York: The League, 1940.

1114.   "Who's Who in the Nursing World (Anna C. Jammé)." *Am J Nurs,*
        21 (Sep 1921), 885.

JELLIFFE, BELINDA

1115.   Jelliffe, Belinda. *For Dear Life*. New York: Charles
        Scribner's Sons, 1936. 355 pp.

JENDRITZA, LORETTA S.

1116.   Gridley, Marion E., ed. *Indians of Today*. n.p. ICFP Inc.,
        1971. p. 50.

JENKINS, MARJORIE

1117.   "Marjorie Jenkins." *Canad Nurs*, 40 (Oct 1944), 767-768.

JOHN GABRIEL, SISTER

1118.   Felton, Margaret. "Sister John Gabriel." *National League of
        Nursing Education: Biographic Sketches, 1937-1940*. New
        York: The League, 1940.

JOHNS, ETHEL

1119.   "A Biography of the Late Ethel Johns, LL.D." *Alum Mag*,
        73(2) (Jul 1974), 25-26.

1120.   Emory, Florence H.M. "The Appointment of an Editor." *Canad
        Nurs*, 27 (Oct 1932), 527.

1121.   Street, Margaret M. *Watch-fires in the Mountains: The Life
        and Writings of Ethel Johns*. Toronto: University of
        Toronto Press, 1973. 336 pp.

JOHNSON, FLORENCE M.

1122.   "Dean of Red Cross Nurses Dies" (news). *Nurs Out*, 2 (Apr
        1954), 218.

1123.   "Obituaries. Florence M. Johnson." *Am J Nurs*, 54 (May 1954),
        556, 558.

1124.   Obituary. *NY Times* (23 Mar 1954), 27; (25 Mar 1954), 29.

1125.   Roberts, Mary M. "The Nurse on the Docks." *Am J Nurs*, 54
        (Jul 1954), 854-857.

JOHNSON, SALLY

1126.   Hall, Carrie M. "Sally Johnson." *National League of Nursing
        Education: Biographic Sketches, 1937-1940*. New York:
        The League, 1940.

JOHNSTON, LILLIAN J.

1127.   "Lillian J. Johnston." *Canad Nurs*, 41 (Sep 1945), 723-724.

JONES, AGNES ELIZABETH

1128.   Cope, Zachary. *Six Disciples of Florence Nightingale*.
         London: Pitman Medical, 1961. pp. 1-9.

1129.   Hallowes, Ruth M. "Distinguished British Nurses." *Nurs
         Mirror*, 100 (7 Jan 1955), 6-7.

1130.   Seymer, Lucy Ridgely. "Agnes Jones, 1832-1932." *Int Nurs
         Rev*, 8 (1933), 43-51; see also *Brit J Nurs*, 81 (Feb 1933),
         38; *Nurs Mirror*, 56 (19 Nov 1932), 149.

1131.   *Una and Her Paupers; Memorials of Agnes Elizabeth Jones by
         Her Sister*. New York: Routledge and Kegan Paul, 1872.

JONES, MARY

1132.   "Our New President." *Nurs Times*, 36 (27 Apr 1940), 447.

JONES, ZILLAH

1133.   Jones, Zillah. *Sister's Log: A Nurse's Reminiscences*.
         London: Gomerion Press, 1964. 145 pp.

JORDEN, ELLA

1134.   Jorden, Ella. *Operation Mercy*. London: F. Muller, 1957.
         210 pp.

JOY, EILEEN M.

1135.   "The New President of the Irish Matrons' Association."
         Brit J Nurs, 50 (25 Jan 1913), 69.

KEO, WEI-HAN

1136.   Henrich, Ruth. *Heroes of the Church Today*. London: Society
         for Propagation of the Gospel, 1948. pp. 45-46.

KARLL, AGNES

1137.   Dock, Lavinia L. "An Appreciation--Sister Agnes Karll."
         Am J Nurs, 27 (May 1927), 357-358.

1138.   Fenwick, Ethel Gordon. "Sister Agnes Karll." *Brit J Nurs*,
         39 (13 Jul 1907), 30; 49 (3 Aug 1912), 83-84; for a note on
         her death, 75 (Mar 1927), 7.

1139.   Fricke, A.   "Agnes Karll."   *Int Nurs Rev*, 14 (Jun 1967),
        43-44.

1140.   Meyer, Helene.   "Agnes Karll."   *Int Nurs Rev*, 12 (Oct 1938),
        321-324.

KEATING, ANNA G.

1141.   Obituary.   *NY Times* (22 May 1955), 88.

KEATON, M.

1142.   Courtney, W.B.   "Angel in Furs: M. Keaton, Sweetheart of
        Alaska."   *Colliers*, 100 (20 Nov 1937), 67ff.

KEEGAN, KATHARINE

1143.   Obituary.   *NY Times* (10 Feb 1950), 23.

KELLER, MANELVA WYLIE

1144.   "Manelva Wylie Keller, B.S., R.N."   *Tr Nurs Hosp Rev*, 84
        (Feb 1930), 210, 217.

KELLETT, ADELAIDE MAUDE

1145.   "Miss Adelaide Maude Kellett, C.B.E., R.R.C."   *Aust Nurs J*,
        43 (May 1945), 57.

KELLEY, FLORENCE

1146.   Goldmark, Josephine.   *Impatient Crusader: Florence Kelley's
        Life Story.*   Urbana, IL: University of Illinois Press, 1953.

KELLY, CORDELIA

1147.   "Those Were the Days."   *Am J Nurs*, 54 (Apr 1954), 452-453.

KELLY, DOROTHY N.

1148.   "Dorothy N. Kelly Accepts Position at N.C.C.N. Headquarters."
        Cath Nurs, 4 (Sep 1955), 31.

KELSO, A.

1149.   Winchester, J.   "Flight Nurse."   *Scholastic*, 67 (6 Oct 1955),
        6.

KENNEDY, JANE

1150.   Snyder, A.   "Singular Woman."   *McCalls*, 98 (Jun 1971), 43.

KENNEDY, MARY

1151.   Obituary. *NY Times* (11 Jun 1955), 15.

KENNY, SISTER

1152.   Kenny, Sister. *And They Shall Walk*. Autobiography. New
         York: Dodd, Mead, 1943. 268 pp.

1153.   "At 59 Sister Kenny is Undaunted." *Life*, 21 (16 Sep 1946),
         82.

1154.   Cohn, Victor. *Sister Kenny--The Woman Who Challenged the
         Doctors*. Minneapolis: University of Minnesota Press, 1975.

1155.   Johns, Ethel M. "It Took Thirty-three Years." *Canad Nurs*,
         39 (Aug 1943), 509-511; another interview, *Tr Nurs*, 109
         (Jul 1942), 36-37.

1156.   "Kenny Fund-raising Scandal." *Life*, 49 (11 Jul 1960), 38.

1157.   Kline, M.L. "Most Unforgettable Character I've Met."
         Read Digest, 75 (Aug 1959), 203-208.

1158.   Levine, Herbert Jerome. *I Knew Sister Kenny; As a Story of
         a Great Lady and Little People*. Boston: Christopher, 1954.
         234 pp.

1159.   McKown, Robin. *Heroic Nurses*. New York: G.P. Putnam's
         Sons, 1966. pp. 189-211.

1160.   Obituary. *Am Ann 1953* (1953), 375; see also *Brit Med J*, 4790
         (6 Dec 1952), 1262; *Colliers Yrbk* (1953), 406; *Cur Biog*, 14
         (Jan 1953), 27; *Cur Biog Yrbk* (Jan 1953), 311; *Illus Lond N*,
         221 (6 Dec 1952), 938; *Lancet*, 263 (6 Dec 1952), 1123;
         NY Times (30 Nov 1952), 1; (1 Dec 1952), 23; *Newsweek*, 40
         (8 Dec 1922), 67; *Time*, 60 (8 Dec 1952), 80ff.

1161.   "The Passing of Sister Elizabeth Kenny." *Brit J Nurs*, 101
         (Jan 1953), 3.

1162.   "Sister Kenny." *Aust Nurs J*, 35 (Jul 1937), 149-150.

1163.   Number deleted.

1164.   "Sister Kenny's New Center." *Newsweek*, 31 (15 Mar 1948), 49-
         50.

1165.   Thomas, Henry, and D.L. Thomas. *50 Great Modern Lives*. New
         York: Hanover House, 1956. pp. 430-438.

1166.   "Why I Left America." *Women's Home Companion*, 78 (19 Mar
         1951), 38ff.

KERR, C.H.

1167.   "Nurses of Note. New Matron-in-Chief (Queen Alexandra's
        Imperial Military Nursing Service." *Brit J Nurs*, 36
        (31 Mar 1906), 251.

KERR, MARGARET

1168.   Lindeburgh, Marion. "The New Editor of the Journal." *Canad
        Nurs*, 40 (May 1944), 310.

KIMBER, DIANA CLIFFORD (SISTER MARY DIANA)

1169.   "Diana Clifford Kimber." *National League for Nursing:
        Leaders of American Nursing (Calendar 1922)*. New York:
        The League, 1921.

KING, SIR TRUBY

1170.   Billing, Armorel. "Centenary of a Great Pioneer, Sir Truby
        King and the Royal New Zealand Society for the Health of
        Women and Children." *Nurs Mirror*, 107 (18 Apr 1958), 192,
        III-IV.

1171.   "Sir Truby King." *Aust Nurs J*, 36 (Feb 1938), 44; also *Nurs
        Mirror*, 66 (19 Feb 1938), 481.

KINNEY, DITA HOPKINS

1172.   "Mrs. Dita H. Kinney." *Am J Nurs*, 1 (Mar 1901), 403-404.

1173.   "Nursing News and Announcements. Deaths. (Dita Hopkins
        Kinney)." *Pac Cst J Nurs*, 17 (Aug 1921, 458; also *Am J
        Nurs*, 21 (Jul 1921), 76.

KUEHN, RUTH PERKINS

1174.   Suhrie, Eleanor Brady. "Evidences of the Influence of Ruth
        Perkins Kuehn on Nursing and Nursing Education." Ph.D.
        dissertation, University of Pittsburgh, 1975. 241 pp.

KUIZON, LUTGARDA

1175.   Nicanor, Precioso M. *Profiles of Notable Filipinos in the
        U.S.A.* New York: Pre-Mer Pub. Co., 1963. Vol. 1, pp. 155-
        158.

LABIN, JOANNE GREEN

1176.   Gridley, Marion E., ed. *Indians of Today*. n.p.: ICFP Inc.,
        1971. p. 133.

LAMB, MARGARET

1177.   "Distinguished Portrait Gallery--7. Miss Margaret Lamb."
         Nurs Mirror, 93 (Aug 1951), 381.

LAMBIE, MARY

1178.   "Distinguished Portrait Gallery--9. Miss Mary Lambie, C.B.E.,
         R.R.C." *Nurs Mirror*, 93 (21 Sep 1951).

1179.   Lambie, Mary. *My Story; Memories of New Zealand Nurse.*
         Christchurch, New Zealand: Peyer, 1956. 189 pp.

1180.   "Miss Mary Lambie." *New Zeal Nurs J*, 24 (Jul 1931), 161.

1181.   "Miss Mary Lambie Strove for Better Conditions." *New Zeal
         Nurs J*, 64 (Mar 1971), 8-10.

LAMONT, MARY

1182.   "Nurses of Note. Miss Mary Lamont." *Brit J Nurs*, 42 (17 Apr
         1909), 307.

LA MOTTE, ELLEN NEWBOLD

1183.   Obituary. *NY Times* (4 Mar 1961), 23.

LANDY, RAE D.

1184.   Obituary. *NY Times* (7 Mar 1952), 23.

LA SOURCE, LAUSANNE

1185.   "La Source, Lausanne 1859-1959." *Nurs Times*, 55 (29 May
         1959), 633-639.

LAWSON, MABEL G.

1186.   "This is Her Job--President, National Council of Nurses."
         Nurs Times, 55 (8 May 1959), 559-560.

LAWSON, MARGARET

1187.   "Midwives of Note. Mrs. Margaret Lawson." *Brit J Nurs*, 47
         (14 Oct 1911), 318.

LEE, ELEANOR

1188.   Obituary. *NY Times* (1 Jun 1967), 43.

LEFEBVRE, SISTER MARIE DENIESE

1189.   "Sister Marie Deniese Lefebvre." *Canad Nurs*, 42 (Oct 1964),
        882-883.

LENNOX, JESSIE

1190.   "David Livingstone and Florence Nightingale--A Nurse (Jessie
        Lennox) Who Worked with Both." *Nurs Mirror*, 32 (19 Feb
        1921), 369.

LENT, MARY E.

1191.   "Who's Who in the Nursing World." *Am J Nurs*, 23 (Mar 1923),
        478.

LIGHTWOOD, TERESA

1192.   Lightwood, Teresa. *My Three Lives*. New York: E.P. Dutton,
        1960. 189pp. Also published as *Teresa of Spain*. London:
        Cassel, 1960. 189pp. Abridged in *Cornet*, 48 (Oct 1960),
        153-158.

LIM, JANET

1193.   Lim, Janet. *Sold for Silver; An Autobiography*. New York:
        World Publishing Co., 1958.

LINDEBURGH, MARION

1194.   Mathewson, Mary S. "The New President of the C.N.A." *Canad
        Nurs*, 38 (Aug 1942), 540-542; see also *Canad Nurs*, 39 (Jul
        1943), 452-453; *Nurs Times*, 40 (May 1944), 372; *Brit J
        Nurs*, 90 (Nov 1942), 143.

1195.   "Nursing Yesterday and Today." *Canad Hosp*, 12 (Dec 1935),
        7-9.

1196.   Obituary. "In Memoriam--Marion Lindeburgh." *Canad Nurs*, 51
        (May 1955), 376-377.

LINDER, ANNA

1197.   Obituary. *Sci*, 113 (16 Feb 1951), 196.

LINTHICUM, BARBARA

1198.   "American Women: Givers, Doers, Changers." *Vogue*, 151 (May
        1968), 204.

LIVERMORE, MARY A.

1199.   Livermore, Mary A. *My Story of the War: A Woman's Narrative of Four Years Experience As A Nurse.* Hartford, CT: A.D. Worthington & Co., 1889.

LIVINGSTON, MARION CHRISTINE

1200.   "Marion Christine Livingston." *Canad Nurs*, 45 (Jan 1949), 50.

1201.   Upton, E. Frances. "Miss Marion Christine Livingston." *Canad Nurs*, 21 (Jun 1925), 295-298.

LLOYD, BARBARA

1202.   "Everybody's Favorite Nurse." *Look*, 24 (15 Mar 1960), 100-104.

LLOYD, DAME HILDA

1203.   "Honor for Dame Hilda Lloyd." *Mid Chron & Nurs Notes*, 66 (Sep 1953), 238.

LLOYD-STILL, ALICIA

1204.   "Nursing Notes, Miss Lloyd Still's U.S.A. Visit." *Nurs Times*, 22 (16 Jan 1926), 48.

LOBO, RACHEL HADDOCK

1205.   "Rachell Haddock Lobo." *Int Nurs Rev*, 9 (1934), 4-5.

LOCH, CATHERINE GRACE

1206.   Bradshaw, A.F. *Catherine Grace Loch, Royal Red Cross Senior Lady Superintendent, Queen Alexandra's Military Nursing Service for India.* London: H. Frowde, 1905.

LOGAN, LAURA R.

1207.   Densford, Katharine J. "Laura R. Logan." *National League of Nursing Education: Biographic Sketches, 1937-1940.* New York: The League, 1940.

1208.   "Who's Who in the Nursing World (Laura R. Logan)." *Am J Nurs*, 22 (Aug 1922), 913.

LOPES PONTES, SISTER DULCE

1209.   McKown, Robin. *Heroic Nurses.* New York: G.P. Putnam's Sons, 1966. pp. 291-309.

LOVERIDGE, EMILY LEMOINE

1210.   "Bellevue (Hospital, New York, N.Y.) Alumnae Honor Miss
        (Emily) Loveridge--Oregon's Most Renowned Woman." *Mod Hosp*,
        27 (Nov 1926), 85-86.

LOWMAN, ISABEL WETMORE

1211.   Howell, Marion G. "Isabel Wetmore Lowman." *Nurs Out*, 3
        (Feb 1955), 79-80.

LOWRY, IVA MARIE

1212.   Lowry, Iva Marie. *Second Landing*. New York: Dorrance, 1974.
        53 pp.

LUARD, K.E.

1213.   Luard, K.E. *Unknown Warriors--Extracts from the Letters of
        K.E. Luard, R.R.C., Nursing Sister in France 1914-1918*.
        London: Chatto & Windus, 1930. 193 pp.

LUCKES, EVA

1214.   Hallowes, Ruth M. "Distinguished British Nurses." *Nurs
        Mirror*, 104 (26 Oct 1956), 3-4.

MAAS, CLARA LOUISE

1215.   Berman, J.K. "Florentia and Clarabellas--A Tribute to Nurses
        (Nightingale, Barton and Maas)." *J Ind State Med Assoc*,
        67 (Aug 1974), 717-719.

1216.   "Clara Louise Maas." *Am J Nurs*, 50 (Jun 1950), 343.

1217.   Cunningham, John T. *Clara Maas: A Nurse, A Hospital, A
        Spirit*. Belleville, NJ: Privately printed, 1968. 96 pp.

1218.   Doctor, Amelia. "She Sacrificed to Serve." *Nurs J India*,
        42 (Sep 1951), 238-239.

1219.   Guinther, Leopoldine. "A Nurse Among the Heroes of the
        Yellow Fever Conquest." *Am J Nurs*, 32 (Feb 1932), 173-176;
        for similar accounts see *Tr Nurs*, 109 (Aug 1942), 94-97;
        121 (Sep 1948), 170; *Hosp Mgmt*, 66 (Oct 1948), 82.

McALLISTER, MARY

1220.   "News From the Nursing World--First Member of Parliament."
        Nurs Mirror, 106 (Mar 1958), 1868; see also *Nurs Times*, 54
        (2 Mar 1958), 321.

McARTHUR, HELEN G.

1221.   "Helen G. McArthur." *Canad Nurs*, 53 (Jul 1957), 626.

1222.   "Helen McArthur, President." *Canad Nurs*, 46 (Aug 1950), 620-
         621.

McBRIDE, GRACE

1223.   Watson, Lila. *Grace McBride, Missionary Nurse.* Illustrated
         by Reed McBride. Nashville: Convention Press, 1958.   131
         pp.

McCARTHY, DAME MAUD

1224.   Biography. *DNB 1941-1950* (1959), 546-547.

McCLEERY, ADA BELLE

1225.   Odell, Elizabeth W. "Ada Belle McCleery." *National League
         of Nursing Education: Biographic Sketches, 1937-1940.*   New
         York: The League, 1940.

McCRAE, ANNABELLA

1226.   Parsons, Sara E. "Anabella McCrae." *National League of
         Nursing Education: Biographic Sketches, 1937-1940.*   New
         York: The League, 1940.

MacDONALD, ISABEL

1227.   "Nurses of Note Who Have Promoted Registration." *Brit J
         Nurs*, 63 (Dec 1919), 360-361.

MacDONALD, MARGARET CLOTILDE

1228.   "Margaret Coltilde MacDonald." *Canad Nurs*, 44 (Dec 1948),
         1005.

MacDONNELL, ANNIE MAUD

1229.   "Nurses of Note." *Brit J Nurs*, 42 (8 May 1909), 369-370.

McFARLAND, DOROTHY FERNE

1230.   "Distinguished Service Awards for 1973." *J Sch Hlth*, 43
         (Dec 1973), 652-653.

McGAHEY, SUSAN B.

1231.   "Miss Susan B. McGahey" (obituary). *Aust Nurs J*, 17 (Dec
         1919), 407-408.

McGEE, ANITA NEWCOMB

1232. "First Superintendent of the Army Nurse Corps Passes." *Am J Nurs*, 40 (Nov 1940), 1308-1309.

1233. Kinney, Dita H. "Anita Newcomb McGee and What She Has Done for the Nursing Profession." *Tr Nurs*, 26 (May 1901), 129-134.

McISAAC, ISABEL

1234. "Hospital and Training School Items (Retirement of Isabel McIsaac)." *Am J Nurs*, 4 (Sep 1904), 955.

1235. National League of Nursing Publications Committee. *Early Leaders of American Nursing (Calendar 1922): Isabel McIsaac.* New York: The League, 1921.

McIVER, PEARL

1236. Biography. *Cur Biog*, 10 (Mar 1949), 25ff.; see also *Cur Biog Yrbk* (1949), 378-380.

MACKENZIE, ELISA

1237. "A Naval Florence Nightingale." *J Roy Brit Nurs*, 2 (Dec 1951), 201-202.

MACKENZIE, MARY ARD

1238. "Miss Mary Ard Mackenzie, R.N." *Canad Nurs*, 9 (Jun 1913), 368-369.

McLAREN, AGNES

1239. Burton, Katherine. *According to the Pattern: The Story of Dr. Agnes McLaren and the Society of Catholic Medical Missionaries.* New York: Longmans, Green and Co., 1946.

MACLEAN, HESTER

1240. "Hester Maclean Memorial Insignia." *New Zeal Nurs J*, 46 (Feb 1953), 2-4.

1241. "Nurses of Note. Hester Maclean." *Brit J Nurs*, 43 (14 Aug 1909), 142-143; see also 49 (28 Sep 1912), 253-254.

1242. Valintine, T.H.A. "In Memoriam--Hester Maclean." *Int Nurs Rev*, 7 (Sep 1932), 19-22; see also *Brit J Nurs*, 80 (Sep 1932), 233.

MacMANUS, EMILY ELVIRA PRIMROSE

1243.   MacManus, Emily Elvira Primrose. *Matron of Guys*. London:
              Melrose, 1956. 228 pp.

MacMASTER, ALENA JEAN

1244.   "Alena Jean MacMaster." *Canad Nurs*, 34 (Oct 1938), 581-582;
              see also 40 (Oct 1944), 792.

McMILLAN, M. HELENA

1245.   "Who's Who in the Nursing World (M. Helena McMillan)." *Am
              J Nurs*, 23 (May 1923), 665.

1246.   National League of Nursing Education. *Early Leaders of
              American Nursing (Calendar 1923)*. New York: The League,
              1922.

McMILLEN, CLARA BARTON

1247.   Obituary. *NY Times* (3 May 1957), 27.

MACNAUGHTON, M.

1248.   "Distinguished Portrait Gallery--15. Miss M. Macnaughton."
              Nurs Mirror, 94 (Nov 1951), 202.

McPHERSON, MARY G.

1249.   Obituary. *NY Times* (9 Apr 1956), 27.

McQUILLEN, FLORENCE

1250.   "Hospital Management Salutes Florence McQuillen." *Hosp Mgmt*,
              88 (Oct 1959), 18.

MacRAE, DOROTHY I.

1251.   "The New Matron in Chief." *Canad Nurs*, 40 (Jun 1944), 403-
              404.

MAHONEY, MARY ELIZA

1252.   Chayer, Mary Ella. "Mary Eliza Mahoney." *Am J Nurs*, 54
              (Apr 1954), 429-431.

MAJOR, A.

1253.   "The Poor Man's Nightingale. Major A." *Queens Nurs J*,
              18(7) (Oct 1975), 198.

MALLORY, EVELYN

1254.   "Evelyn Mallory." *Canad Nurs*, 40 (Oct 1944), 67-68; 42 (Oct 1946), 882-883; 44 (Oct 1948), 832-833.

MALONE, SISTER STANISLAUS

1255.   Doherty, Edward Joseph. *Nun with a Gun: Sister Stanislaus: A Biography.* St. Paul: Bruce Publishing Co., 1960. 194 pp.

MANCE, JEANNE

1256.   Brocard, Jeanne Mance. "The First French Nurse to Go Over to Canada." *Rev Inferm Assoc Soc*, 18 (Oct 1968), 863-864. (Fr)

1257.   Burton, Doris. *Loveliest Flower.* London: Burns & Oates, 1958. 186 pp.; Fresno, CA: Academy Guild Press, 1959.

1258.   Daveluy, Marie-Claire. "Life of Jeanne Mance." *Brit J Nurs*, 87 (Aug 1939), 219-220; (Sep 1939), 247-248; (Nov 1939), 282-283.

1259.   Davidson, Catherine. "Jeanne Mance and Florence Nightingale." *Hosp Nurs*, 18 (Mar 1937), 83-85.

1260.   Emory, Florence H.M. "Yesterday and Tomorrow." *Canad Nurs*, 30 (Aug 1934), 349-352.

1261.   Foran, J.K. *Jeanne Mance.* Montreal: Herald Press, 1931. 192 pp.

1262.   "June 19th, Jeanne Mance Day, Has the Significance." *Canad Hosp*, 12 (Jun 1931), 12.

1263.   Lapointe, G. "Jeanne Mance." *Infirm Can*, 15 (Apr 1973), 24-29. (Fr)

1264.   ————. "Nurses Remember." *Infirm Can*, 13 (Nov 1971). (Fr)

1265.   Lefebvre, Sister Denise. "Jeanne Mance." *Canad Nurs*, 38 (Mar 1942), 164-167.

MANGURN, EMILY (SELLMAN)

1266.   Swann, L. Alline. *Song in the Night: The Story of Dr. and Mrs. Thomas E. Mangurn.* Kansas City, MO: Beacon Hill Press, 1957. 112 pp.

MANN, LADY

1267.   "Distinguihsed Portrait Gallery--1. Lady Mann." *Nurs Mirror*, 93 (4 May 1951), 80.

MANNERHEIM, SOPHIE

1268.   Edelfelt, Berta. "Sophie Mannerheim." *Am J Nurs*, 30 (Oct
        1930), 1318-1319; see also *Brit J Nurs*, 78 (Oct 1930), 270-
        272; *Canad Nurs*, 27 (Jan 1931), 10-12.

1269.   Hallsten-Kallia, Armi. "Tribute to Baroness Sophie Manner-
        heim." *ICN*, 3 (Jan 1928), 2-3. For other obituaries see
        Nurs Times, 24 (14 Jan 1928), 32; *Pub Hlth Nurs*, 20 (Mar
        1928), 109-110; *Am J Nurs*, 28 (Mar 1928), 109-110; *Brit J
        Nurs*, 76 (Feb 1928), 41-42; *Nurs Mirror*, 45 (21 Jan 1928),
        353.

MANSFIELD, BERNICE D.

1270.   Philbrick, J.C. "In Memoriam: Bernice D. Mansfield." *Maine
        Nurs*, 3 (Jan 1972), 6-7.

MANUEL, BENILDA (CASTANEDA)

1271.   Nicanor, Precioso M. *Profiles of Notable Filipinos in the
        U.S.A.* New York: Pre-Mer Pub. Co., 1963, I, 182-184.

1272.   Number deleted.

MARIANNE, MOTHER

1273.   Jacks, L.V. *Mother Marianne of Molokai*. New York: Macmillan
        Co., 1935. 203 pp.

MARKHAM, JOAN

1274.   Markham, Joan. *My Little Black Bag. The Story of a District
        Nurse*. London: Hale, 1973. 176 pp.

1275.   ————. *The Lamp Was Dimmed: The Story of a Nurse's Train-
        ing*. London: Hale, 1975. 204 pp.

MARWICK, S.M.

1276.   "Miss S.M. Marwick." *So Afr Nurs J*, 7 (Sep 1942), 172.

1277.   Number deleted.

MARY OF ETHIOPIA, SAINT

1278.   "District Nurse Miraculous." *Nurs Mirror*, 108 (17 Apr 1959),
        i.

1279.   Number deleted.

MARY PAUL, SISTER

1280.   Mary Paul, Sister, and Edmund C. Fisher. *American Nun in Taiwan*. New York: Doubleday, 1967. 240 pp.

MARY WINIFRED, SISTER

1281.   Young, L. "Unforgettable Sister Winifred." *Read Digest*, 88 (Mar 1966), 173ff.

MASUNAGA, SUMIKO

1282.   "Documentary: The Japanese Midwife. The Life of Mrs. Sumiko Masunaga." *Jap J Mid*, 26 (Dec 1972), 46-50.

MATHEWS, STELLA S.

1283.   MacOwan, Amy. "Who's Who in the Western Nursing World. Stella S. Mathews, R.N." *Pac Cst J Nurs*, 29 (Jun 1933), 343-344.

MATILDA OF SCOTLAND, LADY

1284.   "Royal Nurses, Mold the Good." *J Roy Brit Nurs*, 3 (Dec 1953), 243-246.

MATTHEWS, MARY LATHROP WRIGHT

1285.   Matthews, Alexander. *A Nurse Named Mary*. New York: Pageant, 1957. 155 pp.

MAUDE, SIBYLLA EMILY

1286.   Somers Cocks, Emily May. *Friend In Need: Nurse Maude, Her Life and Work*. Christchurch, N.Z.: Nurse Maud Dist Nursing Assn., 1950. 170 pp.

MAXWELL, ANNA CAROLINE

1287.   "Anna C. Maxwell." *Pac Cst Nurs J*, 11 (Dec 1915), 527-529.

1288.   "Anna Caroline Maxwell, R.N., M.A., 1851-1929." *Am J Nurs*, 29 (Feb 1929), 187-194; see also *Nurs Times*, 25 (26 Jan 1929), 88, 94-95; *New England J Med*, 200 (17 Jan 1929), 155; *Mod Hosp*, 32 (Feb 1929), 108.

1289.   Munck, Charlotte. "Anna Caroline Maxwell." *ICN*, 4 (Jan 1929), 10-12.

1290.   National League of Nursing Education. *Early Leaders of Ameri-can Nursing (Calendar 1920).* New York: The League, 1921.

1291.   "Resignation of Anna C. Maxwell." *Am J Nurs*, 21 (May 1921), 513-514; (Jun 1921), 688; 22 (Mar 1922), 407-409; *Brit J Nurs*, 68 (4 Feb 1922), 71.

1292.   "Who's Who in the Nursing World (Anna C. Maxwell)." *Am J Nurs*, 23 (Jun 1923), 766.

MERRY, E.J.

1293.   "Distinguished Portrait Gallery--3. Miss E.J. Merry, S.R.N., S.C.M." *Nurs Mirror*, 93 (Jun 1951), 174.

MEYER, LUCY RIDER

1294.   Horton, Isabel. *High Adventure. Life of Lucy Rider Meyer.* New York: Methodist Book Concern, 1928.

MIGUEL, CELERINA (FINOS)

1295.   Nicanor, Precioso M. *Profiles of Notable Filipinos in the U.S.A.* New York: Pre-Mer Pub. Co., 1963. I, pp. 198-199.

MILLER, ROBIN

1296.   Miller, Robin. *Flying Nurse.* New York: Taplinger, 1972; London: Hale, 1972. 230 pp.

MILLS, MARY

1297.   "M.C.A. Graduate (Lt. Col. Mary Mills, USPHS) Wins High Honor." *Briefs Maternity Center Assn* (New York), 17 (Apr 1953), 3.

MINDNICK, CHARLOTTE

1298.   Mindnick, Charlotte. *The Memoirs of a Nurse.* New York: Carlton, 1970. 105 pp.

MINNIGERODE, LUCY

1299.   "Lucy Minnigerode." *Am J Nurs*, 35 (May 1935), 499-500; see also *Tr Nurs*, 94 (Apr 1935), 321.

1300.   "Who's Who in the Nursing World." *Am J Nurs*, 24 (Sep 1924), 964.

MITCHELL, F.R.

1301.   "Distinguished Portrait Gallery--14. Mrs. F.R. Mitchell,
             O.B.E." *Nurs Mirror*, 94 (16 Nov 1951), 153.

1302.   "Tribute to a Great Midwife." *Nurs Mirror*, 97 (17 Apr 1953),
             V.

MOAG, MARGARET LAURA

1303.   "Margaret Laura Moag." *Canad Nurs*, 41 (Dec 1945), 982.

MOLLETT, WILHELMINA

1304.   Fenwick, Ethel Gorden. "Resignation of Miss Wilhelmina
             Mollett." *Brit J Nurs*, 46 (Apr 1911), 269.

1305.   Obituary. *Canad Nurs*, 76 (Apr 1928), 100; (Jun 1928), 139-
             140.

MOLTER, DOROTHY

1306.   Hamilton, A. "Loneliest Woman in America." *Sat Eve Post*,
             225 (18 Oct 1952), 37ff.

MOODY, MRS.

1307.   "Pioneer Nursing in Alberta." *Canad Nurs*, 12 (Sep 1916),
             502-508.

MOORE, ELLEN MIAMA

1308.   Furnas, J.C. "House That Saves Lives." *Sat Eve Post*, 225
             (16 May 1953), 22-23.

MOORE, LUCY ELEONORA

1309.   "Lucy Eleonora Moore." *Canad Nurs*, 33 (Mar 1937), 129-130.

MOORE, SAMUEL PRESTON

1310.   Wiese, E. Robert. "Life and Times of Samuel Preston Moore,
             Surgeon-General of the Confederate States of America."
             So Med J, 23 (Oct 1930), 916-921.

MOREHEAD, WILLIE (CARHART)

1311.   *Saving Grace*. New York: Vantage Press, 1953. 57 pp.

MORGAN, EDITH GALT

1312.   Biography. *NCAB*, 55 (1974), 286.

MUHLENBERG, WILLIAM AUGUSTUS

1313.   Ayres, Anne. *The Life and Work of William Augustus Muhlen-
           berg.* New York: Harper & Bros., 1880.

MUNCK, CHARLOTTE

1314.   Funding, Inge. "In Memoriam--Charlotte Munck." *Int Nurs Rev*,
           7 (Sep 1932), 417-419; see also *Brit J Nurs*, 80 (Aug 1932),
           227; *Canad Nurs*, 28 (Sep 1932), 507; *Tr Nurs*, 89 (Oct
           1932), 431.

MUNROE, FANNY

1315.   "Fanny Munroe." *Canad Nurs*, 40 (Aug 1944), 546-547.

MURDOCK, MARGARET

1316.   "Margaret Murdock." *Canad Nurs*, 43 (Apr 1947), 298-299.

MURILLO, AGAPITA

1317.   "Who's Who in the Nursing World." *Filipino Nurs*, 14 (Jul
           1939), 17-19.

MURRAY, EUNICE

1318.   Carpozi, G. "I Was There the Night Marilyn Monroe Died"
           (interview). *Ladies Home J*, 90 (Nov 1973), 54ff.

MUSE, MAUDE B.

1319.   Cunningham, Bess V., and Isabel M. Stewart. "Maud B. Muse--
           Nurse, Educator, Author, and Creative Thinker." *Am J Nurs*,
           56 (Nov 1956), 1434-1436.

MUSSON, DAME ELLEN MARY

1320.   "Dame Ellen M. Musson Celebrating Her 90th Birthday." *Nurs
           Times*, 53 (16 Aug 1957), 909.

1321.   "In Honor of Two Distinguished Nurse-Chairmen of the GNC."
           Nurs Mirror, 100 (14 Jan 1955), i.

1322.   Obituary. *Illus Lond Nurs*, 237 (19 Nov 1960), 909.

1323.   "Prestige." *Brit J Nurs*, 74 (Feb 1926), 23-24; see also
           Nurs Mirror, 42 (23 Jan 1926), 363.

1324.   Wilcox, Barbara M. "Notable People at Home." *Nurs Mirror*, 68 (8 Oct 1938), 39, 58.

MYERS, MARION

1325.   "Marion Myers." *Canad Nurs*, 44 (Oct 1948), 832-835.

NEILL, GRACE

1326.   Campbell, Helen. "Mrs. Grace Neill--Her Life and Work and Her Contribution to Nursing in New Zealand." *New Zeal Nurs J*, 39 (Jun 1949), 146-148.

1327.   "Grace Neill Memorial Trophy." *New Zeal Nurs J*, 46 (Aug 1953), 114-115.

1328.   "Pioneers Who Have Passed On." *ICN*, 2 (Apr 1927), 79-82; see also *Brit J Nurs*, 75 (Jan 1927), 13.

NELSON, SOPHIE C.

1329.   "Ladies With Lamps" (editorial). *New England J Med*, 253 (1 Dec 1955), 989-990.

NELSON, TERESA (LEOPANDO) LUCERO

1330.   Nelson, Teresa (Leopando) Lucero. *White Cap and Prayer.* New York: Vantage Press, 1955. 226 pp.

NERI, ANA

1331.   Paixao, W. "Ana Neri and the Women's International Year." *Rev Enferm Nov Dimens*, 1(5) (Nov-Dec 1975), 223-228. (Por)

NETTLETON, R.

1332.   "A Nurse's Life in the 1900's." *Nurs Times*, 63 (21 Dec 1972), 1615.

NEWMAN, EDNA

1333.   Newman, Edna. *My Nursing Years and In Between.* Torrs Park, Ilfracombe (Gt. Brit.): Stockwell, 1967. 141 pp.

NEWSOM, ELLA K.

1334.   Richard, J.F. *The Florence Nightingale of the Southern Army; Experiences of Mrs. Ella K. Newsom.* New York: Broadway, 1914.

NEWTON, MARY ALICE

1335.   Obituary. *NY Times* (23 Apr 1974), 46.

NICOLAY, MARY ANN

1336.   "Our Pioneer Nurses; Miss Mary Ann Nicolay, 1850 to 1939."
         J West Aust Nurs, 33 (Jul 1967), 14.

NIENHUYS, JANNA

1337.   McKown, Robin. *Heroic Nurses*. New York: G.P. Putnam's Sons,
         1966. pp. 239-265.

NIGHTINGALE, FLORENCE

1338.   Abbott, Maude E. "Portraits of Florence Nightingale." *Bost
         Med Surg J*, 175 (14 Sep 1916), 361-367; (21 Sep 1916), 413-
         422; 175 (28 Sep 1916), 453-457.

1339.   "Address by the Archbishop of York (Florence Nightingale
         Memorial Service)." *Nurs Times*, 66 (21 May 1970), 670.

1340.   *The Adelaide Nutting Historical Collection*. Teachers Col-
         lege, Columbia University, New York, NY at Department of
         Nursing, School of Medicine, Columbia University and at
         School of Nursing, University of Kansas, Kansas City, KS.
         A collection of anecdotes, tributes, and letters relating
         to Miss Nightingale's life and career.

1341.   Agnew, L.R.C. "Florence Nightingale--Statistician." *Am J
         Nurs*, 58 (May 1958), 664-665.

1342.   Aikens, Charlotte A. *Lessons from the Life of Florence
         Nightingale*. New York: Lakeside, 1915. 48 pp.

1343.   Aldis, Mary. *Florence Nightingale*. New York: National
         Organization of Public Health Nursing, 1914. 24 pp.

1344.   Andrews, C.T. "Miss Nightingale at Scutari." *Nurs Times*, 56
         (30 Dec 1960), 1624-1626.

1345.   Andrews, Mary Raymond Shipman. *A Lost Commander*. Garden
         City, NY: Doubleday, 1929. 299 pp.

1346.   ———. "Soldier's Angel." *Great Lives, Great Deeds*.
         Read Digest (1964), pp. 551-556.

1347.   "Angel in War: Miss Nightingale and Her Nurses." *Contemp*,
         106 (Sep 1914), 42-422.

1348.   "Anniversary of Florence Nightingale's Birth." *Med Bull US
         Army* (Europe), 13 (May 1956), 107.

1349. "Anniversary Wreath." *Nurs Mirror*, 97 (28 Aug 1953), i.

1350. Arango, L. "Florence Nightingale: Heroine of Hospitals."
       Epheta, 8 (Oct-Dec 1969), 13-26. (Spa)

1351. Arnstein, Margaret G. "Florence Nightingale's Influence on
       Nursing." *Bull NY Acad Med*, 32 (1956), 540-546.

1352. "At Embley Park and East Wellow." *Nurs Times*, 33 (24 Jul
       1937), 730-731.

1353. "At the Crimean Exhibition. The Florence Nightingale Relics."
       Nurs Mirror, 62 (18 Jan 1936), 299.

1354. Austin, R.F. "Health Contributions of Dr. Joseph Lister and
       Florence Nightingale." *J Med Assoc Ala*, 3 (Oct 1943), 149-
       151.

1355. Ball, Otho F. "Florence Nightingale." *Mod Hosp*, 78 (May
       1952), 88-90, 144.

1356. Baly, M.E. "Florence Nightingale On Nursing Today." *Nurs
       Times*, 65(1) (2 Jan 1969), 1-4.

1357. Barnsley, R.E. "Miss Nightingale and the College (Royal Army
       Medical College)." *J Roy Army Med Cps*, 111(1) (1965), 66-
       73.

1358. Barth, Ramona Sawyer. *Fiery Angel: The Story of Florence
       Nightingale*. Coral Gables: Glade House, 1945. 95 pp.
       Fictionalized biographical sketch.

1359. Baylen, J.O. "The Florence Nightingale-Mary Stanley Contro-
       versy; Some Unpublished Letters." *Med Hist*, 18(2) (Apr
       1974), 186-193.

1360. Bellis, Hannah. *Florence Nightingale*. Women of Renown
       Series. London: Newones, 1953. 48 pp.

1361. Bennett, B.A. "Florence Nightingale as an Educator." *Nurs
       Mirror*, 91 (19 May 1950), 147-148.

1362. Benson, Arthur Christopher, and Viscount Esher, eds. *The
       Letters of Queen Victoria. A Selection from Her Majesty's
       Correspondence Between the Years 1837 and 1861*. 3 vols.
       London: Murray, 1907.

1363. Berkeley, Reginald. *The Lady with the Lamp*. London:
       Gollancz, 1929. 136 pp.

1364. Berman, J.K. "Florentia and the Clarabellas--A Tribute to
       Nurses" (Nightingale, F., Barton, C., Maas, C.) *J Ind
       Med Assoc*, 67 (Aug 1974), 717-719.

1365.   Bishop, William John. *Bio-bibliography of Florence Nightin-*
        gale: Completed by Sue Goldie. London: Dawsons of Pall
        Mall, 1962. 160 pp.

1366.   ————. "Florence Nightingale's Letters." *Am J Nurs,* 57
        (May 1957), 607-609.

1367.   Black, Benjamin W. "A Tribute to Florence Nightingale."
        Pac Cst J Nurs, 35 (Jul 1939), 408-409.

1368.   Blanchard, J.R. "Florence Nightingale--A Study in Vocation."
        New Zeal Nurs, 32 (Jun 1939), 193-197.

1369.   Blanchard, Regina. "Life of Florence Nightingale." *Hosp*
        Prog, 11 (Nov 1930), 490-492.

1370.   Blomquist, R. "Elisabet Dillner and the Uppsala Museum of
        Medicine and Nursing." *News Lett Florence N Int Nurs Assoc*
        (1973), 4-7.

1371.   "Book Reviews and Digests" (Brief Biographies). *Pub Hlth*
        Nurs, 12 (May 1920), 442-448.

1372.   Bower, C. Ruth. "Another Portrait of Miss Nightingale."
        Am J Nurs, 28 (Nov 1928), 1099-1100.

1373.   Bower, Walter Russell. *Women of Light.* New York: Harper and
        Row, 1963. pp. 71-89.

1374.   Bridges, Daisy C. "Florence Nightingale Centenary" (edi-
        torial). *Int Nurs Rev News,* 1 (Apr 1954), 3.

1375.   Broe, Ellen J. "Florence Nightingale and Her International
        Influence." *Int Nurs Rev News,* 1 (Apr 1954), 17-19.

1376.   ————. "Florence Nightingale--International Pioneer." *New*
        Zeal Nurs J, 47 (Apr 1954), 44-47.

1377.   Canning, John, ed. *100 Great Adventures.* New York: Taplin-
        ger, 1969. pp. 346-353.

1378.   "The Carriage Used by Miss Florence Nightingale in the
        Crimean War." *Nurs Notes & Mid Chron,* 46 (Jul 1933), 97.

1379.   "The Celebration of a Great Anniversary (Florence Nightin-
        gale)." *Hellen Adelphe,* 33 (Jul 1970), 2-23. (Gk)

1380.   "Centenary and Golden Jubilee." *Nurs Mirror,* 99 (21 May
        1954), 498-499, 510.

1381.   "Centenary Celebrations" (Florence Nightingale). *Nurs Times,*
        50 (5 Nov 1954), 1213-1214.

1382.   Chavez, Neyra. "Florence Nightingale; Her Life and the
        Projection of Her Work in Modern Nursing." *Enfermeras,* 14
        (Jan-Jun 1967), 28-36. (Sp)

1383.   Clayton, R.E. "Florence Nightingale's Work in India." *Nurs J India*, 65 (Oct 1974), 261ff.

1384.   Colby-Monteith, Mary. "The Angel of the Crimea and More." *Pac Cst J Nurs*, 33 (May 1937), 284-286.

1385.   Collins, William J. "Florence Nightingale and District Nursing." *Nurs Mirror*, 81 (12 May 1945), 74.

1386.   Columbia University. *Catalog of the Florence Nightingale Collection*. New York: Dept. of Nursing Alumnae Assn., 1956. 79 pp.

1387.   Cook, Edward. "Florence Nightingale." *Nurs Times*, 50 (2 Jan 1954), 4-6 through (24 Dec 1954), 1438-1439.

1388.   ————. *The Life of Florence Nightingale*. 2 vols. London: Macmillan & Co., 1913-1914.

1389.   Cope, Zachary. "Florence Nightingale and District Nursing." *Dist Nurs*, 1 (Nov 1958), 179-180.

1390.   ————. "Florence Nightingale and Nurses' Duties." *Dist Nurs*, 1 (Dec 1958), 213-214.

1391.   ————. "Florence Nightingale and Her Nurses." *Nurs Times*, 56 (13 May 1960), 597-598.

1392.   ————. *Florence Nightingale and the Doctors*. Philadelphia: J.B. Lippincott, 1958. 163 pp.

1393.   ————. "John Shaw Billings, Florence Nightingale and the Johns Hopkins Hospital." *Med Hist*, 1 (1957), 367-368.

1394.   ————. *Six Disciples of Florence Nightingale* . London: Pitman Medical, 1961. 74 pp.

1395.   Coxhead, E. "Miss Nightingale's Country Hospital." *Country Life*, 152 (23 Nov 1972), 1362-1364.

1396.   "A Criticism of Miss Florence Nightingale" (editorial). *Nurs Times*, 3 (2 Feb 1907), 89.

1397.   "The Death of Florence Nightingale." *Am J Nurs*, 10 (Sep 1910), 919-920; see also *Bost Med Surg J*, 163 (25 Aug 1910), 335.

1398.   Deen, Edith (Alderman). *Great Women of the Christian Faith*. Harper and Row, 1959. pp. 214-217.

1399.   Deniz, E. "Florence Nightingale." *Turk Hemire Derg*, 20 (Apr-Jun 1970), 5-8. (Turk)

1400.   Dilworth, Ava S., ed. "Florence Nightingale Bibliography." *Nurs Res*, 5 (Oct 1956), 85-88.

1401.   Dock, Lavinia L. "English Letter." *Am J Nurs*, 14 (Jun 1914),
        728-730.

1402.   Draper, Jennie M. "A Brief Sketch of the Life of Florence
        Nightingale." *Tr Nurs*, 38 (Jan 1907), 1-4.

1403.   Dunbar, Virginia M. "Florence Nightingale's Influence on
        Nursing Education." *Int Nurs Rev*, 1 (Oct 1954), 17-23.

1404.   Dwyer, Bessie Agnes. "The Mother of Our Modern Nursing
        System." *Filipino Nurs*, 12 (Jan 1937), 8-10.

1405.   Ellett, E.C. "Florence Nightingale." *Tr Nurs*, 32 (May 1904),
        305-310.

1406.   Elton, Lord. "Florence Nightingale." *Nurs Times*, 35 (2 Dec
        1939), 1442-1443.

1407.   Emerson, Haven. "Miss Nightingale: R.N., U.S.A." *Survey*, 50
        (1 May 1923), 184-185.

1408.   "An Evening with Florence Nightingale." *Hosp Prog*, 4 (Mar
        1924), 163-165; 3 (Apr 1923), 202-204; 1 (May 1920), 51-53.

1409.   "Everybody's Opinion. Memorial to Florence Nightingale."
        Nurs Mirror, 94 (12 Oct 1951), 34.

1410.   Fink, Leo Gregory. "Catholic Influences in the Life of
        Florence Nightingale." *Hosp Prog*, 15 (Dec 1934), 482-489.

1411.   Fleming, T.J. "Beauties Who Changed the Course of History."
        Cosmopolitan, 140 (Jun 1956), 24.

1412.   "F.N." *Am J Nurs*, 36 (Nov 1937), 1198-1200.

1413.   "Florence Nightingale." *Am J Nurs*, 35 (May 1935), 402; see
        also *Aust Nurs J*, 6 (Feb 1908), 48; *Hosp* (London), 31
        (Feb 1935), 50; editorial *Med Dial*, 5 (Jul 1903), 122-124;
        Nurs J India, 1 (Sep 1910), 162-166; *Nurs Mirror*, 99 (7 May
        1954), viii; 103 (11 May 1956), i; *Nurs Times*, 30 (3 Nov
        1934), 997; *Pac Cst J Nurs*, 19 (May 1923), 281-287.

1414.   "Florence Nightingale, May 12, 1820--August 13, 1910." *Pub
        Hlth Nurs*, 23 (May 1931), 232; see also 24 (May 1932), 252;
        25 (May 1933), 25.

1415.   "Florence Nightingale and Red Cross Day." *Nurs Notes & Mid
        Chron*, 42 (1930).

1416.   "Florence Nightingale as a Leader in the Religious and Civic
        Thought of Her Time." *Hosp*, 10 (Jul 1936), 78-84.

1417.   "Florence Nightingale as a Young Woman--Born May 12, 1820."
        Nurs Mirror, 95 (9 May 1952), i.

1418.   "Florence Nightingale at 73" (editorial). *Nurs Times*, 24
        (3 Nov 1928), 1330.

1419.   "The Florence Nightingale Bibliography." *So Afr Nurs J*, 22
        (Apr 1956), 16.

1420.   "Florence Nightingale Bibliography is Compiled" (news). *Mod
        Hosp*, 36 (May 1931), 126.

1421.   "Florence Nightingale Celebration in New York." *Johns Hop
        Nurs Alum Mag*, 9 (Jun 1910), 66-68.

1422.   "The Florence Nightingale Centenary May 12, 1820--May 12,
        1920" (editorial). *Pac Cst J Nurs*, 16 (May 1920), 266-269.

1423.   "Florence Nightingale Centenary Service" (editorial). *Brit
        J Nurs*, 102 (Dec 1954), 133-134.

1424.   "Florence Nightingale Commemorative Plaque in British Ceme-
        tery, Istanbul (Turkey)." *Nurs Mirror*, 99 (11 Jun 1954),
        698.

1425.   "The Florence Nightingale Lamp" (editorial). *Prac Nurs Dig*,
        1 (Jul 1954), 26.

1426.   "Florence Nightingale Medal." *Rev Int Croix Rge*, 37 (Nov
        1955), 730-736.

1427.   "Florence Nightingale Memorial Service" (editorial). *Pac
        Cst J Nurs*, 19 (Jun 1923), 330-332.

1428.   "Florence Nightingale, O.M." *Brit J Nurs*, 45 (20 Aug 1910),
        141-147.

1429.   "Florence Nightingale Pledge for Nurses." *Nurs Mirror*, 99
        (7 May 1954), 40.

1430.   "Florence Nightingale--Supposed Portrait." *Nurs Mirror*, 59
        (28 Apr 1954), 63.

1431.   "Florence Nightingale's Letter of Advice to Bellevue (Hospital
        School of Nursing, New York, N.Y.)." *Am J Nurs*, 11 (Feb
        1911), 361-364.

1432.   "Florence Nightingale's Voice." *Am J Nurs*, 35 (Oct 1935),
        958.

1433.   "Florence Nightingale's War Cart." *Nurs Mirror*, 52 (22 Nov
        1930), 155.

1434.   "Florence Nightingale's Work for Public Health" (editorial).
        Am J Pub Hlth, 4 (Jun 1914), 510-511.

1435.   Folendorf, Gertrude R.   "Florence Nightingale, Her Service
        to Mankind." *Pac Cst J Nurs*, 35 (Jul 1939), 406-407.

1436.   Foley, Edna L. "A Pilgrimage to the Shrines." *Am J Nurs*, 20
        (Dec 1919), 232-234.

1437.   Frankenstein, Luise. "The Lady With a Lamp." *Red Cr Courier*,
        16 (Dec 1936), 15-17.

1438.   French, Y. *Florence Nightingale, 1820-1910*. London: Hamish
        Hamilton, 1954.

1439.   "From the Journal 50 Years Ago." *Am J Nurs*, 54 (May 1954),
        591.

1440.   "Fynes-Clinton Memorial Lecture. Florence Nightingale."
        Nurs Notes & Mid Chron, 46 (Jul 1933), 97.

1441.   Gill, Frederick Cyril. "Glorious Company." *Epworth*, 1
        (1958), 132.

1442.   Goldsmith, Margaret. *Florence Nightingale. The Woman and
        the Legend*. London: Hodder & Stoughton, 1937. 320 pp.

1443.   Goldwater, S.S. "Seeing Hospitals with Florence Nightingale."
        Mod Hosp, 35 (Sep 1930), 57-59.

1444.   Gonzalez, M. Rivera. "Florence Nightingale." *Salub y assist*,
        5 (Jan-Feb 1946), 103-109. (Sp)

1445.   Gordon, Richard. *The Private Life of Florence Nightingale*.
        London: William Heinemann, 1978.

1446.   Gottstein, Werner K. "Miss Nightingale's Personality."
        RN, 19 (May 1956), 58-60, 80, 82.

1447.   Gould, M. "A Woman of Parts. F. Nightingale." *News Lett
        Florence N Int Nurs Assoc*, 21 (Autumn 1970), 4.

1448.   ————, and C. Gamlen. "A Woman of Parts (F. Nightingale)."
        Nurs Times, 66 (7 May 1970), 606-607.

1449.   Grant, Duff. "British Nurse in Turkey--1954." *Nurs Mirror*,
        99 (7 May 1954), 367.

1450.   "Greatness in Little Things. Some Unpublished Letters of
        Florence Nightingale with Comments by David Cleghorn
        Thomson." *Nurs Times*, 50 (8 May 1954), 508-510.

1451.   Greenleaf, W.H. "Biography and the Amateur Historian: Mrs.
        Woodham-Smith's Florence Nightingale." *Victorian Stud*, 3
        (1959), 190-202.

1452.   Greenwood, Major. *Some British Pioneers of Social Medicine*.
        London: Oxford University Press, 1948. pp. 98-106.

1453.   Grigson, Geoffrey, and C.H. Gibbs-Smith. *People*. New York:
        Hawthorn, 1956. p. 306.

1454.   Grunnston, David. "Pioneers in the Art of Healing. 1.
        Florence Nightingale ..." *Brit J Nurs*, 100 (Oct 1952),
        103-104; 100 (Dec 1952), 123; 101 (Jan 1953), 101-108.

1455.   Guzman, Gregoria de. "Florence Nightingale." *Filipino Nurs*,
        10 (Jul 1935), 10-14.

1456.   Haldane, Elizabeth. *Mrs. Gaskell and Her Friends*. New York:
        Appleton, 1931. 318 pp.

1457.   Hall, Eleanor Frances. *Florence Nightingale*. New York:
        Macmillan Co., 1920. 84 pp.

1458.   Hallock, Grace T., and Clair E. Turner. *Florence Nightin-
        gale*. New York: Metropolitan Life Ins. Co., 1928. 24 pp.

1459.   —————. *Florence Nightingale and the Founding of Profes-
        sional Nursing*. New York: Metropolitan Life Ins. Co.,
        1959. 24 pp.

1460.   Hallowes, Ruth. "Distinguished British Nurses—14. Florence
        Nightingale." *Nurs Mirror*, 105 (27 Sep 1957), viii-x.

1461.   Hamesh, Dash D.M. "Florence Nightingale's Writings." *Nurs
        J India*, 63 (May 1972), 149 *passim*.

1462.   Harding, W.G. "Florence Nightingale's Lamp." *Ohio St Med J*,
        56 (1960), 176.

1463.   Haydon, A.L. *Florence Nightingale: A Heroine of Mercy*.
        London: Andrew Melrose, 1908. 107 pp.

1464.   Hearn, Mary J. "Florence Nightingale." *Quart J Chin Nurs*, 1
        (Apr 1920), 12-14.

1465.   "Her Letters (Florence Nightingale)." *Nurs J India*, 46 (Jun
        1955), 210; 46 (Jul 1955), 236; 46 (Aug 1955), 268; (Oct
        1955), 326.

1466.   "Historic Carriage." *So Afr Nurs J*, 20 (May 1954), 23.

1467.   Holmes, Marion. *Florence Nightingale: A Cameo Life-Sketch*.
        London: Women's Freedom League, 1912. 20 pp.

1468.   "Honouring Florence Nightingale." *Nurs Times*, 50 (12 Nov
        1954), 1243-1244.

1469.   "House Party at Embley Park." *Nurs Mirror*, 103 (31 Aug 1956),
        viii-x.

1470.   Houstoun, John Fleming. *Names of Renown*. Glasgow: Gibson,
        1954. pp. 166-177.

1471.   Hubble, A. "William Ogle of Derby and Florence Nightingale."
        Med Hist, 3 (Jul 1959), 201-211.

1472.   Hurd, Henry M. "Florence Nightingale--A Force in Medicine."
        Johns Hop Nurs Alum Mag, 9 (Jun 1910), 68-81.

1473.   Huxley, E. *Florence Nightingale*. New York: G.P. Putnam's
        Sons, 1975. 254 pp.

1474.   "In Nightingale's Footsteps." *Red Cr Bull*, 4 (24 May 1920),
        8.

1475.   Inoue, N. "Life of Florence Nightingale and Effects of Her
        Teachings." *Kango*, 16 (May 1972), 14-20. (Jap)

1476.   Isler, Charlotte N. "Florence Nightingale. The Call to War."
        RN, 33 (May 1970), 42, 45, 74; "The Early Years." 33 (May
        1970), 39, 41; "The Final Years." 33 (May 1970), 50, 52;
        "The Great Experiment." 33 (May 1970), 46, 49; "Rebel
        with a Cause." 33 (May 1970), 35, 37.

1477-
1480.   Numbers deleted.

1481.   Jake, D.G. "Florence Nightingale ... Mission Impossible."
        Ariz Med, 32(11) (Nov 1975), 894-895.

1482.   James, Anna C. "Florence Nightingale. The Great Teacher of
        Nurses." *Pac Cst J Nurs*, 16 (May 1920), 282-285.

1483.   ————. *Is That Lamp Going Out? To the Heroic Memory of
        Florence Nightingale*. New York: Hodder & Stoughton, 1911.
        48 pp.

1484.   Jaro, H.J.A. "Florence Nightingale. A Life of Wisdom and
        Courage at the Service of Justice and Mercy." *J Int Coll
        Surg*, 34(6) (1960), Sect. 2, 13-15.

1485.   Jones, Harold Wellington. "Some Unpublished Letters of
        Florence Nightingale." *Bull Hist Med*, 8 (Nov 1940), 1389-
        1396.

1486.   Karman, T. "Florence Nightingale, Pioneer of Public Health
        Statistics." *Orv Hetil*, 112 (4 Apr 1971), 813-815. (Hun)

1487.   Kerling, N.J. "Letters from Florence Nightingale." *Nurs
        Mirror*, 143(1) (1 Jul 1976), 68.

1488.   Kim, Y.M. "Florence Nightingale." *Korean Nurse*, 6 (1967),
        174-176. (Kor)

1489.   King, Frank A. "Miss Nightingale and Her Ladies in the
        Crimea." *Nurs Mirror*, 100 (22 Oct 1954), 11-12; 100 (29 Oct
        1954), 8-9; 100 (5 Nov 1954), 5-6; 100 (12 Nov 1954), 10-11.

1490.   Kominami, Y. "Literature on Florence Nightingale." *Compr
        Nurs Q*, 7 (Summer 1972), 25-54.

1491.   Konderska, Z. "The Birthday of Nursing (Florence Nightingale)." *Pieleg Polozna*, 8 (Oct 1971), 12-13. (Pol)

1492.   Konstantinova, Miss. "Student Nurses' Page. In the Cradle of Nursing." *Am J Nurs*, 24 (Oct 1923), 47-49.

1493.   Kovacs, A.R. "The Personality of Florence Nightingale." *Int Nurs Rev*, 20 (May-Jun 1973), 78-79 *passim*.

1494.   Kroksnes, I. "Florence Nightingale--Fearless, Well-informed Nursing Administrator." *Kroksnes I Sykepleien*, 62(9) (5 May 1975), 378-379. (Nor)

1495.   "The Lady with a Lamp." *Nurs Times*, 25 (9 Feb 1929), 154; *Pub Hlth Nurs*, 21 (May 1929), 227-229.

1496.   "Lady with a Lamp and a Purpose." *Mod Hosp*, 36 (May 1931), 126.

1497.   "The Lady with a Lamp. A Noble Tribute to a Noble Woman." *Mid Chron & Nurs Notes*, 64 (Oct 1951), 304-305.

1498.   Lammond, D. *Florence Nightingale*. London: Duckworth, 1935. 144 pp.

1499.   Lear, Edward. "Nightingale, Florence--Drawings Made at Scutari." *Med Press*, 241 (1959), 89.

1500.   Lee, Eleanor. "A Florence Nightingale Collection." *Am J Nurs*, 38 (May 1938), 555-561.

1501.   Leslie, Shane. *Henry Edward Manning, His Life and Labours*. 2nd ed. London: Burns, Oates & Washbourne, 1921. 520 pp.

1502.   "The Letters of Florence Nightingale." *Dist Nurs*, 1 (May 1958), 37-38; (Jun 1958), 61-63.

1503.   Levine, M.E. "Florence Nightingale. The Legend That Lives." *Compr Nurs Q*, 6 (Fall 1971), 38-46.

1504.   Levy, Goldie. *Arthur Hugh Clough, (1819-1961)*. London: Sidgwick, 1938. 236 pp.

1505.   Linden, Kathryn. "Florence Nightingale is Placed Among Mankind's Benefactors." *Am J Nurs*, 50 (May 1950), 265.

1506.   Litchfield, Henrietta, ed. *Emma Darwin. A Century of Family Letters, 1792-1896*. London: Murray, 1915.

1507.   "Literature on Florence Nightingale." *Hosp Prog*, 12 (Apr 1931), 188.

1508.   MacDonnell, Freda. *Miss Nightingale's Young Ladies. The Story of Lucy Osburn and Sydney Hospital*. Sydney: Angus & Robertson, 1970.

1509.   McInnes, E.M. "Florence Nightingale and the Goddess (Letters
        from Florence Nightingale to Rachel Williams Recently Pre-
        sented to St. Thomas's)." *St Thom Hosp Gaz*, 61 (1963),
        73-74.

1510.   McKee, E.S. "Florence Nightingale and Her Followers."
        Washville J Med Surg, 103 (Sep 1909), 385-392.

1511.   Mackie, Thomas T. "Florence Nightingale and Tropical and
        Military Medicine." *Am J Trop Med*, 22 (Jan 1942), 1-8.

1512.   Marks, Geoffrey, and W.K. Beatty. *Women in White*. New York:
        Charles Scribner, 1971. pp. 161-174.

1513.   "Mary Baker Eddy Mentioned Them." *Christian Science Sentinel*.
        Boston: Christian Science Pub., 1961. pp. 160-161.

1514.   Masson, Flora. *Victorians All*. London: Chambers, 1931.
        128 pp.

1515.   Matensen, R. "Nightingale--No Rebel Behind the Myth."
        Sykepleien, 64 (1977), 1022-1024. (Nor)

1516.   "Materials for the Study of Florence Nightingale." *Tr Nurs*,
        86 (May 1931), 656-657.

1517.   Matheson, Annie. *Florence Nightingale. A Biography*. London:
        Nelson, 1913. 374 pp.

1518.   Maxwell, J. Preston. "Florence Nightingale." *Quart J Chin
        Nurs*, 11 (Jan 1930), 16-25.

1519.   "A Memorable Date, August 20, 1910." *Brit J Nurs*, 82 (Sep
        1934), 231-232.

1520.   "Memories of Florence Nightingale." *Brit J Nurs*, 101 (9 Jan
        1953), 7.

1521.   "Memories of Florence Nightingale." *Nurs Times*, 35 (12 Aug
        1939), 1008.

1522.   Miller, Basil William. *Florence Nightingale, The Lady and
        the Lamp*. Grand Rapids: Zondervan Pub House, 1950.

1523.   "Military Nursing. Florence Nightingale--Military Nurse."
        J Am Med Assoc, 187 (1964), 672-673.

1524.   "Miscellany. Florence Nightingale's Medals." *Bos Med &
        Surg J*, 165 (7 Sep 1911), 391.

1525.   "Miss Florence Nightingale: Signatures of 650 St. Thomas
        Nurses." *Nurs Mirror*, 28 (19 May 1900), 95.

1526.   "Miss Goodrich's Nightingale Tribute." *Tr Nurs Hosp Rev*, 97
        (Aug 1936), 130.

1527. "Miss Nightingale, Minister of Health." *Nurs Times*, 27
       (9 May 1931), 529-530.

1528. Monteiro, L. "Letters to a Friend (Florence Nightingale,
       Catherine Marsh)." *Nurs Times*, 69 (8 Nov 1973), 1474-1476.

1529. Morney, Peter de. *Best Years of Our Lives.* New York: Cen-
       tury Press, 1955. pp. 88-100.

1530. Mosby, C.V. *A Little Journey to the Home of Florence
       Nightingale.* St. Louis: C.V. Mosby, 1938. 38 pp.

1531. Muir, Charles Stothard. *Women, The Makers of History.* New
       York: Vantage Press, 1956. pp. 162-166.

1532. Murrow, Edward Roscoe. *This I Believe: 2.* New York: Simon &
       Schuster, 1954. pp. 204-206.

1533. Murthi, A.N.S. *Names You Should Know.* Ambala, Cantt., India:
       Army Educ. Stores, 1954. pp. 65-73.

1534. Nagatoya, Y. "Publication on History of Nursing and Florence
       Nightingale. Additional Notes." *Jap J Nurs Educ*, 11 (Mar
       1970), 60-63. (Jap)

1535. Naree-Rochanapuranada (nfn). "Florence Nightingale and Modern
       Nursing." *Thai Nurs Assoc J*, 3 (Jul 1965), 185-190. (Thai)

1536. Nash, Rosalind, ed. *Florence Nightingale to Her Nurses.*
       London: Macmillan & Co., 1914. 147 pp.

1537. ————. *A Short Life of Florence Nightingale: Abridged from
       the Life by Sir Edward Cook.* New York: Macmillan Co.,
       1925. 404 pp.

1538. ————. *A Sketch of the Life of Florence Nightingale.*
       London: Soc. for Promoting Christian Knowledge, 1937.
       32 pp.

1539. National League for Nursing Education. *Early Leaders of
       Nursing Education (Calendar 1921).* New York: The League,
       1920.

1540. ————. *Early Leaders of Nursing Education (Calendar 1931).*
       New York: The League, 1930.

1541. Neagle, Anna. "Portraying Florence Nightingale." *Nurs
       Mirror*, 93 (18 May 1951), 121-122.

1542. Nelson, J. "Florence, The Legend." *Nurs Mirror*, 142(20)
       (13 May 1976), 40-41.

1543. Newman, George. *The Commemoration of Florence Nightingale.*
       London: International Council of Nurses, 1937. 16 pp.

1544. ———. "The Commemoration of Florence Nightingale" (reprint).
       Int Nurs Rev, 1 (Oct 1954), 4-10.

1545. ———. "Florence Nightingale and Hospital Services." *Nurs
       Mirror*, 58 (17 May 1934), 476; (24 Mar 1934), 491; (31 May);
       (7 Apr), 10.

1546. Newman, T.R. "Florence Nightingale (1820-1910)." *Nurs Times*,
       45 (4 Feb 1950), 121-123.

1547. Newton, Mildred E. "The Power of Statistics." *Pub Hlth Nurs*,
       43 (Sep 1951), 502-505.

1548. "The Nightingale Bibliography" (editorial). *Am J Nurs*, 57
       (May 1957), 585.

1549. "Nightingale Centenary." *Am J Nurs*, 20 (Apr 1920), 527-528.

1550. "Nightingale Centennial." *Pub Hlth Nurs*, 12 (May 1920),
       360-384.

1551. *Nightingale (Florence) at Harley Street; Her Reports to the
       Governors of Her Nursing Home.* London: Dent, 1970. 197 pp.

1552. "Nightingale Letter to Alice Fisher in Philadelphia." *Am
       Nurs*, 8(2) (31 Jan 1976), 2.

1553. "Nightingaliana." *J Roy Brit Nurs*, 2 (Sep 1950), 145.

1554. Nolan, Jeannette Covert. *Florence Nightingale.* New York:
       Junior Literary Guild & Messner, 1946. 209 pp.

1555. "No Other Earth." *Today's Hlth*, 40 (Nov 1962), 63.

1556. Noyes, Clara D. "Florence Nightingale--Sanitarian and
       Hygienist." *Red Cr Courier*, 10 (Jan 1931), 41-42.

1557. "Nursing Conventions and Nightingale Anniversary." *Survey*,
       24 (4 Jun 1910), 363-365.

1558. "Nursing Echoes." *Brit J Nurs*, 100 (Apr 1952), 36.

1559. "Nursing News and Announcements. Florence Nightingale
       Exhibit." *Am J Nurs*, 10 (Jul 1910), 766-770. Exhibit was
       forerunner of Adelaide Nutting Historical Collection.

1560. "Nurse's Service." *Brit J Nurs*, 102 (Jun 1954), 65-67.

1561. Nutting, M. Adelaide. *Adelaide Nutting Historical Collec-
       tion.* Teachers College and the School of Nursing, Columbia
       University, New York, NY; School of Nursing, University of
       Kansas, Lawrence, KS.

1562. ———. "Florence Nightingale as a Statistician." *Pub Hlth
       Nurs*, 19 (May 1927), 207.

1563.   O'Malley, Ida Beatrice. *Florence Nightingale, 1820-1856.* London: Thornton Butterworth, 1931. 416 pp.

1564.   ————. "Florence Nightingale After the Crimean War (1856-1861)." *Tr Nurs*, 94 (May 1935), 401-407.

1565.   Oman, Carola. "Florence Nightingale as Seen by Two Biographers." *Nurs Mirror*, 92 (17 Nov 1950), 30-31.

1566.   Osborne, James Insley. *Arthur Hugh Clough.* Boston: Houghton Mifflin, 1920. 191 pp.

1567.   Osvath, Z. "Florence Nightingale (1820-1910)." *Orv Hetil*, 111 (22 Feb 1970), 455-457. (Hun)

1568.   Pace, Dixie Ann. *Valiant Women.* New York: Vantage Press, 1972. pp. 61-62.

1569.   Parker, E. Catherine. "The Contributions of the Writings of Florence Nightingale." *Am J Nurs*, 31 (May 1931), 619-622.

1570.   "The Passing of Florence Nightingale." *Nurs J Pac Cst*, 6 (Nov 1910), 481-519.

1571.   Paull, Edith. "Florence Nightingale. A Brief Sketch of Her Life and Work." *Nurs J India*, 44 (May 1953), 113-114.

1572.   Pearce, Evelyn C. "The Influence of Florence Nightingale on the Spirit of Nursing." *Int Nurs Rev*, 1 (Apr 1954), 20-22.

1573.   Peter, Mary. "A Personal Interview with Florence Nightingale." *Pac Cst J Nurs*, 32 (May 1936), 270-271.

1574.   Petroni, A. "Florence Nightingale." *Munca Sanit*, 15 (Jul 1967), 434-438. (Rum)

1575.   Phelps, George Allison. *Holidays and Philosophical Biographies.* Los Angeles: House-Warven, 1951. pp. 79-86.

1576.   Phillips, Elsie Courrier. "Florence Nightingale--A Study." *Pac Cst J Nurs*, 16 (May 1920), 272-274.

1577.   Pickering, G. "Letter: Florence Nightingale's Illness." *Brit Med J*, 4(5945) (14 Dec 1974), 656.

1578.   Number deleted.

1579.   Pollard, Eliza F. *Florence Nightingale, The Wounded Soldiers' Friend.* London: Partridge, 1902. 160 pp.

1580.   Presbyterian Hospital School of Nursing (New York City). *Catalogue of the Florence Nightingale Collection.* New York: School of Nursing, Presbyterian Hospital, 1937. 63 pp.

1581.   "Public Health Nursing (Florence Nightingale as a Consultant)."
        Pac Cst J Nurs, 16 (May 1920), 299-300.

1582.   Rao, G.A. "Florence Nightingale." *Nurs J India*, 62 (Jun
        1971), 179.

1583.   Rasmussen, I.F. *Nightingale (Royal United Services Institu-
        tion, London)*. Copenhagen: T. Sygepler, 1960. No. 24 in
        Kopenhagen University Med Hist Mus Ars (1959-1961).

1584.   Rees, R. "Two Women Mystics." *20th Cent*, 164 (Aug 1958),
        101-102.

1585.   Reid, Edith C. *Florence Nightingale: A Drama*. New York:
        Macmillan Co., 1922. 118 pp.

1586.   Rhynas, Margaret. "Intimate Sketch of Life of Florence
        Nightingale." *Canad Nurs*, 27 (May 1931), 229-231; see also
        Canad Hosp, 14 (May 1937), 13-16.

1587.   Richards, Laura E. *Florence Nightingale: Angel of the Crimea*.
        New York: Appleton, 1909. 167 pp.

1588.   ————, ed. "Letters of Florence Nightingale." *Yale Rev*,
        24 (1934), 326-347.

1589.   Richards, Linda. "Foreign Department. Recollections of
        Florence Nightingale." *Am J Nurs*, 20 (May 1920), 649.

1590.   Number deleted.

1591.   Robinson, Grace B. "Centenary of Florence Nightingale, Fore-
        runner of the Trained Nurse." *Tr Nurs*, 64 (May 1920),
        404-410.

1592.   "The Romantic Florence Nightingale." *Canad Nurs*, 64 (May
        1968), 57-59.

1593.   Ross, Margaret. "Miss Nightingale's Letters." *Am J Nurs*,
        53 (May 1953), 593-594.

1594.   Roxburgh, R. "Miss Clough, Miss Nightingale and the Highland
        Brigade." *Victorian Stud*, 15 (Sep 1971), 75-79.

1595.   ————. "Miss Nightingale and Miss Clough: Letters from
        Crimea." *Victorian Stud*, 13 (Sep 1969), 71-89.

1596.   Ruebner, B. "Florence Nightingale, Pioneer of Public Health
        and Medical Statistics." *N S Med Bull*, 36 (1957), 375-376.

1597.   Rundall, Francis B.A. "Florence Nightingale's Place in
        British History." *Bull of New York Acad Med*, 32 (1956),
        536-539.

1598.   Sabatini, Rafael. *Heroic Lives--Richard I; Saint Francis of
        Assissi; Joan of Arc; Sir Walter Raleigh; Lord Nelson;
        Florence Nightingale.* Boston: Houghton Mifflin, 1934. 416
        pp. See pp. 363-416.

1599.   "St. Paul's--May 12 1954." *Nurs Times*, 50 (22 May 1954), 545.

1600.   Schuyler, Constance Bradford. "Molders of Modern Nursing:
        Florence Nightingale and Louisa Schuyler." Ed.D. disser-
        tation, Columbia University Teachers College, 1975. 351 pp.

1601.   Scovil, Elisabeth R. "Florence Nightingale and Her Nurses."
        Am J Nurs, 15 (Oct 1914), 13-18.

1602.   ———. "Florence Nightingale's Notes on Nursing." *Am J
        Nurs*, 27 (May 1927), 355-357.

1603.   ———. "The Later Activities of Florence Nightingale."
        Am J Nurs, 20 (May 1920), 609-612.

1604.   ———. "Florence Nightingale." *Am J Nurs*, 14 (Oct 1913),
        28-32.

1605.   ———. "The Life Story of Florence Nightingale." *Am J
        Nurs*, 17 (Dec 1916), 209-212.

1606.   ———. "Personal Recollections of Florence Nightingale."
        Am J Nurs, 11 (Feb 1911), 365-368.

1607.   Sedan, F. "Florence Nightingale and Turkish Education."
        Pub Hlth Nurs, 39 (Jun 1947), 349.

1608.   "A Service of Rededication to Nursing--Suitable for Florence
        Nightingale's Birth, May 12." *Nurs Mirror*, 95 (25 Apr
        1952), 75-76.

1609.   "Seven Hundred Nurses in Colorful Ceremony (Florence Nightin-
        gale Memorial)." *Irish Nurs News*, 4 (Aug-Sep 1954), 6-7.

1610.   Seymer, Lucy Ridgeley (Buckler). *Florence Nightingale.* New
        York: Macmillan Co., 1950. 154 pp.

1611.   ———. "Florence Nightingale." *Nurs Mirror*, 99 (2 Apr
        1954), 34-36.

1612.   ———. *Florence Nightingale.* London: Faber and Faber,
        1950. 154 pp.

1613.   ———. "Florence Nightingale at Kaiserwerth." *Am J Nurs*,
        51 (Jul 1951), 424-426.

1614.   ———. *Florence Nightingale's Nurses. The Nightingale
        Training School, 1860-1960.* London: Pitman, 1960.

1615.   ————. "Florence Nightingale Oration." *Int Nurs Bull*, 3
         (Sep 1947), 12-17.

1616.   ————. "The Nightingale Jewel." *Am J Nurs*, 55 (May 1955),
         549-550.

1617.   ————. "A Nursing Centenary for July, 1951." *Nurs Mirror*,
         93 (20 Jul 1951), 277-278.

1618.   ————. *Selected Writings of Florence Nightingale.* New York:
         Macmillan Co., 1954.   396 pp.

1619.   Shalders, G.M. "A Few Memories of Miss Nightingale." *Queens
         Nurs Mag*, 27 (Mar 1934), 38-39.

1620.   Shibata, T. "Introduction and a Study of Reference Materials
         Concerning the Life of Florence Nightingale. A Section of
         the Diary of Miss Umeko Tsuda on Her Visit to Miss Nightin-
         gale." *Jap J Nurs Educ*, 15 (Apr 1974), 272-279. (Jap)

1621.   ————. "Introduction and a Study of Reference Materials
         Concerning the Life of Florence Nightingale. II. Nightin-
         gale and the Nightingale Training School." *Jap J Nurs Educ*,
         15 (Feb 1974), 116-121. (Jap)

1622.   ————. "The Literature on Nightingale: Introduction and
         Comments. I. The First Edition of the Notes on Nursing and
         Its Japanese Translation." *Jap J Nurs Educ*, 15 (Jan 1974),
         119-166. (Jap)

1623.   ————. "On a Visit to Sites Associated with Florence
         Nightingale." *Jap J Nurs Educ*, 37 (May 1973), 588-594.
         (Jap)

1624.   ————. "On Visiting Places Associated with Florence
         Nightingale." *Jap J Nurs Educ*, 37 (Aug 1973), 1006-1010;
         (Sep 1973), 1180-1184. (Jap)

1625.   Shonan, Y. "Trip to Embley. A Visit to Nightingale's Tomb."
         Compr Nurs Q, 8 (Spring 1973), 94-99. (Jap)

1626.   Simpson, Cora E. "International Hospital Day." *Quart J Chin
         Nurs*, 9 (Feb 1928), 13-14.

1627.   Skvortso, K.A. "Florence Nightingale, Nurse." *Klin Med*
         (Mosk), 54(2) (Feb 1976), 147-149. (Rus)

1628.   "Some Letters from Florence Nightingale." *Hosp* (London), 30
         (Dec 1934), 335-336.

1629.   "Some Nursing Treasures." *Am J Nurs*, 37 (May 1937), 476-479.

1630.   Sotejo, J.V. "Florence Nightingale--Nurse for All Seasons."
         ANPHI Pap, 5 (Apr-Jun 1970), 4.

1631.   "South Africa Has a Florence Nightingale Festival." *Nurs Mirror*, 100 (10 Dec 1954), i.

1632.   Stedman, Amy. *The Story of Florence Nightingale*. New York: Frederick A. Stokes Co., 1926. 63 pp.

1633.   Stephen, Barbara. "Florence Nightingale's Home." *Int Nurs Rev*, 11 (Jul 1937), 331-334.

1634.   Stewart, Isabel Maitland. "Florence Nightingale--Educator." *Teach Coll Rec*, 41 (Dec 1939), 208-223.

1635.   Strachey, L. "Florence Nightingale." In *Adventures in Modern Literature*. 3rd ed. Edited by Ruth Matilda Stauffer and others. New York: Harcourt, Brace & World, 1951. pp. 332-361.

1636.   ———. "Strongest Will Be Wanted at the Washtub." In *Turning Point*. Edited by Philip Dunaway and George DeKay. New York: Random House, 1958. pp. 55-68.

1637.   ———. *Eminent Victorians: Cardinal Manning, Florence Nightingale, Dr. Arnold, General Gordon*. New York: G.P. Putnam's Sons, 1918. 310 pp. Many editions.

1638.   Sullivan, Howard A. *Florence Nightingale Collection at Wayne State University: An Annotated Bibliography*. Detroit: Wayne State University Library, 1963. 20 pp.

1639.   Talbott, John H. *Biographical History of Medicine*. New York: Grune & Stratton, 1970. pp. 806-808.

1640.   Tarrant, W.G. *Florence Nightingale as a Religious Thinker*. London: British & Foreign Unitarian Assn., 1920. 32 pp.

1641.   Thomas, Henry, and D.L. Thomas. *50 Great Modern Lives*. New York: Hanover House, 1956. pp. 210-218.

1642.   Tooley, Sarah A. *The Life of Florence Nightingale*. 5th ed. London: S.H. Bousfield, 1904. 344 pp. 6th ed. New York: Macmillan Co., 1905. 347 pp.

1643.   Tracy, Margaret Anthony. "Florence Nightingale and Her Influence on Hospitals." *Pac Cst J Nurs*, 36 (Jul 1940), 406-407.

1644.   "Trois Anniversaires (The Deaths of Florence Nightingale, Gustave Moynier and Henry Dunant)." *Rev Int Croix R*, 42 (1960), 656-672.   (Fr)

1645.   Tuulio, Tino. "Florence Nightingale ..." *League Red Cr Soc Mth Bull*, 20 (Feb 1939), 27-28.

1646.   Usui, H. "Notes on Notes on Nursing." *Compr Nurs Q*, 9(2) (Summer 1974), 68-76.   (Jap)

1647.   ———. "Notes on Notes on Nursing by Nightingale." *Compr Nurs Q*, 8 (Winter 1973), 39-50.   (Jap)

1648.   ———. "Observations on Notes on Nursing by Florence Nightingale." *Compr Nurs Q*, 11(T) (1976), 55-66.   (Jap)

1649.   ———. "Remarks on Notes on Nursing by Nightingale." *Compr Nurs Q*, 8 (Summer 1973), 15-26.   (Jap)

1650.   Van Doren, Charles, ed. *Letters to Mother*. Great Neck, NY: Channel, 1959. pp. 252-254.

1651.   Verney, Harry. "The Complete Aunte (Florence Nightingale)." *Osterr Schwesternztg*, 24 (May 1971), 130-133.   (Ger)

1652.   ———. *Florence Nightingale at Harley Street: Her Reports to the Governors of Her Nursing Home, 1853-1854*. London: J.M. Dent & Sons, 1970.

1653.   ———. "The Perfect Aunt--FN 1820-1910." *News Lett Florence N Int Nurs Assoc*, 70 (Spring 1970), 13-16.

1654.   Verney, Parthenope. "A Crimean Bed Time Story." *Nurs Mirror*, 99 (7 May 1954), 7-13.

1655.   Verney, R. "Florence Nightingale: By Her God-daughter." *Nurs J India*, 68 (1977), 123-125.

1656.   Walton, P. "The Lady with the Lamp (Florence Nightingale)." *Phlp J Nurs*, 41 (Jan-Mar 1972), 11-12.

1657.   Watkin, B. "Notes on Nightingale." *Nurs Mirror*, 142(19) (6 May 1976), 42.

1658.   West, Roberta Mayhew. "Florence Nightingale Memorial Service." *Am J Nurs*, 31 (Jun 1931), 710-712.

1659.   "Westminster Abbey, Florence Nightingale Commemoration Service Tuesday, May 12th, 1970 at 6:30 p.m. the 150th Anniversary of Her Birth." *News Lett Florence N Int Nurs Assoc* (Autumn 1970), 19-20.

1660.   "White Angel." *Am J Nurs*, 36 (Jun 1936), 574-575.

1661.   White, Francis S. "At the Gate of the Temple." *Pub Hlth Nurs*, 15 (Jun 1923), 279-283.

1662.   "Who Is Mrs. Nightingale?" *London Times* (30 Oct 1854).

1663.   Widmer, Carolyn Ladd. "Grandfather and Florence Nightingale." *Am J Nurs*, 55 (May 1955), 569-571.

1664.   Williams, John Hargreaves Harley. *Healing Touch*. Springfield, IL: Charles C Thomas, 1951. pp. 157-217.

1665. Willis, Irene Cooper. *Florence Nightingale*. New York: Coward-McCann, 1931. 275 pp.

1666. Winchester, J.H. "Tough Angel of the Battlefield: The Real Florence Nightingale." *Today's Hlth*, 45 (May 1967), 30ff.

1667. Winslow, Charles-Edward A. "Florence Nightingale and Public Health Nursing." *Pub Hlth Nurs*, 38 (Jul 1946), 330-332.

1668. Wintle, W.J. Florence. *Florence Nightingale and Frances E. Willard. The Story of Their Lives*. London: Sunday School Union, 1912.

1669. Wolstenholme, G.E. "Florence Nightingale: New Lamps for Old." *Proc R Soc Med*, 63 (Dec 1970), 1282-1288; see also *Sogo Kango*, 12 (1977), 59-78. (Jap)

1670. Woodham-Smith, Mrs. Cecil. *Florence Nightingale, 1820-1910*. London: Constable, 1950. 615 pp.; New York: McGraw-Hill, 1951.

1671. ———. "Florence Nightingale 1820-1910" (abridged). *Read Digest*, 59 (Aug 1951), 145-168.

1672. ———. *Florence Nightingale 1820-1910*. New ed. abr. London: Collins, 1964. 445 pp.

1673. ———. "Florence Nightingale as a Child." *Nurs Mirror*, 85 (10 May 1947), 91-92.

1674. ———. "Florence Nightingale's Pet Owl." In *Saturday Book*. New York: McMillan Co., 1949. pp. 171-179.

1675. ———. "Florence Nightingale Revealed." *Am J Nurs*, 52 (May 1952), 570-572.

1676. ———. "The Greatest Victorian." *Nurs Times*, 50 (10 Jul 1954), 738-741.

1677. ———. *Lady-in-Chief*. London: Methuen, 1956. 210 pp.

1678. ———. "They Stayed in Bed." *Harper's*, 212 (Jun 1956), 41.

1679. Worchester, Alfred. "Florence Nightingale, May 12, 1820-1920." *Bost Med Surg J*, 183 (12 Aug 1920), 193-201.

1680. Wren, David. *They Enriched Humanity*. London: Skilton, Ltd., 1948. pp. 106-130.

1681. Yen, Victoria Pon. "Florence Nightingale." *Nurs J China*, 15 (Jul 1933), 98-100, 118-120.

1682. Yoshioka, S. "Florence Nightingale Biography." *Jap J Nurs Educ*, 30 (Feb 1966), 86-87. (Jap)

1683.   Yumaki, M. "Discussion: Nursing Described by Nightingale and
        Modern Nursing--Thoughts on Nursing After Completion of
        Translation of Nightingale's Writings." *Compr Nurs Q*, 9(2)
        (Summer 1974), 77-84.

1684.   ————. "Notes from the Editor of the Collection of Florence
        Nightingale's Writings." *Compr Nurs Q*, 10(2) (15 May 1975),
        64-65. (Jap)

NORTH, SADIE

1685.   "Life Visits a 77-Year-Old Dynamo." *Life*, 33 (8 Sep 1952),
        149-150.

NOTHARD, C.A.

1686.   "Retirement of South African Military Nursing Service Matron-
        in-Chief, C.A. Nothard." *So Afr Nurs J*, 12 (Feb 1946), 5.

NOYES, CLARA DUTTON

1687.   Biography. *DAB* sup. 2 (1958), 494-495.

1688.   Fitzgerald, Alice A. "Clara D. Noyes--An Appreciation." *Tr
        Nurs*, 97 (Jul 1936), 18-21.

1689.   "The Passing of a Great Leader." *Red Cr Courier*, 16 (Jul
        1936), 11-12.

1690.   Roberts, Mary M. "Clara Dutton Noyes." *Proceedings, 30th
        Convention, American Nursing Association.* New York: The
        Association, 1936. pp. 527-529.

NUTTING, MARY ADELAIDE

1691.   "The Adelaide Nutting Historical Collection." *Nurs Educ Bull*,
        2 (Winter 1929-1930), 4-5.

1692.   ————. "Hopkins Pioneers in Nursing: Isabel Hampton Robb
        and Mary Adelaide Nutting." *Alum Mag* (Baltimore), 72(2)
        (1976), 37-41.

1693.   Christy, Teresa E. "Portrait of a Leader: M. Adelaide Nut-
        ting." *Nurs Out*, 17 (1969), 20.

1694.   Columbia University, Teachers College, Department of Nursing
        Education. *The Adelaide Nutting Historical Collection.*
        New York: Bureau of Publications, Teachers College, 1929.
        68 pp.

1695.   Gardner, Mary Sewall. "Miss (M. Adelaide) Nutting's Resig-
        nation." *Pub Hlth Nurs*, 17 (Mar 1925), 115-116; see also
        Am J Nurs, 25 (Mar 1925), 201; *Mod Hosp*, 24 (Jun 1925),
        535-536; *Pac Cst J Nurs*, 21 (Aug 1923), 493-494.

1696.   Goodsell, Willystine. "Mary Adelaide Nutting--Educator and
         Builder." *Teach Coll Rec*, 27 (Jan 1926), 382.

1697.   Goostray, Stella. "Mary Adelaide Nutting." *Am J Nurs*, 58
         (Nov 1958), 1524-1529.

1698.   Marshall, Helen E. *Mary Adelaide Nutting: Pioneer of Modern
         Nursing.* Baltimore: Johns Hopkins Press, 1972.

1699.   "Mary Adelaide Nutting--1858-1948; Julia Catherine Stimson--
         1881-1948." *Am J Nurs*, 48 (Nov 1948), 675-676.

1700.   National League of Nursing Education. *Early Leaders of
         American Nursing (Calendar 1923)--(Mary Adelaide Nutting).*
         New York: The League, 1922.

1701.   Noyes, Clara D. "M. Adelaide Nutting. Some Reminiscences."
         Red Cr Courier, 4 (15 Jun 1925), 13-14.

1702.   Obituary. *NY Times* (5 Oct 1948), 25; see also *Sch & Soc*, 68
         (16 Oct 1948), 266.

1703.   Roberts, Mary M. "The Immortality of Influence." *Am J Nurs*,
         58 (Nov 1958), 1523.

1704.   Russell, J.E. "M. Adelaide Nutting as Known by Friends,
         Students, and Co-workers." *Am J Nurs*, 25 (1925), 445.

1705.   Stewart, I.M. "Mary Adelaide Nutting 1858-1948." *Teach Coll
         Rec*, 50 (Dec 1948), 199-201.

1706.   "Teachers College (Columbia University, New York, N.Y.)
         Receives a Portrait of Adelaide Nutting." *Teach Coll Rec*,
         33 (Mar 1932), 481-482.

1707.   "Tribute to Mary Adelaide Nutting." *Am J Nurs*, 16 (16 Jan
         1916), 363-371; see also *Brit J Nurs*, 74 (Apr 1926), 71.

OCHIAL, H.

1708.   "Documentary: Japanese Midwives. Life of Mrs. Nami Murakami."
         Jap J Mid, 27 (Mar 1973), 48-52. (Jap)

O'DONNELL, MARY AGNES

1709.   "Mary Agnes O'Donnell, Pioneer Educator in the South." *Tr
         Nurs & Hosp Rev*, 101 (Aug 1938), 136-139.

O'FLYNN, MARGARET

1710.   "New President of the Irish Nurses' Association." *Brit J
         Nurs*, 58 (31 Mar 1917), 226.

O'HARA, DOLORES

1711.   McDonnell, Virginia B. *Dee O'Hara. Astronauts' Nurse: The
          Complete Life Story of the First Aerospace Nurse.* Edin-
          burgh: Thomas Nelson, 1965. 126 pp.

1712.   "People on the Way Up." *Sat Eve Post*, 235 (30 Jun 1962), 26.

1713.   "Nursing Profiles, Agnes Ohlson." *Canad Nurs*, 53 (Oct 1957),
          921.

OLIVIA, SISTER MARY

1713.1 Somers, Mary A. "Sister Mary Olivia." *National League of
          Nursing Education: Biographic Sketches, 1937-1940.* New
          York: The League, 1940.

OLNHANSEN, BARONESS VON

1714.   Worcester, Alfred. "The Baroness von Olnhansen." *Bost Med &
          Surg J*, 136 (1922), 135-138.

OLSEN, BETTY ANNE

1715.   Enloe, C.F., Jr. "Story of Michael Benge, Betty Ann Olsen
          and Henry Blood." *Sat Eve Post*, 245 (Nov 1973), 42ff.

OSBOURN, LUCY

1716.   "Portrait of Lucy Osbourn. Matron of Sydney Hospital."
          Aust Nurs J, 51 (Dec 1953), i.

1717.   Bowd, D.G. *Founder of the Nightingale System of Nursing of
          Sydney Hospital.* Sydney: Hawkesberry Press, 1969.

1718.   Cope, Zachary. *Six Disciples of Florence Nightingale.*
          London: Pitman Medical, 1961.

1719.   MacDonnell, Freda. *Miss Nightingale's Young Nurses: The Story
          of Lucy Osbourn and Sydney Hospital.* Sydney: Angus, 1970.

1720.   Salmon, Mary. "A Pioneer of Trained Nurses." *Aust Nurs J*, 9
          (Nov 1911), 364-366.

1721.   Susman, M.P. "Lucy Osbourn and Her Five Nightingale Nurses."
          Med J Aust, 1 (1965), 633-642.

OSLER, WILLIAM

1722.   Abbott, Maude E. *Sir William Osler Memorial Number. Bull
          #19 Internat'l Assn of Medical Muse and Jnl of Technical
          Methods.* Toronto: Murray Print Co., 1926.

1723. "Centenary of Sir William Osler (1849-1919)." *Nurs Mirror*, 89 (9 Jul 1949), 225.

1724. Cushing, Harvey W. *Life of Sir William Osler.* Oxford: Clarendon Press, 1952.

1725. "Sir William Osler Memorial Meeting." *Med & Chirurgical Fac of Maryland Bull*, 12 (Jan 1978), 59-78.

OSTLAND, SIRI

1726. "I've Had a Thousand Babies; As Told to J. Ellison." *Sat Eve Post*, 225 (6 Jun 1953), 22ff.

OTTLEY, L.J.

1727. "The New President." *Nurs Times*, 48 (24 May 1952), 505-506.

PACIS, ESCOLASTICA

1728. Nicanor, Precioso M. *Profiles of Notable Filipinos in the U.S.A.* New York: Pre-Mer Pub. Co., 1963. vol. 1. pp. 235-237.

PAGET, KATHLEEN

1729. "Honour for our Chairman." *Mid Chron & Nurs Notes*, 69 (May 1956), 117.

PAGET, ROSALIND

1730. Biography. *DNB 1941-1950.* (1959), 646-647.

1731. Hallowes, Ruth M. "Distinguished British Nurses: Rosalind Paget." *Nurs Mirror*, 99 (3 Sep 1954), xii-xiv.

1732. "A Notable Cèntenerary." *Mid Chron & Nurs Notes*, 68 (Jun 1955), 8.

1733. "Notable People at Home." *Nurs Mirror*, 68 (29 Oct 1938), 160.

1734. Obituary. *NY Times* (21 Aug 1948), 15.

1735. Pye, E.M. "Rosalind Paget." *Mid Chron & Nurs Notes*, 48 (Jul 1935), 108.

PALMER, SOPHIA F.

1736. Christy, T.E. "Portrait of a Leader: Sophia F. Palmer." *Nurs Out*, 23 (Dec 1975), 746-751.

1737. "Nursing Echoes." *Brit J Nurs*, 89 (Aug 1941), 131.

1738.   "Try to Remember Our Heritage." *Bull Texas Nurs Assoc*, 40
         (Nov-Dec 1966), 3.

PAMBRUN, ANDRA MARIE

1739.   Diamonstein, Barbaralee. *Open Secrets*. New York: Viking,
         1972.

1740.   Gridley, Marion E. *Indians of Today*. n.p.: ICEP, Inc.,
         1971. pp. 399-400.

PAQUETTE, GEORGINA S.

1741.   Paquette, Georgina S. *My Book*. (Autobiography.) New York:
         Exposition Press, 1949. 32 pp.

PARLIAMENT, JOAN

1742.   "A Nurse and A Secret Service Agent of Cromwell's Parliament."
         J R Brit Nurs Assoc, 4 (Mar 1956), 117-119.

PARSONS, SARA ELIZABETH

1743.   "Who's Who in the Nursing World." *Am J Nurs*, 24 (Mar 1924),
         460.

PASSAVANT, W.A.

1744.   Heberding, G.H. *Life and Letters of W.A. Passavant*. 3rd ed.
         Greenville, PA: Young Lutheran Co., 1906.

PATTERSON, FLORENCE

1745.   "The Resignation of Miss Florence Patterson." *Pub Hlth Nurs*,
         14 (Jan 1922), 1-2.

PATTERSON, LILLIAN B.

1746.   "Lillian B. Patterson." *Am Nurs J*, 54 (Oct 1954), 1198-1200.

1747.   Obituary. *NY Times* (10 Sep 1954), 23.

PATTISON, DOROTHY WYNDLOW

1748.   "Homage to a Nurse. Birthday Celebrations at Sister Dora
         Statue." *Nurs Mirror*, 106 (31 Jan 1958), vi.

1749.   Manton, J. *Sister Dora: The Life of Dorothy Pattison*.
         London: Methuen, 1971. 380 pp.

1750.   Price, Millicent. *'In As Much As ...' The Story of Sister
         Dora of Walsall*. London: SPCK, 1952. 65 pp.

PEABODY, CLAIR

1751. Peabody, Clair. *Singing Sales*. Caldwell, ID: Caxton, 1950.
        197 pp.

PEARCE, EVELYN

1752. "Distinguished Portrait Gallery--6. Miss Evelyn Pearce."
        Nurs Mirror (Aug 1951), 336.

PENSE, E.P.

1753. "Miss E.P. Pense." *Brit J Nurs*, 88 (Jul 1940), 115.

PERCY, PIERRE FRANÇOIS

1754. Bett, W.R. "Pierre Baron Percy (1754-1825)." *Nurs Mirror*,
        100 (29 Oct 1954), iv.

PERRY, MURIEL HAIDÉE

1755. Petre, Diana. *Secret Orchard of Roger Ackerly*. New York:
        George Braziller, 1975. 182 pp.

PETER, PAULINE W.

1756. "Nurses of Note. Miss Pauline W. Peter." *Brit J Nurs*, 35
        (2 Dec 1905), 454.

PETERKIN, A.M.

1757. "A Great Day." *Queen's Nurs Mag*, 25 (Jun 1932), 231-233.

PETRY, LUCILE

1758. "Our Lady Admiral of Public Health." *Coronet* (Jan 1953),
        102-105.

PETTIGREW, LILLIAN ETHEL

1759. "Lillian Ethel Pettigrew." *Canad Nurs*, 42 (Oct 1946), 882-
        883.

PFEFFERKORN, BLANCHE

1760. "The National League of Nursing Education Appoints a New
        Executive Secretary." *Am J Nurs*, 24 (Dec 1923), 204.

1761. "Tribute to Blanche Pfefferkorn." *Am J Nurs*, 49 (Sep 1949),
        607.

PHILLIPS, ELSIE COURRIER

1762.   Pottenger, Catherine Caldwell. "Tribute to Elsie Courrier
        Phillips." *Pac Cst J Nurs*, 8 (Aug 1912), 350-351.

PHILLIPS, HARRIET

1763.   "Miscellany. Do You Know? (First Diploma in Nursing)." *New
        England J Med*, 215 (12 Nov 1936), 946.

1764.   Large, J.T. "Harriet Newton Phillips, The First Trained
        Nurse in America." *Image*, 8 (1976), 49-51.

PHILLIPS, MARY G.

1765.   Gove, G.F. "Specialists in Personnel." *Ind Woman*, 30 (Feb
        1951), 36ff.

PILCHER, CAROLINE

1766.   Bower, C. Ruth. "Caroline Pilcher." *Am J Nurs*, 35 (Mar
        1935), 217-221.

PIRQUET, CLEMENS

1767.   Fitzgerald, Alice. "An Appreciation of the Late Professor
        Pirquet." *ICN*, 4 (Apr 1929), 122-124.

POHJALA, KYLLIKKI

1768.   "Finish Nurse Solon Lectures in U.S." *Am J Nurs*, 56 (Mar
        1956), 274.

PORTER, ELIZABETH (KERR)

1769.   *Cur Biog*, 13 (Oct 1952), 54-56; see also *Cur Biog Yrbk 1952*
        (1953), 475-477.

POTTER, MARY

1770.   Hallowes, Ruth. "Distinguished British Nurses. 13. Mary
        Potter." *Nurs Mirror*, 105 (31 May 1957), 6-9.

POWELL, LOUISE M.

1771.   Wayland, Mary Marvin. "Louise M. Powell." *National League
        of Nursing Education: Biographic Sketches, 1937-1940*. New
        York: The League, 1940.

1772.   "Who's Who in the Nursing World." *Am J Nurs*, 24 (Jan 1924),
        289.

PREECE, ELIZABETH

1773.   "Distinguished British Nurses of the Past. 4. Mrs. Elizabeth Preece." *Mid Hlth Visit*, 11 (Jul 1973), 218-223.

PRINGLE, ANGELIQUE LUCILLE

1774.   Cope, Zachary. *Six Disciples of Florence Nightingale*. London: Pitman, 1961. pp. 35-46.

PURTELL, SISTER REGINA

1775.   Obituary. *NY Times* (25 Oct 1950), 35.

RAND, WINFRED

1776.   Vincent, Elizabeth Lee. "It Is Children with Whom We Are Concerned." *Am J Nurs*, 35 (Feb 1935), 141-144.

RANDAL, HELEN

1777.   "A Fine Record." *Canad Nurs*, 37 (Apr 1941), 257-258.

RATHBONE, WILLIAM

1778.   Rathbone, Eleanor F. *William Rathbone, A Memoir*. New York: Macmillan Co., 1905.

1779.   "William Rathbone: The Founder of District Nursing." *Hosp* (London), 38 (13 May 1905), 112.

REDELSTEIN, ELIZABETH

1780.   Ogale, Mary S. *China Nurse: The Life Story of Elizabeth Redelstein*. n.p.: Pacific, 1974. 118 pp.

REEVES, ALICE

1781.   "New President of the Irish Nurses' Association. Miss Alice Reeves." *Brit J Nurs*, 62 (12 Apr 1919), 243.

REID, ELIZABETH MILLS

1782.   "Elizabeth Mills Reid." *Am J Nurs*, 31 (Jun 1931), 716-717.

REIMANN, CHRISTINE

1783.   "An International Marriage." *Am J Nurs*, 34 (Dec 1934), 1176.

1784.   "Christine Reimann, Internationalist." *Am J Nurs*, 25 (Jul 1925), 571.

1785.   Dock, Lavinia. "The Open Form: An Appreciation." *Am J Nurs*, 26 (Sep 1926), 721.

RICHARDS, LINDA A.J.

1786.   Alford, Marion. "Students Page. Linda Richards." *Pac Cst J Nurs*, 22 (May 1926), 296-297.

1787.   Baker, Rachel. *America's First Trained Nurse: Linda Richards*. New York: Julian Messner, 1959. 192 pp.

1788.   Brent, K.A. "Story of Linda Richards--America's First Trained Nurse." *Hosp Mgmt*, 66 (Nov 1948), 31-33.

1789.   Carbary, L.J. "America's First Trained Nurse." *J Prac Nurs*, 23 (Oct 1973), 22ff.

1790.   Collins, David R. *Linda Richards: First American Trained Nurse*. Champaign, IL: Garrard Pub. Co., 1973.

1791.   Hughes, Wilkie. "Linda Richards." *Am J Nurs*, 41 (Apr 1941), 437.

1792.   Jones, Pilani. "Miss Linda Richards--A Sketch." *Pac Cst J Nurs*, 3 (Mar 1907), 106-109.

1793.   Joynes, Agnes B. "Linda Richards as I Knew Her." *Am J Nurs*, 21 (Nov 1920), 72-77.

1794.   Kleinert, M.N. "Linda Richards and the New England Hospital." *J Am Med Wom Assoc*, 23 (Sep 1968), 828ff.

1795.   "Linda A.J. Richards--Pioneer." *Am J Nurs*, 30 (May 1930), 639-642.

1796.   Muson, Helen W. "Linda Richards." *Am J Nurs*, 48 (Sep 1948), 551-556.

1797.   National League of Nursing Education. *Early Leaders of American Nursing (Calendar 1922) Linda Richards*. New York: The League, 1921.

1798.   Popiel, E.S. "Linda Richards Pioneered. Try to Remember Our Heritage." *Colo Nurs*, 66 (Nov 1966), 7-10.

1799.   "Report on Graduation Exercises at Massachusetts General Hospital Training School." *Bost Med & Surg J*, 192 (22 Jan 1925), 197-198.

1800.   "Resignation of Linda Richards." *Am J Nurs*, 9 (Jul 1909), 789.

1801.   Richards, Linda. "Early Days in the First American Training School for Nurses." *Am J Nurs*, 16 (Dec 1915), 174-179.

1802.   ————. "Recollections of a Pioneer Nurse." *Am J Nurs*, 3
         (Jan 1903), 245-252.

1803.   ————. *Reminiscences*. Boston: Hitcomb & Barrows, 1911.
         117 pp.; Philadelphia: J.B. Lippincott, 1949. 121 pp.

1804.   Sloan, Isabel W. *America's First Trained Nurse*. Boston:
         School of Nursing, New England Hospital for Women and
         Children, 1941. 15 pp.

1805.   Thomas, Margaret. "Linda Richards. Our First Graduate
         Nurse." *Red Cr Courier*, 4 (May 1925), 11-12.

1806.   Townsend, Adelaide. "Concerning Miss (Linda) Richards."
         Am J Nurs, 26 (Apr 1926), 323-324.

RIDDELL, MARION SCOTT

1807.   "Retirement of Miss Marion Scott Riddell." *Nurs Mirror*, 58
         (Oct 1933), 9-10.

RIDDLE, ESTELLE MASSEY

1808.   Haupt, Alma C. "A Pioneer in Negro Nursing." *Am J Nurs*, 35
         (Sep 1935), 875-879.

RIDDLE, MARY MARGARET

1809.   "Mary M. Riddle." *Am J Nurs*, 37 (Jan 1937), 112-113.

1810.   "Miss Mary Riddle Broadens Her Field of Work." *Am J Nurs*, 14
         (Feb 1914), 333-334.

1811.   National League of Nursing Education. *Early Leaders of
         American Nursing (Calendar 1923)*. New York: The League,
         1922.

1812.   "Who's Who in the Nursing World: Mary M. Riddle." *Am J Nurs*,
         21 (Jun 1921), 619.

RISTORI, BRIDGET

1813.   Ristori, Bridget. *Patients In My Care: The Autobiography of
         a Nurse*. London: Paul Elek Books, Ltd., 1967. 190 pp.

ROBB, ISABEL HAMPTON

1814.   Christy, Theresa E. "Hopkins Pioneers in Nursing: Isabel
         Hampton Robb and M. Adelaide Nutting." *Alum Mag*, 75 (Jul
         1976), 37-41.

1815.   ————. "Portrait of a Leader: Isabel Hampton Robb." *Nurs Out*, 17 (1969), 26.

1816.   Draper, Edith A.   "Isabel Hampton Robb." *Am J Nurs*, 2 (Dec 1901), 243–245.

1817.   "In Memoriam, Isabel Hampton Robb." *Am J Nurs*, 10 (May 1910), 531–532.

1818.   "In Memoriam Mrs. Isabel Hampton Robb." *Nurs J India*, 1 (Jun 1910), 108.

1819.   "Memorial Services for Isabel Hampton Robb, Who Died April 15, 1910 Cleveland, Ohio." *Bull Johns Hop Hosp*, 21 (Aug 1910), 251–257.

1820.   "Memorial Sketches of Isabel Hampton Robb." *Am J Nurs*, 11 (Oct 1910), 9–32.

1821.   Moody, Selma. "Isabel Hampton Robb—Her Contribution to Nursing." *Am J Nurs*, 38 (Oct 1938), 1131–1139.

1822.   National League of Nursing Education. *Early Leaders of American Nursing (Calendar 1923)*. New York: The League, 1922.

1823.   "Nursing Notes. Isabel Hampton Robb." *Nurs Times*, 3 (5 Oct 1907), 862.

1824.   Obituary. *Brit J Nurs*, 44 (23 Apr 1910), 330; 44 (7 May 1910), 378.

1825.   Popiel, E.S. "Isabel Hampton Robb Organized. Try to Remember Our Heritage." *Colo Nurs*, 67 (Jan 1967), 3–6.

ROBERTS, MARY M.

1826.   Best, Ella. "Miss Mary M. Roberts—An Appreciation." *Int Nurs Rev*, 6 (Apr 1959), 16.

1827.   DeWitt, Katharine. "Mary M. Roberts." *National League of Nursing Education: Biographic Sketches, 1937-1940*. New York: The League, 1940.

1828.   "Executive Edition of the American Journal of Nursing— Company-Friend-Nurse-Teacher." *Nurs Out*, 5 (Jun 1957), 342–343.

1829.   "In Memoriam—Mary M. Roberts." *Canad Nurs*, 55 (May 1959), 240.

1830.   Lewis, Edith Patton. "Mary M. Roberts—Spokesperson for Nursing." *Am J Nurs*, 59 (Mar 1959), 336–343.

1831. "Mary M. Roberts." *Am J Nurs*, 59 (Mar 1959), 344-345; see also *Nurs Out*, 7 (Feb 1959), 72-74; *Nurs Res*, 8 (Winter 1959), 3.

1832. "Mary M. Roberts Retires as Editor." *Am J Nurs*, 49 (May 1941), 621-622.

1833. Obituary. *NY Times* (12 Jan 1959), 39.

1834. "Two National Editors." *Pac Cst J Nurs*, 32 (Apr 1936), 208-209.

ROBINSON, M.O.

1835. "Distinguished Portrait Gallery--13. Miss M.O. Robinson, O.B.E." *Nurs Mirror*, 94 (26 Oct 1951), 88.

ROME, SHERIFF

1836. "Mrs. Sheriff Rome, R.R.C.: An Appreciation." *Nurs Times*, 34 (11 Jun 1938), 609.

ROMIG, EMILY CRAIG

1837. Romig, Emily Craig. *Pioneer Woman in Alaska*. Caldwell, ID: Caxton Printers, 1948. 140 pp.

RORKE, MELINA

1838. *Melina Rorke--Her Amazing Experiences in the Stormy Nineties of South Africa's Story--As Told by Herself*. London: George G. Harrop, 1939.

ROSENKELDE, ANNA

1839. Hamilton, A. "Wonder Scene of Salt Lake City." *Coronet*, 29 (Apr 1951), 32-35.

ROWE, HELEN

1840. "Distinguished Portrait Gallery--18. Miss Helen Rowe, S.R.N., S.C.M." *Nurs Mirror*, 94 (28 Dec 1951), 282.

RUNDLE, MARY

1841. "Retirement of Miss Mary Rundle." *Nurs Mirror*, 58 (20 Jan 1934), 317-318.

RUSSELL, JAMES EARL

1842. "One Who Had Faith." *Am J Nurs*, 27 (Nov 1927), 899-900.

RUSSELL, MARJORIE GORDON

1843.   "Across the Desk. Chief of R.C.N. Nursing Service." *Canad Hosp*, 21 (Mar 1944), 12.

RUSSELL, MARTHA MONTAGUE

1844.   "Who's Who in the Nursing World. Martha Montague Russell." *Am J Nurs*, 23 (Aug 1923), 938.

RUTH, SISTER

1845.   Hall, V.C. *Sister Ruth*. London: Spearman, 1968.

SANDERS, FLORA

1846.   Laffin, John. *Women in Battle*. New York: Abelard, 1968. pp. 151-162.

SANDERSON, KATHLEEN I.

1847.   "Kathleen Sanderson." *Canad Nurs*, 34 (Oct 1938), 581-582.

SANGER, MARGARET

1848.   Dash, Joan. *A Life of One's Own: Three Gifted Women and the Men They Married*. New York: Harper & Row, 1973. pp. 69-113.

1849.   Douglas, Emily T. *Pioneer of the Future: Margaret Sanger*. New York: Holt, Rinehart and Winston, 1970.

1850.   Hersey, Harold. *Margaret Sanger: The Biography of the Birth Control Pioneer*. New York: Sovereign House, 1938.

1851.   Kennedy, David M. *Birth Control in America: The Career of Margaret Sanger*. New Haven: Yale University Press, 1970.

1852.   Lader, Lawrence. *The Margaret Sanger Story*. New York: Doubleday, 1955.

1853.   Reed, James. *From Private Vice to Public Virtue: The Birth Control Movement and American Society Since 1830*. New York: Basic Books, 1978.

1854.   Sanger, Margaret. *An Autobiography*. New York: W.W. Norton, 1938. Reprint. New York: Dover Publications, 1971.

1855.   ———. *My Fight for Birth Control*. New York: Farrar & Rinehart, 1931.

1856.   ———. Personal Papers. There are approximately 500 boxes of papers divided between the Library of Congress, the

Sophia Smith Collection at Smith College, and the Houghton Library in Cambridge, Mass. The journal literature is voluminous but deals only indirectly with nursing.

SAYER, JOHN

1857.   "Distinguished Portrait Gallery--12. Mr. John Sayer, M.B.E., S.R.N., D.N." *Nurs Mirror*, 94 (12 Oct 1951), 36.

SCHNALL, SUSAN LEVENE

1858.   Streshinsky, S. "Court-martial of Lt. Susan Schnall." *Redbook*, 134 (Nov 1969), 78-79.

SCHRADERS, CATHARINA GEERTRUIDA

1859.   Marchetti, Andrew A. "Catharina Geertruida Schraders and Her Diary." *Am J Obstet Gyn*, 50 (Aug 1945), 160-167.

SCHRIEVER, AUGUSTE

1860.   Sticker, A. "Auguste Schriever 1877-1963." *Deutsch Schwesternzeitung*, 18 (10 Oct 1965), 376-379. (Ger)

SCHULTZE, MARIE A.

1861.   Romero, D. "Saint of Santiago." *Read Digest*, 60 (Oct 1955), 163-166.

SCHUTT, BARBARA G.

1862.   "Barbara Schutt to Become Journal Editor." *Am J Nurs*, 58 (Aug 1958), 1114; see also *Am J Nurs*, 59 (Jan 1959), 22; *Am Nurs*, 55 (Jul 1959), 637.

SCHUYLER, LOUISA LEE

1863.   Goodrich, Annie Warburton. "Louisa Lee Schuyler--An Appreciation." *Am J Nurs*, 15 (Sep 1915), 1078-1082.

SCHWARZENBERG, ANNA MARIA

1864.   "Death of Miss Anna Schwarzenberg." *Nurs Mirror*, 98 (29 Jan 1954), 1115.

1865.   "Miss Anna Schwarzenberg." *Int Nurs Rev*, 1 (Apr 1954), 16.

1866.   "News Highlights. Obituaries. Anna Maria Schwarzenberg." *Am J Nurs*, 54 (May 1954), 558-559.

1867.   "The Passing Bell. Miss Anna Maria Schwarzenberg." *Brit J Nurs*, 102 (Feb 1954), 19.

SCOTT, ALMA H.

1868.   American Nurses' Association. "Tribute to Alma H. Scott."
         Am J Nurs, 50 (Dec 1950), 789.

1869.   Clarke, Ethel P. "Alma Ham Scott." *National League of
         Nursing Education: Biographic Sketches, 1937-1940.* New
         York: The League, 1940. See also *Am J Nurs*, 36 (Feb 1936),
         149-152.

SCOVIL, ELISABETH ROBINSON

1870.   White, G.C.M. "Miss Elisabeth Scovil." *Canad Nurs*, 20
         (Jul 1924), 393-397.

SEACOLE, MARY

1871.   Gordon, J.E. "Mary Seacole--A Forgotten Nurse Heroine of the
         Crimea." *Mid Hlth Visit*, 11(2) (Feb 1975), 47-60.

1872.   Vernon, C. "The Story of Mary Seacole; the Florence Nightin-
         gale of Jamaica." *Jamaican Nurs*, 9 (Dec 1969), 19.

SEAGRAVE, GORDON

1873.   Seagrave, Gordon. *Burma Surgeon.* New York: W.W. Norton,
         1943.

SEIFERT, HETTIE W.

1874.   Obituary. *NY Times* (6 Mar 1956), 31.

SELL, FRANCIS D.

1875.   Obituary. *NY Times* (26 Jul 1948), 17; see also *Sch & Soc*, 68
         (31 Jul 1948), 74.

SETON, ELIZABETH R.

1876.   Allen, Stephen. "Sainthood for Blessed Elizabeth Seton."
         Hosp Prog (Sep 1975), 36-44.

1877.   Burns, Arthur J. "New Light on Mother Seton." American
         Catholic Historical Society, *Record*, 22 n.s. (1905).

1878.   Dirvin, Joseph I. *Blessed Elizabeth Ann Seton.* New York:
         Farrar, Straus & Cudahy, 1963.

1879.   ———. Mrs. Seton, *Foundress of the American Sisters of
         Charity.* New York: Farrar, Straus & Cudahy, 1962.

1880.   Seton, Elizabeth A. *Memoir, Letters and Journals of Eliza-
         beth Seton.* Edited by Robert Seton. 2 vols. New York:
         O'Shea, 1869.

1881.   White, Charles. *Mother Seton; Mother of Many Daughters.*
        Emmitsburg, MD: Mother Seton Guild, 1949.

SHARPE, GLADYS

1882.   "Gladys Sharpe, President." *Canad Nurs*, 50 (Sep 1954), 702-
        703.

SHAW, FLORA MADELINE

1883.   "Canadian Nurses Association President." *Brit J Nurs*, 74
        (Dec 1926), 278.

1884.   Reed, Francis L.   "Flora Madeline Shaw: From National to
        International and Onward." *ICN*, 2 (Oct 1927), 260-261;
        see also *Brit J Nurs*, 75 (Sep 1927), 206; *Nurs Times*, 23
        (10 Sep 1927), 1065.

SHAW, MAUD

1885.   Shaw, Maud. *White House Nannie: My Years with Caroline and
        John Kennedy, Jr.* New York: New American Library, 1966.
        205 pp.   Abridged in *Ladies' Home J*, 82 (Dec 1965), 82-85;
        83 (Jan 1966), 69-70; (Feb 1966), 68ff.

SHEAHAN, MARION W.

1886.   "Miss Sheahan--The New President." *Am J Pub Hlth*, 50 (Nov
        1960), 1807-1808.

SHERWOOD, GEORGINA EVELINE

1887.   Romilly, G.   "Strange Case of Miss Sherwood." *New Stsm &
        Nat*, 36 (24 Jul 1948), 71-72.

SIEVEKING, AMELIA WILHEMINA

1888.   Hoyer, Ernst-Fritz.   "Amelia Wilhemina Sieveking." *Tr Nurs*,
        42 (Apr 1909), 231-233.

1889.   Poel, Emma. *Life of Amelia Wilhemina Sieveking.*   London:
        Longmans, 1863.

SIMMONS, LEO W.

1890.   "Dr. Simmons to Teachers College." *Nurs Res*, 8 (Summer
        1959), 180.

SIMPSON, CORA E.

1891.   "Cora E. Simpson, General Secretary Emeritus of the Nurses
        Association of China." *Brit J Nurs*, 96 (Jun 1948), 71-72.

SIMPSON, MARJORIE

1892.   "Focus on a Pioneer." *Nurs Times*, 70 (4 Apr 1974), 518-519.

SIMPSON, RUBY M.

1893.   "Ruby M. Simpson." *Canad Nurs*, 30 (Feb 1934), 53-56; (Aug
         1934), 353; 41 (Jun 1945), 458.

SIRCH, MARGARET ELLIOTT FRANCES

1894.   "In Memory of Our First Editor." *Nurs World*, 128 (Sep 1954),
         17.

SLEEPER, RUTH

1895.   Biography. *Cur Biog*, 13 (Oct 1952), 56-58; see also *Cur Biog
         Yrbk 1952* (1953), 543-555.

SMELLIE, ELIZABETH L.

1896.   "Elizabeth L. Smellie." *Canad Nurs*, 30 (Feb 1934), 53-56;
         34 (Jun 1938), 291-293; 34 (Oct 1938), 581-582; 36 (Aug
         1940), 497-498; 38 (Jul 1942), 471-472; 42 (Aug 1946), 670;
         43 (Jun 1947), 462; 45 (Jan 1949), 52.

1897.   "Miss Elizabeth L. Smellie for V.O.N." *Canad Nurs*, 20 (Jan
         1924), 787.

1898.   Moag, Margaret L. "Setting a Precedent." *Canad Nurs*, 35
         (Dec 1939), 645.

1899.   "Nurses of Note. Elizabeth L. Smellie." *Brit J Nurs*, 74
         (Jun 1926), 123.

1900.   Upton, E. Frances. "Whom the King Delighteth to Honor."
         Canad Nurs, 40 (May 1944), 327-328.

SMITH, ADAH B. THOMS

1901.   "Mrs. Adah B. Thoms Smith." *Tr Nurs*, 110 (Mar 1943), 213.

SMITH, DOROTHY M.

1902.   "In Honour of Two Distinguished Nurse-chairmen of the GNC."
         Nurs Mirror, 100 (4 Jan 1955), 1.

SMITH, EMMA M.

1903.   "Nurses of Note. Emma M. Smith." *Brit J Nurs*, 44 (23 Apr
         1910), 326.

SMITH, LAURA D.

1904. Obituary. *NY Times* (21 Nov 1961), 39.

SNIVELY, MARY AGNES

1905. Browne, Jean E. "Agnes Mary Snively." *INT Nurs Rev*, 9 (1934), 1-3.

1906. ————. "A Daughter of Canada (Mary Agnes Snively)." *Canad Nurs*, 20 (Oct 1924), 617-620; 20 (Nov 1924), 681-684; 20 (Dec 1924), 734-736.

1907. "Doyenne of Canadian Nursing." *Brit J Nurs*, 43 (18 Dec 1909), 503.

1908. Emory, Florence H.M. "Yesterday and Tomorrow." *Canad Nurs*, 30 (Aug 1934), 349-352.

1909. "A Great Canadian Nurse." *Canad Nurs*, 6 (Jan 1910), 1-4.

1910. "Miss Mary Agnes Snively." *Canad Nurs*, 29 (Nov 1933), 567.

1911. "Miss Mary Agnes Snively and the Story of Nursing." *Nurs J Pac Cst*, 6 (Apr 1910), 160-162.

1912. Whitton, Charlotte. "The Trumpet in the Dust." *Canad Nurs*, 46 (Sep 1950), 699-712.

SOTEJO, JULITA V.

1913. Aragon, Leonor Malay. "Julita V. Sotejo." *Filipino Nurs*, 17 (Oct 1948), 321-322.

SOULE, ELIZABETH STERLING

1914. "Goodbye Messrs Chips." *Time*, 56 (3 Jul 1950), 60.

1915. Leahy, Kathleen M. "Elizabeth Sterling Soule." *National League of Nursing Education: Biographic Sketches, 1937-1940.* New York: The League, 1940.

1916. Loughran, Henrietta Adams. "Mrs. Soule of Washington. Part I --Her Early Career in Nursing. Part II--The University of Washington School of Nursing." *Nurs Out*, 4 (Sep 1956), 492-496; (Oct 1956), 567-572.

1917. Number deleted.

SOYER, ALEXIS

1918. "Alexis Soyer--Chef in the Crimea. Centenary of Collaborator with Florence Nightingale." *Nurs Mirror*, 107 (29 Aug 1958), 1633.

1919.   Morris, Helen. *Portrait of a Chef*. London: Cambridge, 1938.
         221 pp.

1920.   Prichard, M.F. Lloyd. "Alex Soyer at Scutari. Side-Light on
         the Crimea." *Nurs Times*, 47 (22 Sep 1951), 934-939.

SPARSHOTT, M.E.

1921.   "Miss M.E. Sparshott." *Nurs Times*, 25 (13 Apr 1939), 437.

SPOELSTRA-DECKER, B.C.

1922.   Winberg, L. "Farewell Interview with Mrs. B.C. Spoelstra-
         Decker. I Had to Mold." *Tijdschr Ziekenverpl*, 24 (27 Apr
         1971), 407-414. (Dut)

SPRAGUE, ELFREDA

1923.   Neal, H.E. "Adventure--In Bold Relief." *Ind Woman*, 26
         (Sep 1947), 251ff.

STEPHENSON, ELSIE

1924.   "Director. Nursing Teaching Unit, University of Edinburgh."
         Nurs Times, 52 (20 Apr 1956), 299-300.

STEVENS, ANNE A.

1925.   "Miss (Anne A.) Stevens Resigns." *Pub Hlth Nurs*, 17 (Sep
         1925), 442.

STEVENS, LEONARD F.

1926.   "Top Man in a Woman's World." *Life*, 40 (14 May 1956), 115ff.

STEVENSON, BEATRICE V.H.

1927.   Obituary. *NY Times* (14 May 1948), 72.

STEWART, ISABEL MAITLAND

1928.   Christy, Teresa E. "Portrait of a Leader: Isabel Maitland
         Stewart." *Nurs Out*, 17 (Oct 1969), 44-48.

1929.   "A Distinguished Visitor Isabel Stewart." *Pac Cst J Nurs*, 30
         (Jan 1934), 21.

1930.   Goostray, Stella. "Isabel Maitland Stewart. The Story of a
         National and International Leader in Nursing Education."
         Am J Nurs, 54 (Mar 1954), 302-306.

1931.   "Nurses of Note. Isabel Maitland Stewart." *Brit J Nurs*, 75
         (Apr 1927), 79.

1932.   Obituary. *NY Times* (7 Oct 1963), 31.

1933.   Taylor, Effie Jane. "Isabel Maitland Stewart." *National
         League of Nursing Education: Biographic Sketches, 1937-1940.*
         New York: The League, 1940.

1934.   ————. "Isabel Maitland Stewart, Educator." *Am J Nurs*, 36
         (Jan 1936), 38-41.

1935.   "Try to Remember Our Heritage." *Colo Nurs*, 67 (Dec 1967),
         3-6.

1936.   "Who's Who in the Nursing World." *Am J Nurs*, 22 (Apr 1922),
         543.

STEWART, ISLA

1937.   Breay, Margaret. "Banquet to Miss Isla Stewart." *Brit J
         Nurs*, 41 (4 Jul 1908), 3-9.

1938.   "Centenary of a Scottish Nurse." *Nurs Mirror*, 101 (26 Aug
         1955), 1460.

1939.   Dock, Lavinia L. "Miss (Isla) Stewart's Work." *Am J Nurs*,
         10 (May 1910), 579-580.

1940.   "In Memoriam, Isla Stewart." *Brit J Nurs*, 44 (12 May 1910),
         201.

1941.   "In Memoriam. Miss Isla Stewart." *Nurs J India*, 1 (May
         1910), 80.

1942.   Strong, Mrs. Rebecca. "Nurses of Note." *Brit J Nurs*, 72
         (Jan 1924), 3.

STILL, ALICIA LLOYD

1943.   Armstrong, Katharine F. "Dame Alicia Lloyd Still, O.B.E.,
         R.R.C." *Nurs Times*, 40 (29 Jul 1944), 515; see also *Nurs
         Times*, 33 (4 Dec 1937), 1225; *Canad Nurs*, 34 (Feb 1938),
         79; *Nurs Notes*, 51 (Jan 1938), 5; *So Afr Nurs J*, 3 (Feb
         1938), 133.

1944.   Hallowes, Ruth M. "Distinguished British Nurses." *Nurs
         Mirror*, 104 (7 Dec 1956), 5-6, 8.

STIMSON, JULIA CATHERINE

1945.   "Major (Julia C.) Stimson Resigns from the Army Corps."
         Tr Nurs & Hosp Rev, 98 (May 1937), 500.

1946.   National League of Nursing Education.   *Biographic Sketches,*
        1937-1940 (Julia Catherine Stimson).   New York: The League,
        1940.

1947.   Obituary.   *Cur Biog*, 9 (Nov 1948), 49; see also *Cur Biog Yrbk*
        1948 (1949), 601-602; *NY Times* (1 Oct 1948), 2-6.

1948.   "Who's Who in the Nursing World (Julia Catherine Stimson)."
        Am J Nurs, 24 (Oct 1924), 1030.

STOBO, ELIZABETH

1949.   "Distinguished Service Awards."   *J Sch Hlth*, 37 (Nov 1967),
        421.

STOPES, MARIE C.

1950.   Aylmer, Maude.   *The Authorized Life of Marie C. Stopes*.
        London: Williams & Norgate, 1924.   226 pp.

STRONG, ANNE HERVEY

1951.   Goldmark, Josephine, and Henry Lefavour.   "Anne Hervey Strong
        --Died June 17, 1925."   *Pub Hlth Nurse*, 17 (Oct 1925), 516-
        519.

1952.   Weston, Alice A.   "Anne Hervey Strong."   *Tr Nurs*, 85 (Aug
        1930), 187-189.

STRONG, REBECCA

1953.   Cope, Zachary.   *Six Disciples of Florence Nightingale*.
        London: Pitman, 1961.   pp. 25-34.

1954.   "The Doyenne of the Nursing Profession (Mrs. Rebecca Strong)."
        Brit J Nurs, 87 (Feb 1939), 31.

1955.   Gordon, J.E.   "Distinguished British Nurses of the Past.   6.
        Mrs. Rebecca Strong."   *Med Hlth Visit*, 11 (Dec 1975), 395-
        398, 409.

1956.   Hallowes, Ruth M.   "Distinguished British Nurses."   *Nurs*
        Mirror, 102 (25 Nov 1955), 11-13.

1957.   Strong, Rebecca.   *Reminiscences*.   Edinburgh: Douglas &
        Foulis, 1935.   11 pp.

STREET, EMELINE AMELA

1958.   Obituary.   *NY Times* (7 Sep 1963), 19.

SWAIN, GLADYS PERERS

1959. Swain, Gladys Perers. *Stewart Island Days; A District Nurse Looks Back*. Duneden: The author, 1970. 112 pp.

SWIFT, SARAH

1960. "Dame Sarah Swift, O.B.E., R.R.C." *Nurs Times*, 33 (3 Jul 1937), 647-648.

SWISSHELM, JANE GREY (CANNON)

1961. Thorp, Margaret (Farrand). *Female Persuasion*. New Haven: Yale University Press, 1949. pp. 56-106.

SWOPE, ETHEL

1962. Jammé, Anna C. "Ethel Swope." *Tr Nurs*, 98 (Aug 1937), 130-131.

TAMM, AUGUSTA

1963. McCallen, Katherine Boies. *By Dim and Fearing Lamps*. New York: Vantage Press, 1964. 143 pp.

TATE, BARBARA L.

1964. "New Editor Appointed for Nursing Research" (news). *Am J Nurs*, 59 (Apr 1959), 464-466.

1965. "Nursing Profiles. Barbara Tate." *Canad Nurs*, 59 (Jul 1959), 637.

1966. "Research Reporter: Editor Appointed for Nursing Research." *Nurs Res*, 8 (Winter 1959), 36.

TATTERSHALL, LOUISE M.

1967. "Next Steps for Miss Tattershall." *Pub Hlth Nurs*, 26 (Mar 1934), 163-164.

TAYLOR, EFFIE JANE

1968. "Effie Jane Taylor." *Am J Nurs*, 34 (May 1934), 476.

1969. "Effie Jane Taylor, R.N." *Am J Nurs*, 39 (Jul 1939), 733-737.

1970. "Items of Interest (Effie J. Taylor)." *Am J Nurs*, 23 (Mar 1923), 483.

1971. "Professor of Nursing" (editorial). *Am J Nurs*, 27 (Jan 1927), 43.

1972.   "Who's Who in the Nursing World (Effie J. Taylor)." *Am J
         Nurs*, 24 (Aug 1924), 890.

TAYLOR, SUSIE KING

1973.   "Nurse and Teacher." In *Growing Up Female in America*. Edited
         by Eve Merriam. Garden City, NY: Doubleday, 1971. pp. 161-
         174.

1974.   Taylor, Susie King. *Reminiscences of My Life in Camp*. New
         York: Arno Press, 1968. 82 pp.

1975.   "Teenage Civil War Nurse: Susie King Taylor." *Ebony*, 25
         (Feb 1970), 96ff.

TEBO, JULIE C.

1976.   Celestine, Sister. "Julia C. Tebo, R.N." *Am J Nurs*, 34
         (Sep 1934), 887-888.

TERROT, SARAH ANNE

1976.1   *Nurse Sarah Anne: With Florence Nightingale at Scutari*.
         Edited with introduction and notes by R.G. Richardson.
         London: Murray, 1977. 183 pp.

THIELBAR, FRANCES CHARLOTTE

1977.   Obituary. *NY Times* (24 Mar 1962), 25.

THOMPSON, DORA E.

1978.   Stimson, Julia C. "Army Nurse Corps." *Am J Nurs*, 20 (Feb
         1920), 421-422.

THOMPSON, SARAH

1979.   Hoehling, A.A. In *Women Who Spied*. New York: Dodd Mead,
         1967. pp. 18-44.

THOMSON, DAME ANNE

1980.   "Distinguished Portrait Gallery--10. Dame Anne Thomson,
         D.B.E., R.R.C., K.H.N.S." *Nurs Mirror*, 93 (28 Sep 1951),
         490.

THOMSON, ELIZABETH MCKECHNIC

1981.   Pott, Emily G. "Elizabeth McKechnic Thomson (Mrs. E.H.
         Thomson), the Pioneer Nurse in China." *Quart J Chin Nurs*,
         3 (Oct 1922), 5-8.

THOMSON, ELNORA E.

1982.   Obituary. *NY Times* (27 Apr 1957), 19.

1983.   "Portraits and Biographical Notes of Nurse Leaders--Elnora E. Thomson." *Brit J Nurs*, 78 (Oct 1930), 257.

1984.   Soule, Elizabeth Sterling. "Elnora E. Thomson." *National League of Nursing Education: Biographic Sketches, 1937-1940.* New York: The League, 1940.

THORPE, JANE WINIFRED

1985.   "Passing Bell. Another Tragedy." *Brit J Nurs*, 44 (25 Jun 1910), 511.

1986.   Tippetts, L.M. "In Memoriam. Miss Jane Winifred Thorpe." *Nurs J India*, 1 (Jul 1910), 113.

THURINGEN, E. VON

1987.   Dorgen, J.A. von. "The Life of Elizabeth von Thuringen." *Tijdschrs Ziekenverpl*, 23 (Nov 1970), 1198-1199. (Dut)

TINAWIN, MARIA L.

1988.   Sotejo, Julita V. "Maria L. Tinawin, Officer of the F.N.A." *Filipino Nurs*, 18 (Apr 1949), 98.

TIPPETTS, LILIAN M.

1989.   "Nurses of Note. Miss Lilian M. Tippetts." *Brit J Nurs*, 46 (24 Jun 1911), 493-494.

TODD, MARGARET STRATHIE

1990.   Obituary. *NY Times* (29 Jul 1949), 21.

TOMASGAARD, J.T.

1991.   "Norway's Mother Gulberg." *T Sygepl*, 53 (15 Mar 1966), 158-159. (Nor)

TOMPKINS, SALLY

1992.   Somerville, M. "Sally Tompkins, Nurse and the Cavalry Captain." *RN*, 20 (Oct 1957), 74ff.

TRACY, MARGARET A.

1993.   "Margaret A. Tracy." *Pac Cst J Nurs*, 30 (Jan 1934), 13.

TREACY, KILDARE

1994.   "A Grievous Loss." *Brit J Nurs*, 48 (24 Feb 1912), 148.

TREMBLE, JOHN

1995.   "Dr. John Tremble." *So Afr Nurs J*, 9 (Dec 1943), 19-20.

TSCHERNING, HENNY

1996.   Lütken, Cecil. "In Memoriam--Henny Tscherning." *Int Nurs Rev*, 7 (Sep 1932), 416-417; see also *Brit J Nurs*, 80 (Sep 1932), 251; *Canad Nurs*, 28 (Sep 1932), 507.

TSHAI, PRINCESS

1997.   "A Nurse's Hospital." *Nurs Times*, 41 (25 Aug 1945), 557, 559.

TUCKER, KATHARINE

1998.   Gardner, Mary Sewall. "Katharine Tucker." *National League of Nursing Education: Biographic Sketches, 1937-1940*. New York: The League, 1940.

1999.   Hansen, Anne L. "Katharine Tucker." *Pub Hlth Nurs*, 21 (Jan 1929), 1-2.

2000.   Obituary. *NY Times* (7 Jun 1957), 23.

TURKINGTON, FLORENCE

2001.   "Col. Florence Turkington, Salvation Army." *Hosp Topics*, 35 (Aug 1957), 3.

TURNER, DAME MARGOT

2002.   Smyth, Sir John George. *Will to Live: The Story of Dame Margot Turner; With a Foreword by Barbara Gordon*. London: Cassell, 1970. 176 pp.

TWINING, LOUISA

2003.   "Passing Bell. Louisa Twining." *Brit J Nurs*, 49 (5 Oct 1912), 275.

UDELL, F.

2004.   "Distinguished Portrait Gallery--17. Miss F. Udell, O.B.E." *Nurs Mirror*, 94 (14 Dec 1951), 246.

URCH, DAISY DEAN

2005. Domitilla, Sister Mary. "Daisy Dean Urch." *National League of Nursing Education: Biographic Sketches, 1937-1940*. New York: The League, 1940.

UTINSKY, PEGGY DOOLIN

2006. Furnas, H. "Miss U." *Colliers*, 117 (5 Jan 1946), 34.

VAN DER VELDEN, LOUISE MATHIA

2007. Van Der Velden, Louise Mathia. *My Journey Through Hell*. New York: Vantage Press, 1975. 511 pp.

VAN KOOG, CORNELIA

2008. Wisconsin State Historical Society. *Dictionary of Wisconsin Biography*. Madison, WI: The Society, 1960. 359 pp.

VAN LANSCHOT-HUBRECHT, J.C.

2009. "Passing Bell. J.C. Van Lanschot-Hubrecht." *Brit J Nurs*, 61 (23 Nov 1918), 323.

VARLEY, MARGARET LIVINGSTON

2010. Knox, C.A. *Passing Years*. Ilfracombe, Gt. Britain: Stockwell, 1967. 47 pp.

2011. Obituary. *NY Times* (9 Nov 1960), 35.

VILLASENOR, E.

2012. Nicanor, Precioso M. *Profiles of Notable Filipinos in the U.S.A.* New York: Pre-Mer Pub. Co., 1963. Vol. 1, pp. 313-315.

VINCENT DE PAUL, SAINT

2013. Coste, Pierre. *The Life and Works of Saint Vincent De Paul.* 3 vols. London: Bates & Washbourne, 1934.

2014. Oddie, W.A. "St. Vincent de Paul." *Nurs Mirror*, 108 (20 Feb 1959), 1585.

VINEY, HESTER

2015. "Miss Hester Viney." *Nurs Times*, 55 (2 Jan 1959), 3.

2016. Number deleted.

WALD, LILLIAN

2017.   Beatty, J.   "She Never Gave Up; Lifesafer Lillian Wald."
        Forum, 96 (Aug 1936), 70-73; see also *Read Dig*, 29 (Aug
        1936), 42-46.

2018.   Block, Irvin. *Neighbor to the World; The Story of Lillian
        Wald (Woman of America)*. New York: Thomas Y. Crowell,
        1969.   313 pp.

2019.   Biography. *DAB*, Sup. 2 (1958), 687-688.

2020.   Christy, T.E.   "Portrait of a Leader: Lillian D. Wald."
        Nurs Out, 18 (Mar 1970), 50-54.

2021.   Davis, Mac. *Jews at a Glance*. New York: Hebrew Publishing
        Co., 1956.   212 pp.

2022.   Duffus, R.L.   *Lillian Wald: Neighbor and Crusader*. New
        York: Macmillan Co., 1938.

2023.   "Forty Years of Service to the Sick and the Poor." *Am J
        Nurs*, 33 (Apr 1933), 326. For later tributes see *Tr Nurs*,
        92 (Mar 1934), 278; *Pac Cst J Nurs*, 35 (Jun 1939), 333-335.

2024.   Hill, R.W.   "Papers of Lillian D. Wald (1867-1940)." *Spc
        Serv R*, 36 (Dec 1962), 462-463.

2025.   Kelly, D.N.   "A Nurse in the Hall of Fame." *Superv Nurs*, 3
        (Nov 1971), 9-11.

2026.   Levitan, Tina. *Jews in American Life*. New York: Hebrew
        Publishing Co., 1969. pp. 135-137.

2027.   "Lillian D. Wald; Social Worker and Philanthropist." *Hosp
        Topics*, 5 (Jul 1927), 506, 526.

2028.   "Looking Back--Jane Addams and Lillian Wald." *Nurs Out*, 8
        (Sep 1960), 492.

2029.   National League of Nursing Education. *Early Leaders of
        American Nursing (Calendar 1923) (Lillian Wald)*. New York:
        The League, 1922.

2030.   "Nurses of Note. Lillian D. Wald, LL.D." *Brit J Nurs*, 50
        (Jan 1913), 11.

2031.   "Our First Public Health Nurse." *Nurs Out*, 19 (Oct 1971),
        659-660.

2032.   Popiel, E.S.   "Lillian Wald, Community Nurse. Try to Remember
        Our Heritage." *Colo Nurs*, 68 (Jan 1968), 3-5.

2033.   "Record of a Remarkable Woman." *Am J Pub Hlth*, 48 (May
        1958), 631.

2034.   Reznick, Allen E. Lillian D. Wald: *The Years at Henry Street*.
        Ph.D. dissertation, University of Wisconsin, 1973.

2035.   Vorspan, Albert. *Grants of Justice*. New York: Thomas Y.
        Crowell, 1960. pp. 58-75.

2036.   Wald, Lillian. *House on Henry Street*. New York: Holt, 1915.
        Other editions available.

2037.   ————. *Windows on Henry Street*. Boston: Little, Brown &
        Co., 1934.

2038.   "Wald Papers Presented to New York Library" (news). *Nurs Out*,
        6 (Apr 1958), 208.

WALSH, AGNES MARION MCLEAN (GIBSON)

2039.   Walsh, Agnes. *Life in Her Hands: The Matron Walsh Story Told
        to Ruth Allen*. London: Georgian House, 1955. 139 pp.

WARDROPER, SARAH

2040.   "Distinguished British Nurses of the Past. 5. Mrs. Sarah
        Wardroper--Florence Nightingale's Collaborator." *Mid Hlth
        Visit*, 11(9) (Sep 1975), 203-301.

2041.   "Florence Nightingale Writes (in *Nursing Mirror*, December
        1892) on Sarah Wardroper, First Lady Superintendent,
        Nightingale School." *Nurs Mirror*, 107 (9 May 1958), iv.

2042.   Hallowes, Ruth. "Distinguished British Nurses. 12. Mrs.
        Sarah Wardroper, Matron, St. Thomas' Hospital, London 1854-
        1887." *Nurs Mirror*, 105 (May 1957).

2043.   Hone, Henry E. "The Wardroper Family." *Nurs Mirror*, 107
        (16 May 1958), xvi.

2044.   McInnes, E.M. "Our Forerunners, Mrs. Sarah Elizabeth Ward-
        roper, Matron of St. Thomas Hospital 1854-1887." *St
        Thomas Hosp Gaz*, 60 (1962), 91-93.

WARNER, LENA A.

2045.   Obituary. *NY Times* (20 Aug 1940), 17.

WATKIN, B.

2046.   "Retrospect, One Pair of Feet." Part 1, *Nurs Mirror*, 119
        (18 Dec 1964), 265ff.

2047.   "Six Months' Hard." Part 2, *Nurs Mirror*, 119 (25 Dec 1964),
        295ff.

WATKINS, RHODA

2048.   Carterer, Helen. *Foreigner in Kiveilin: The Story of Rhoda Watkins, South Australian Nursing Missionary.* London: Epworth, 1966. 150 pp.

WATT, DAME KATHERINE CHRISTIE

2049.   Obituary. *Illus Lord News*, 243 (9 Nov 1963), 783.

WELCH, WILLIAM H.

2050.   Carr, Ada M. "William H. Welch and Nursing." *Int Nurs Rev*, 5 (Sep 1950), 447-449.

2051.   "Dr. William Henry Welch." *Am J Nurs*, 30 (May 1930), 607-608.

2052.   Emerson, Charles P. "William H. Welch, M.D." *Pub Hlth Nurs*, 17 (May 1925), 232-233.

2053.   Welch, William H. *Papers and Addresses*. 3 vols. Baltimore: Johns Hopkins Press, 1920.

WELLIN, BERTHA

2054.   Lind, Elisabet. "Bertha Wellin." *Int Nurs Rev*, 5 (Sep 1930), 444-447.

WERLEY, HARRIET H.

2055.   "Nursing Research Department at Walter Reed Has Fulltime Director" (news). *Am J Nurs*, 58 (Jun 1958), 784.

WEST, JESSE (STEVENSON)

2056.   Obituary. *NY Times* (24 May 1976), 32.

WESTPHOL, LILLIAN

2057.   Pirhalla, J. "Wentworth's Happy Museum." *Hobbie*, 59 (Mar 1954), 30-31.

WHEELER, CLARIBEL A.

2058.   Deming, Dorothy. "Claribel A. Wheeler Retires." *Pub Hlth Nurs*, 34 (Sep 1942), 519.

2059.   Robson, Emilie G. "Claribel A. Wheeler." *Am J Nurs*, 36 (Mar 1936), 226-229.

WHEELER, MARY CURTIS

2060. "Who's Who in the Nursing World (Mary Curtis Wheeler)." *Am J Nurs*, 23 (Oct 1922), 33-34.

WHITAKER, JUDITH GAGE

2061. "Mrs. Whitaker to Succeed Miss Best in 1958." *Am J Nurs*, 57 (Mar 1957), 305.

WHITE, JEANETTE V.

2062. Faddis, Margene O. "Jeanette V. White, 1908-1957." *Am J Nurs*, 57 (Apr 1957), 461.

2063. "Nursing Profiles. Jeanette V. White." *Canad Nurs*, 53 (Jan 1957), 35.

WHYTE, ROBERTA

2064. "New Year Honors (Elizabeth Cockayne, Roberta Whyte and Others)." *Nurs Times*, 51 (7 Jan 1955), 3.

WILKENDEN, ELMIRA W. (BEERS)

2065. "Defense of Nation's Health." *Pub Hlth Nurs*, 33 (Oct 1941), 612.

2066. "Well Done." *Time*, 50 (29 Sep 1947), 25.

WILCOX, MABEL L.

2067. Smyth, Mabel L. "Public Health Nursing in Hawaii; A Tribute to Mabel L. Wilcox." *Pac Cst J Nurs*, 31 (Jun 1935), 297-298.

WILKINSON, KITTY

2068. Rathbone, Winifred R. *The Life of Kitty Wilkinson*. Liverpool: Henry Young & Sons, 1910. 67 pp.

WILKINSON, LOUISA J.

2069. "The New President" (editorial). *Nurs Times*, 44 (26 Jun 1948), 453-454.

2070. "The War. The New Matron-in-Chief, O.A.I.M.N.S." (Queen Alexandria's Imperial Nursing Service). *Brit J Nurs*, 92 (Aug 1944), 91.

WILLIAMS, A.E.

2071.   Wakeford, J.   "Address Given to Commemorate the 70th Anniver-
           sary of the First Rhodesian Trained Nurse (Annie Ella Bea-
           trice Williams)."   *Rhod Nurs*, 5 (Jun 1972), 7-10.

WILLIAMS, GLADYS VIRGINIA (LYONS)

2072.   "Distinguished Service Awards for 1973."   *J Sch Hlth*, 43
           (Dec 1973), 653-654.

WILLIAMS, RACHEL

2073.   Cope, Zachary.   *Six Disciples of Florence Nightingale*.
           London: Pitman Medical, 1961.   pp. 47-56.

2074.   McInnes, E.M.   "Florence Nightingale and the Goddess.
           (Letters from F.N. to Rachel Williams)."   *St Thomas Hosp
           Gaz*, 61 (1963), 73-74.

WILLIAMSON, ANNE H.

2075.   Williamson, Anne H.   *50 Years In Starch*.   London: Murray &
           Gee, 1948.   245 pp.

WILLMS, EMILIE

2076.   Beer, Ethel S.   *The Greek Odyssey of an American Nurse;
           Adapted from the Unfinished Autobiography of Emilie
           Willms*.   Mystic, CT: Verry, 1972.

WILLS, EFFIE GILLETT

2077.   Wills, N.   "Portrait of an Australian (Effie Gillett Wills)."
           Lamp, 27 (Nov 1970), 27-32.

WILSON, JEAN S.

2078.   "Convention Personalities--Jean S. Wilson."   *Canad Nurs*, 54
           (Apr 1958), 332-334.

2079.   Simpson, Ruby M.   "Jean Wilson Retires."   *Canad Nurs*, 39
           (Oct 1943), 655-656; for early accounts see *Am J Nurs*, 33
           (1933), 1062; *Brit J Nurs*, 81 (Nov 1933), 300-301; *Tr Nurs*,
           91 (Oct 1933), 333.

WINSLOW, CHARLES-EDWARD AMORY

2080.   "Dr. C-E. A. Winslow" (editorial).   *Am J Nurs*, 57 (Mar 1957),
           299.

2081. "We Pay Tribute to Charles-Edward Amory Winslow." *Nurs Out*, 5 (1957), 155.

2082. Roberts, Mary M. "We Pay Tribute to Charles-Edward Amory Winslow." *Nurs Out*, 5 (Mar 1957), 155-156.

2083. Watkins, Eleanor M., and Jean H. Nelbach, comps. "Bibliography of Charles-Edward Amory Winslow." *Yale J Biol Med*, 19 (Mar 1947), 779-800.

WINTERNITA, MILTON C.

2084. Goodrich, Annie W. "An Attempt to Interpret a Great Scientist's Contribution to Humanity Through Medicine and Nursing." *Yale J Biol Med*, 22 (Jul 1950), 605-610.

WOLCOTT, DELPHINE (WILDE)

2085. Obituary. *NY Times* (26 Sep 1964), 23.

WOLF, ANNA D.

2086. Frost, Harriet. "Anna D. Wolf." *National League of Nursing Education: Biographic Sketches, 1937-1940*. New York: The League, 1940.

WOOD, HELEN

2087. Reid, Grace L. "Helen Wood." *National League of Nursing Education: Biographic Sketches, 1937-1940*. New York: The League, 1940.

WOODWARD, LUCIA F.

2088. Abbott, E. Stanley. "A Pioneer in Mental Nursing." *Am J Nurs*, 36 (Feb 1936), 147-148.

WOOLSEY, GEORGEANNE

2089. Austin, Anne L. *The Woolsey Sisters of New York: 1860-1900*. Philadelphia: American Philosophical Society, 1971.

YMAKI, M.

2090. "Growing Pains--A Personal Recollection." *Sogo Kango*, 13(2) (1978), 104-115. (Jap)

YOUNG, HELEN

2091. Lee, Eleanor. "Helen Young." *National League of Nursing Education: Biographic Sketches, 1937-1940*. New York: The League, 1940.

2092.   Obituary. *NY Times* (25 Nov 1966), 37.

ZABRISKIE, LOUISE

2093.   "Louise Zabriskie." *Am J Nurs*, 58 (Jun 1958), 802-804.

ZAKRZEWSKA, MARIE ELIZABETH

2094.   New England Hospital for Women and Children, Boston, Mass.
         Marie Elizabeth Zakrzewska 1829-1902. Boston: The Hospital,
         1903.   30 pp.

2095.   Vietor, Agnes C., ed. *A Woman's Quest*. New York: Appleton,
         1924.   514 pp.

8. GOVERNMENT, MILITARY, AND WARTIME NURSING

UNITED STATES

2096. Adams, George Worthington. *Doctors in Blue*. New York: Henry Schuman, 1952; New York: Collier Books, 1961.

2097. Alcott, Louisa May. *Hospital Sketches*. Boston: James Redpath, 1863. Reprint., New York: Sagamore Press, 1957.

2098. Allison, Grace E. "Some Experience in Active Service: France." *Am J Nurs*, 19 (Feb 1919), 268-272, 354-359.

2099. "American Nurses in Five Wars." *Clin Excerpts*, 18 (1944), 163-173.

2100. Andrews, Matthew Page. *The Woman of the South in War Times*. Baltimore: Norman Remington, 1927.

2101. "Angels." *Am Mag*, 132 (Nov 1941), 92-93.

2102. "Angels of Saigon: Two Army Nurses." *Ebony*, 22 (Aug 1966), 44-46.

2103. Armstrong, O.K. "GIs Guardian Angel." *Read Digest*, 60 (Jan 1952), 135-138.

2104. "The Army Nurse Corps Celebrates 44th Anniversary." *Army Nurs*, 2 (Feb 1945), 2-3.

2105. "Army Nurses in ETO." *Am J Nurs*, 45 (May 1945), 386-387.

2106. "Army's First Man Nurse." *Scholastic*, 67 (20 Oct 1955), 15.

2107. Austin, Anne L. "Nurses in American History: Wartime Volunteers--1861-1865." *Am J Nurs*, 75 (May 1975), 816-881.

2108. Aynes, Edith A. *From Nightingale to Eagle: An Army Nurse's History*. Englewood Cliffs, NJ: Prentice-Hall, 1973.

2109. Bachman, Walter J. *Souvenir Roster and History of Evacuation Hospital No. 15 with the Story of Verdun and the Argonne Drive*. n.p., 1919.

2110. Bacon, Deborah. "Letters from an Army Nurse." *Mich Alum*, 59 (1953), 101-103, 246-255.

2111.   Beaton, Mama K.M. "Victorial Order of Nurses: Serving Since
        1898." *Dimens Hlth Serv*, 52 (Mar 1975), 22-23.

2112.   Bellows, Henry Whitney. *Report Concerning the Women's Central
        Association of Relief at New York to the United States
        Sanitary Commission.* New York: Bryant, 1861.

2113.   Bolton, Frances P. "Bolton Act--Implications for the Present
        and Future." *Mod Hosp*, 61 (Sep 1943), 59-60.

2114.   ————. "Report to Congress on the Nursing Shortage: Crisis
        in Health Care." *Hosp*, 28 (Apr 1954), 83-85.

2115.   Bowman, J. Beatrice. "The History and Development of the
        Navy Nurse Corps." *Am J Nurs*, 25 (May 1925), 356-360.

2116.   ————. "History of Nursing in the Navy." *US Nav Med Bull*,
        26 (Jan 1928), 123-131.

2117.   ————. "Public Health Nursing in the Navy." *Am J Nurs*, 17
        (May 1927), 541-542.

2118.   "Brief Outline of the Organizing of the U.S. Army Nurse
        Corps." *Pac Cst J Nurs*, 8 (Dec 1912), 561-562.

2119.   Brockett, Linus Pierpont, and M.C. Vaughn. *Women's Work in
        the Civil War: A Record of Heroism, Patriotism and Patience.*
        Philadelphia: Zeigler, McCurdy & Co., 1867.

2120.   Bucklin, Sophronia F. *In Hospital and Camp.* Philadelphia:
        J.E. Potter, 1869.

2121.   Bullough, Bonnie. "Nurses in American History: The Lasting
        Impact of World War II on Nursing." *Am J Nurs*, 76 (Jan
        1976), 118-120.

2122.   ————, and Vern Bullough. "The Origins of Modern Nursing:
        The Civil War Era." *Nurs Forum*, 2 (1963), 13-27.

2123.   Burrage, Thomas J. "An American World War Hospital Centre
        in France." *Military Surg*, 80 (May 1937), 332-360.

2124.   Bytheway, Ruth Evon. *History of the Development of the
        Nursing Service of the Veterans Administration Under the
        Direction of Mrs. A. Hickey, 1919-1942.* New York: Columbia
        University Press, 1972.

2125.   Cabell, Julian M. *A Brief Sketch of Base Hospital No. 41 by
        the Commanding Officer.* Washington, D.C.: n.p., 1925.
        29 pp.

2126.   "A Call for Women to Volunteer." *Lit Digest*, 57 (22 Jun
        1918), 30.

2127.   "Civil War Nurses, North and South." *RN*, 34 (Apr 1971),
        46-47.

2128. Clappison, Gladys Bonner. *Vassar's Rainbow Division*. Lake
       Mills, IA: The Graphic Publishing Co., 1964.

2129. Clarke, Alice R. "Thirty-Seven Months as Prisoners of War."
       Am J Nurs, 45 (May 1945), 342-345.

2130. Clymer, George, ed. *The History of U.S. Army Base Hospital
       No. 6 and Its Part in the American Expeditionary Forces*.
       Boston: n.p., 1924.

2131. Combs, Josiah H. *Siege of Salisbury Court Which Chronicles
       the Feat of Base Hospital 40 Winning the War*. Lexington,
       KY: Hurst & Byars, 1923.

2132. Commanger, H.S. "Women in War 1861-1865." *Scholastic*, 46
       (2 Apr 1945), 7ff.

2133. Cooper, Alice E., ed. *A History of the United States Army
       Base Hospital No. 36*. Detroit: n.p., 1922.

2134. Cooper, Page. *Navy Nurse*. New York: McGraw-Hill Book Co.,
       1946.

2135. Coplin, W.N.L. *American Red Cross Base Hospital No. 38 in
       the World War*. Philadelphia: n.p., 1923.

2136. Cumming, Kate. *Kate: The Journal of a Confederate Nurse*.
       Edited by Richard Barksdale Harwell. Baton Rouge, LA:
       Louisiana State University Press, 1959.

2137. Cunningham, H.H. *Doctors in Gray: The Confederate Medical
       Service*. Baton Rouge, LA: Louisiana State University
       Press, 1958.

2138. Cutbush, Edward. *Observations on the Means of Preserving
       the Health of the Soldiers and Sailors and on the Duties
       of the Medical Department of the Army and Navy with Remarks
       on Hospitals and Their Internal Enlargement*. Philadelphia:
       Dobson, 1808.

2139. Dannett, Sylvia G. "Lincoln's Ladies in White." *NY State J
       Med*, 61 (1961), 1944-1952.

2140. ————. *Noble Women of the North*. New York: Thomas Yoseloff,
       1959.

2141. Darnall, J.R. "War Service Within Evacuation Hospital."
       Military Surg, 80 (Apr 1937), 261-276.

2142. Delano, J.A. "How American Nurses Helped Win the War." *Mod
       Hosp*, 12 (1919), 7.

2143. Dennie, F. "The Experience of an Army Nurse." *Tr Nurs &
       Hosp Rev*, 22 (1899), 111.

2144. DiMeglio, John E. "Calamity and Sanitation: Medical Affairs
       in the Union in the Early War Years." *Soc Stud*, 65 (Feb
       1974), 75-82.

2145. *The Documents of the United States Sanitary Commission.*
       3 vols. New York: United States Sanitary Commission, 1866–
       1871.

2146. Donald, W.J. "Alabama Confederate Hospitals: Part II."
       Alabama R, 16(1) (1963), 64–78.

2147. Drake, K. "Our Flying Nightingales in Vietnam." *Read Digest*,
       91 (Dec 1967), 73–79.

2148. Dreeves, Katherine Densford. "Vassar Training Camps for
       Nurses." *Am J Nurs*, 75 (Nov 1975), 2000–2002.

2149. Edmonds, Emma E. *Nurse and Spy in the Union Army.* Hart-
       ford, CT: W.S. Williams & Co., 1865.

2150. Fisher, Pearl C. "First U.S. Army Nurses Got $50 Per Month
       and Maintenance." *Hosp Mgmt*, 55 (Nov 1943), 58, 60, 62,
       64–68.

2151. Fleeson, D. "Within Sound of the Guns, Italian War Front."
       Woman's Home Companion, 71 (Jan 1944), 4ff.

2152. Flikke, Julia O. *Nurses in Action.* Philadelphia: J.B.
       Lippincott, 1943.

2153. ———. "Nurses in Bataan." *Am Mag*, 134 (Sep 1942), 4.

2154. "Flying Nurses Aid U.S. African Campaign." *Life*, 14 (19 Apr
       1943), 41–42.

2155. Foisie, J. "Angels of Anzio; U.S. Army Nurses." *NY Times
       Mag* (25 Jan 1959), 30ff.

2156. Geisinger, Joseph F., ed. *History of the U.S. Army Base Hos-
       pital No. 45 in the Great War (Medical College of Virginia
       Unit).* Richmond, VA: William Byrd Press, 1924.

2157. Goodnow, Minnie. *War Nursing; A Textbook for the Auxiliary
       Nurse.* Philadelphia and London: W.B. Saunders Co., 1917.

2158. Goodrich, Annie Warburton. "Nursing and National Defense."
       Am J Nurs, 42 (Jan 1942), 11–16.

2159. ———. "Miss Goodrich Called to Service." *Brit J Nurs*, 60
       (13 Apr 1918), 257.

2160. Greenbie, Marjorie L. Barstow. *Lincoln's Daughters of Mercy.*
       New York: G.P. Putnam's Sons, 1944.

2161. Griffith, William, and Richard Newcomb. "The Nurse in
       America: The Image of a Century." *RN*, 33 (Feb 1970), 37.

2162. ———. "Nurses in Peace." *RN*, 33 (Feb 1970), 38–47.

2163. ————. "Nurses in War." *RN*, 33 (Feb 1970), 48-57.

2164. Guyot, Sister Henrietta. "The Nurse in Civil War Literature."
       Nurs Out, 10(5) (May 1962), 311-314.

2165. H, Mrs. *Three Years in Field Hospitals of the Army of the
       Potomac*. Philadelphia: J.B. Lippincott, 1967.

2166. Hamesseley, M.L. "Cadets March." *Am J Nurs*, 76 (Feb 1976),
       243-244.

2167. Hammerlund, Mabel. "The United States Army Nurse in Korea."
       Nurs Out, 3(4) (Apr 1955), 208-210.

2168.-
 2169. Hasson, Esther V. See 2179.1.

2170. Hasson, Esther V. "The Navy Nurse Corps." *Am J Nurs*, 9
       (Nov 1908), 91-92.

2171. Haupt, Alma C. "Our War Nursing Program." *Am J Nurs*, 42
       (Dec 1942), 1381-1385.

2172. *History and Roster of the United States Army General Hospital
       No. 16*. New Haven: Yale University Press, 1919.

2173. *History of the Base Hospital No. 18, American Expeditionary
       Forces*. Baltimore: Base Hospital No. 18 Association, 1919.

2174. *History of Base Hospital No. 53, Advance Section, Services of
       Supply*. Langres, Haute-Marne: 29th Engineers Printing
       Plant, 1919.

2175. *The History of Evaluation Hospital No. 6 United States Army,
       1917-1919*. Poughkeepsie, NY: n.p., 1931.   39 pp.

2176. *History of the Pennsylvania Hospital Unit (Base Hospital
       No. 10, U.S.A.) in the Great War*. New York: P.B. Hoeber,
       1921.

2177. *A History of the Work of the New York Hospital Unit (Base
       Hospital No. 9, U.S.A.) During Two Years of Active Service:
       Written by the Padre*. New York: n.p., 1920.

2178. *A History of U.S.A. Base Hospital No. 115*. Memphis, TN: Toof,
       1919.

2179. Hitz, Benjamin D., ed. *A History of Base Hospital 32 (In-
       cluding Unit R)*. Indianapolis: n.p., 1922.

2179.1 Holcomb, Richmond Cranston. *A Century with Norfolk (Va.)
       Naval Hospital 1830-1930*. Portsmouth, Va.: Printcraft,
       1930.   See the section on nursing by Esther V. Hasson.

2180. Holland, Mary A. Gardiner, comp. *Our Army Nurses: Interesting Sketches, Addresses and Photographs of Nearly 100 of the Noble Women Who Served in Hospitals on Battlefields During Our Civil War.* Boston: B. Wilkins & Co., 1895.

2181. Jacoby, A. "Bataan Nurses; Condensation of Reports by Two Army Nurses." *Life*, 12 (15 Jun 1942), 16ff.

2182. Jolly, Ellen R. *Nuns of the Battlefield*. Providence, RI: Providence Vistor Press, 1927.

2183. Jones, G.M. "Women of the A.E.F." *Ladies Home J*, 45 (16 Dec 1928), 8-9.

2184. Jones, Katherine M. *Heroines of Dixie*. New York: Bobbs-Merrill, 1955.

2185. Kaletzki, Charles H., ed. *Official History of U.S.A. Base Hospital No. 31 of Youngstown, Ohio and Hospital Unit "G".* Syracuse, NY: Syracuse University Press, 1919.

2186. Kalisch, Beatrice J., and Philip A. Kalisch. "Be a Cadet Nurse ... The Girl with a Future." *Nurs Out*, 21 (Jul 1973), 444-449.

2187. ———. "Nurses in American History. The Cadet Nurses Corps in World War II." *Am J Nurs*, 76(2) (Feb 1976), 240-242.

2188. Kalisch, Philip A. "Heroines of '98: Female Army Nurses in the Spanish American War." *Nurs Res*, 24 (Nov-Dec 1975), 411-429.

2189. ———. "How Army Nurses Became Officers: One Bar on a Shoulder Strap is Worth Two Regulations in a Book." *Nurs Res*, 25(3) (May-Jun 1976), 164-177.

2190. ———. "Nurses Under Fire: An Analysis of the World War II Experience of Military Nurses on Bataan and Corregidor." *Nurs Res*, 25 (Nov-Dec 1976), 409-429.

2191. ———. "Untrained but Undaunted: The Women Nurses of the Blue and Grey." *Nurs Forum*, 15 (1976), 4.

2192. ———. "The Women's Draft. An Analysis of the Controversy Over the Nurses' Selective Service Bill of 1945." *Nurs Res*, 22 (Sep-Oct 1973), 402-413.

2193. Keen, W.W. "Civil War Medicine." *AORN J*, 18 (Sep 1973), 637ff.

2194. Kenneally, C.M. "Nurses and Nursing in the Confederacy." *Southern Hospital* (Apr 1942).

2195. Kirk, N.T. "Girls in the Foxholes." *Am Mag*, 137 (May 1944), 17.

2196. Laurence, E.C. *A Nurse's Life in War and Peace*. London: Smith, Elder, 1912.

2197. "Life Visits U.S. Army Nurse in New Caledonia." *Life*, 13 (5 Oct 1942), 126-131.

2198. Livermore, Mary A. *My Story of the War: A Woman's Narrative of Four Years Personal Experience as a Nurse in the Union Army*. Hartford, CT: A.D. Worthington, 1889.

2199. Longest, Virginia. "Expanded Roles for VA Nurses." *Am J Nurs*, 73 (Dec 1973), 2087-2089.

2200. Lowenfels, Walter. *Walt Whitman's Civil War*. New York: Alfred A. Knopf, 1961.

2201. McCaul, E. "Army Nursing." *19th Cent*, 49 (Apr 1901), 580-587.

2202. MacCracken, H.N. "Girls Who Want to Go to France; Vassar College Training Camp for Nurses." *Ind*, 94 (11 May 1918), 248.

2203. McDougall, Grace. *A Nurse at War*. New York: McBride, 1917.

2204. McGee, A.N. "The Army Nurse Corps in 1899." *Tr Nurs & Hosp Rev*, 24 (1900), 119.

2205. McKown, Robin. *Heroic Nurses*. New York: G.P. Putnam's Sons, 1956.

2206. *Mademoiselle Miss: Letters from an American Girl Serving with the Rank of Lieutenant in a French Army Hospital at the Front*. Boston: W.A. Butterfield, 1916.

2207. Marshall, Mary Louise. "Nurse Heroines of the Confederacy." *Bull M Library A*, 45 (1957), 319-336.

2208. Martin, Anita M. "We Earn Our Wings." *Am J Nurs*, 57 (Jul 1957), 894-896.

2209. Martin, L.G. "Angels of Vietnam: U.S. Military Nurses." *Today's Hlth*, 45 (Aug 1967), 16-23.

2210. Martin, R. "They Served the Sick, in North and South." *Military Med*, 126 (1961), 547-550.

2211. Massey, Mary Elizabeth. *Bonnet Brigade*. New York: Alfred A. Knopf, 1966.

2212. Matheson, Martin. *48: An Informal and Mostly Pictorial History of U.S. Base Hospital 48, 1918-1919*. New York: Veterans U.S. Base Hospital No. 48, 1939.

2213.   Maxwell, William Quentin. *Lincoln's Fifth Wheel: The Politi-
        cal History of the United States Sanitary Commission.* New
        York: Longmans, Green & Co., 1956.

2214.   "Military Rank for Army Nurses." *Survey*, 40 (21 Sep 1918),
        698.

2215.   Millard, Shirley. *I Saw Them Die: Diary and Recollections of
        Shirley Millard.* Edited by Adele Comandini. New York:
        Harcourt, Brace, 1936.

2216.   Miller, Jean Dupont. *Shipmates in White.* New York: Dodd,
        Mead, 1944.

2217.   Moore, Frank. *Women of the War: The Heroism and Self-
        Sacrifices.* Hartford, CT: S.S. Scranton & Co., 1866.

2218.   Mortimer, M. "What a Nurse Will Find at the Front." *Ladies
        Home J*, 34 (Oct 1917), 18.

2219.   Munger, Donna B. "Base Hospital 21 and the Great War."
        Missouri Hist Rev, 70 (Apr 1976), 272-290.

2220.   Needham, M.M. "What a War Nurse Saw." *Ind*, 83 (23 Aug
        1915), 258-260.

2221.   Newell, Hope. *The History of the National Nursing Council.*
        New York: National Organization for Public Health Nursing,
        1951.

2222.   "The Nurse and the Nation." *Survey*, 40 (18 May 1918), 194-
        195.

2223.   "The Nurses' Contribution to American Victory: Facts and
        Figures from Pearl Harbor to V-J Day." *Am J Nurs*, 45
        (Sep 1945), 683-686.

2224.   "Nurse's Experiences--Incidents of Life in a French Hospital."
        Cur Opin, 64 (Feb 1918), 136.

2225.   "Nurses of Five Wars." *NY Times Mag* (21 Jun 1942), 18-19.

2226.   "Nursing Council on National Defense." *Am J Nurs*, 40
        (Sep 1940), 1913.

2227.   "Nursing in the Spanish American War." *Tr Nurs & Hosp Rev*,
        63 (Sep 1919), 125-128.

2228.   Nutting, Mary Adelaide. "Relation of the War Program to
        Nursing in Civil Hospitals." *Teach Coll Rec*, 20 (Jun 1919),
        66-78.

2229.   Olnhausen, Mary Phinney. *Adventures of an Army Nurse in 2
        Wars.* Edited from the diary and correspondence of Mary
        Phinney, Baroness von Olnhausen, by James Phinney Monroe.
        Boston: Little, Brown & Co., 1903.

2230.   *On Active Service with Base Hospital 46, U.S.A., Mar 20, 1918
         to May 25, 1919*. Portland, OR: Arcady Press, 1919.

2231.   *The Patriot Daughters of Lancaster Hospital Scenes after the
         Battle of Gettysburg, July, 1863*. Philadelphia: Ashmead,
         1864.

2232.   Patton, James Welch, and Francis Butler Simkins. *The Women
         of the Confederacy*. Richmond: Garrett & Massie, 1936.

2233.   Petersen, Annabelle. "The Nurses' Fight for Military Rank."
         Tr Nurs & Hosp Rev, 109 (1942), 98-100.

2234.   Petry, Lucile. "The U.S. Cadet Nurse Corps: A Summing Up."
         Am J Nurs, 45 (Dec 1945), 1027-1028.

2235.   Pitts, Edmund M., William T. Bauer, and Malcolm G. Saisser,
         eds. *Base Hospital 34 in the World War*. Philadelphia:
         Lyon & Armor, 1922.

2236.   Popiel, E.S. "The ARC Nursing Service." *Colo Nurs*, 67 (Mar
         1967), 5-8.

2237.   ―――. "The Army Nurse Corps: Try to Remember Our Heritage."
         Colo Nurs, 67 (Feb 1967), 5-9.

2238.   ―――. "The Navy Nurse Corps." *Colo Nurs*, 67 (Apr-May
         1967), 5-7.

2239.   Pottle, Frederick A. *Stretchers: The Story of a Hospital
         Unit on the Western Front*. New Haven: Yale University
         Press, 1929.

2240.   Raven, C. "Achievements of Women in Medicine, Past and
         Present--Women in Medical Corps of the Army." *Military
         Med*, 125 (1960), 105-111.

2241.   Redmond, Juanita. *I Served on Bataan*. Philadelphia: J.B.
         Lippincott, 1943.

2242.   Reed, William Howell. *Hospital Life in the Army of the
         Potomac*. Boston: Spencer, 1866.

2243.   Reedy, M.J. "Army Surgeon General Annual Reports--50 Years
         in Retrospect." *Military Med*, 127 (1962), 1020-1026.

2244.   Richard, J. Fraise, comp. *The Florence Nightingale of the
         Southern Army. Experiences of Mrs. Ella K. Newsom, Con-
         federate Nurse in the Great War, 1861-65*. New York:
         Broadway Publishing Co., 1914.

2245.   Roberts, Mary M. *Yesterday, Today: (The Army Nurse Corps)*.
         Washington, D.C.: U.S. Army Nurse Corps, 1955.

2246.   Ross, Ishbel. *Angel of the Battlefield*. New York: Harper
         and Row, 1956.

2247.   Sabine, L. "Evolution of Nurse in Government Service."
        Tr Nurs, 80 (1928), 729-774.

2248.   Salter, L.C. "Epics of Courage; How American Nurses Are
        Serving Our Fighting Men and America." *Hygeia*, 22 (Feb
        1944), 116, 171.

2249.   "Samaritans on Wings; Nurses Fly Transoceanic Missions
        Evacuating Injured GI's from Vietnam." *Ebony*, 25 (May
        1970), 60ff.

2250.   Senn, N. "Nursing and Nurses in War." *J Am Med Assoc*, 32
        (1899), 155.

2251.   Shirley, Arthur M., and Agnes T. Considine. *The Officers and
        Nurses of Evacuation Eight*. New Haven: Yale University
        Press, 1929.

2252.   Sinai, Nathan, and Odin W. Anderson. *Emergency Maternity and
        Infant Care*. Ann Arbor, MI: University of Michigan Press,
        1948.

2253.   Slatterley, L.C. "Air Force Nurses Progress Towards the
        Space Age." *Military Med* (Jul 1960), 482-488.

2254.   Smith, Adelaide W. *Reminiscences of an Army Nurse During the
        Civil War*. New York: Greaves Publishing Co., 1911.   263 pp.

2255.   Stern, Madeleine. "Civil War Nurse." *Americana*, 37 (1943),
        296-325.

2256.   Stevenson, Isobel. "Nursing in the Civil War." *Ciba Sym-
        posia*, 3 (1941), 919-924.

2257.   Stewart, Aileen Cole. "Ready to Serve: A Nurse Recalls Her
        Experience During the First World War." *Am J Nurs* (Sep
        1963), 85-87.

2258.   Stimson, Julia C. "The Army Nurse Corps." *The Medical
        Department of the U.S. Army in the World War*. Vol. 13,
        Part 2. Washington, D.C.: U.S. Surgeon General's Office,
        U.S. Government Printing Office, 1927.

2259.   ———. "Earliest Known Connection of Nurses with Army Hos-
        pitals in the United States." *Am J Nurs*, 25 (Jan 1925), 18.

2260.   ———. *Finding Themselves: The Letters of an American
        Army Chief Nurse in a British Hospital in France*. New
        York: Macmillan Co., 1918.

2261.   ———. "The Forerunners of the American Army Nurse."
        Military Surg, 58 (Feb 1926), 133-141.

2262.   ———. "History and Manual of the Army Nurse Corps." *Army
        Med Bull*, 41 (1937).

2263.   ———. "Women Nurses with the Union Forces During the
         Civil War." *Military Surg* (Jan-Feb 1928).

2264.   Stuart, F.S. "Invasion by Angel: U.S. Army in England."
         Rotarian, 65 (Aug 1944), 14-16.

2265.   Sutherland, Dorothy J. "Nursing in the Peace Corps." *Nurs
         Out* (Dec 1963), 888-890.

2266.   Swan, John M., and Mark Heath. *A History of United States
         Army Base Hospital No. 19*. Rochester, NY: Wegman-Walsh
         Press, 1922.

2267.   Thompson, Dora E. "How the Army Nursing Service Met the
         Demands of War." *Twenty-fifth Annual Report of the Nation-
         al League of Nursing Education*. New York: The League,
         1919. 116 pp.

2268.   Trenchard, Edward. *The Service and Sacrifices of the
         Daughters of the Republic During the Civil War*. New York:
         Knickerbocker Press, 1912. 207 pp.

2269.   "Trojans of the Civil War." *Lit Digest*, 44 (10 Feb 1912),
         307-308.

2270.   U.S. Army AEF Base Hospital No. 4. *Album de la Guerre*.
         Cleveland: Scientific Illustrating Studios, 1919.

2271.   U.S. Army Medical Department. *The Tradition and Destiny of
         the U.S. Army Nurse Corps*. Washington, D.C.: U.S. Army
         Recruiting Publicity Bureau, 1949.

2272.   U.S. Army Nurse Corps. *The Army Nurse*. Washington, D.C.:
         U.S. Government Printing Office, 1944.

2273.   U.S. Army Nurse Corps. See 2277.

2274.   U.S. Navy Nurse Corps. *White Task Force*. Washington, D.C.:
         U.S. Government Printing Office, 1943.

2275.   U.S. Sanitary Commission. *Account of the Field Relief Corps
         of the U.S. Sanitary Commission in the Army of the Potomac*.
         New York: The Commission, 1863.

2276.   "U.S. Student Nurse Reserve." *Sch & Soc*, 8 (27 Jul 1918),
         108-109.

2277.   U.S. Surgeon General's Office, Department of the Army.
         Highlights in the History of the Army Nurse Corps. Wash-
         ington, D.C.: U.S. Government Printing Office, 1958.

2278.   Valentin, E.R. "Our Nurses on the World's Fronts." *NY Times
         Mag* (13 Sep 1942), 12ff; reply by D. Sutherland (27 Sep
         1942), 4.

2279. Vaultier, R. "La Medecine Militaire en 1870." *Presse Med*,
       65 (1957), 2203-2207. (Fr)

2280. Vreeland, Ellwynne M. "Fifty Years of Nursing in the Federal
       Government Nursing Services." *Am J Nurs*, 50 (Oct 1950),
       626-631.

2281. Winter, Francis A. "The Army Nurse in the Past." *Military
       Surg*, 65 (Jul 1929), 133-137.

2282. Wittenmyer, Annie T. *Under the Guns: A Woman's Reminiscences
       of the Civil War*. Boston: E.B. Stillings & Co., 1895.
       272 pp.

2283. Wormeley, Katharine Prescott. *The Other Side of the War with
       the Army of the Potomac*. Boston: Ticknor, 1889; later
       published as *The Cruel Side of War*. Boston: Roberts, 1898.

2284. Worthington, C.G. *The Women in Battle*. Hartford, CT:
       T. Belknap, 1876.

OTHER COUNTRIES

2285. Alice Regina, Sister. "Nursing Service to the Nation."
       Hosp Prog, 22 (1941), 194-197.

2286. Aloysius, Sister Mary. See 2343.1.

2287. Australian Army Nursing Service. *Lest We Forget*. Melbourne:
       The Australian Army Nursing Service, 1944.

2288. Azkle, A. "The Indian Army Nursing Service." *Brit J Nurs*,
       (6 Sep 1902), 196-197.

2289. Beaton, Marmak M. "The U.D.N. (Victorial Order of Midwives)."
       Dimens Hlth Serv, 52 (Mar 1975), 22-23.

2290. Beauchamp, Pat. *Fanny Went to War*. London: Routledge &
       Kegan Paul, 1940.

2291. Beith, J.H. *100 Years of Army Nursing: The Story of the
       British Army Nursing Service from the Time of Florence
       Nightingale to the Present Day*. London: Cassell, 1953.

2292. Bernardine, Sister. "The Crusades and Nursing." *Tomorrow's
       Nurse*, 3 (Dec-Jan 1962-1963), 21ff.

2293. Berny, Frank B. "Florence Nightingale's Influence on Mili-
       tary Medicine." *Bull NY Acad Med*, 32 (1956), 547-553.

2294. Bigué, Marie. "Diary of a Nurse at the Battle Front, 1914-
       1918." *Infirm Canad*, 12 (Nov 1970), 20-25.

2295.   Bolster, Evelyn. *The Sisters of Mercy in the Crimean War*.
         Cork: Mercier Press, 1964.

2296.   Bowden, Jean. *Grey Touched with Scarlet: The War Experiences
         of the Army Nursing Sisters*. London: Hale, 1959.

2296.1   Bowser, Thelka. *Britain's Civilian Volunteers*. New York:
         Moffat, Yard & Co., 1917.

2297.   ————. *The Story of the British V.A.D. Work in the Great
         War*. London: Melrose, 1917.

2298.   Brodrick, A.L. "Correspondence Between Miss Brodrick and the
         War Office on the Shortage of Trained Nurses for the
         Troops." *Brit J Nurs* (5 Jun 1915), 482-483.

2299.   "Caring for the Sick and Wounded Sailor." *Nurs Mir Mid J*,
         114 (14 Sep 1962), 5ff.

2300.   Cilento, Raphael. "Wartime Problems in Health." *Aust Nurs J*,
         40 (Sep 1942), 129-134; (Oct 1942), 143-148.

2301.   Clint, M.B. *Our Bit: Memories of War Service by a Canadian
         Nursing Sister*. Montreal: Royal Victoria Hospital, 1934.

2302.   "Crimean Hospitals." *Brit Med J* (23 Jan 1960), 268.

2303.   Croy, Princess Marie de. *War Memories*. London: Macmillan,
         1932.

2304.   Curtis, John Shelton. "Russian Sisters of Mercy in the
         Crimea, 1854-1855." *Slavic Rev*, 35 (1966), 84-100.

2305.   Dearmer, M. *Letters from a Field Hospital; With a Memoir of
         the Author by Stephen Gwynn*. London: Macmillan, 1915.

2306.   "Diary of Captivity by a Polish Nurse; Seizure of a First-
         line Polish Hospital by Bolsheviks." *Atlan*, 165 (Feb-Mar
         1940), 217-231, 347-360.

2307.   *Diary of a Nursing Sister on the Western Front, 1914-1915*.
         Edinburgh and London: William Blackwood and Sons, 1915.

2308.   Dobson, J. "Army Nursing Service in 18th Century." *Ann Roy
         Coll Surg Eng*, 14 (Jun 1954), 417-419.

2309.   Edge, G., and M.E. Johnston. *The Ships of Youth: The Ex-
         periences of Two Army Nursing Sisters on Board the Hospital
         Carrier "Leinster."* London: Hodder & Stoughton, 1945.

2310.   Elder, A.T. "Social and Preventive Medicine in Civil and
         Military Life." *Pub Hlth* (London), 62 (Jan 1949), 73-78.

2311.   Evatt, G.J.H. "A Corps of Volunteer Female Nurses for Service
         in the Army Hospitals in the Field, with Suggestions as to
         the Incorporation of the Nursing Profession." *Nurs Rec*
         (4 Aug 1900), 95-96; (11 Aug 1900), 112-122.

2312.   Evelyn, G.P. *A Diary of the Crimea*. Edited by Cyril Falls.
        London: Duckworth, 1954.

2313.   Farmborough, Florence. *Nurse at the Russian Front: A Diary
        1914-1918*. London: Constable, 1974.

2314.   Fenwick, Ethel Gordon. "Memories of Queens." *Brit J Nurs*,
        74 (Jul 1926), 145-146; 74 (Aug 1926), 179-181; 74 (Oct
        1926), 222-223.

2315.   Fletcher, N. Corbet, comp. *The St. John Ambulance Associa-
        tion: Its History and Its Part in the Ambulance Movement*.
        London: St. John Ambulance Assn., 1929. 116 pp.

2316.   Gemell, Arthur A. "One Hundred Years Ago." *Nurs Mirror*, 100
        (15 Oct 1954), 182-184; (22 Oct 1954), 253-255, 256.

2317.   Gowing, Timothy. *Voice from the Ranks; A Personal Narrative
        of the Crimean Campaign by a Sergeant of the Royal Fusiliers*.
        London: Folio Society, 1954.

2318.   Haldane, Elizabeth S. *The British Nurse in Peace and War*.
        London: Murray, 1923. 282 pp.

2319.   ————. "Sick Nursing in the Territorial Army." *Contemp*, 94
        (Sep 1908), 356-363.

2320.   Haliburton, M.F. "Sisters in Service: War-Time Experiences
        of a Canadian Nursing Sister." *Canad Med*, 80 (Oct 1933),
        8ff.

2321.   Hargreaves, R. "The Feminine Touch (Military and Naval
        Nursing Apart from the Crimean War)." *Practitioner*, 193
        (1964), 689-697.

2322.   Harrison, Ada, ed. *Grey and Scarlet: Letters from the War
        Areas by Army Nursing Sisters on Active Service*. London:
        Hodder & Stoughton, 1944.

2323.   Hawkins, Doris M. *Atlantic Torpedo: The Record of Twenty-
        seven Days in an Open Boat Following a U-boat Sinking*.
        London: Gollancz, 1943.

2324.   Hay, Ian (pseud. for J.H. Beith). *100 Years of Army Nursing:
        The Story of the British Army Nursing Services from the
        Time of Florence Nightingale to the Present Day*. London:
        Cassell & Co., 1953.

2325.   Hayes, Margaret. "Prisoner of the Congolese Rebel Army."
        Nurs Mirror (3 Dec 1965), 327-331.

2326.   Henrietta, Sister. "War Nursing in South Africa, 1901."
        Brit J Nurs (27 Sep 1902), 254-256.

2327.   "Home Defense Nursing Plans." *Survey*, 38 (9 Jun 1917), 247-
        248.

2328. Hughes, Sister Marie Jeanne d'Arc. *Crimean Diary of Mother M. Francis Bridgman*. Doctoral dissertation, Catholic University of America.

2329. Hunt, Lieutenant Colonel Dorothy. "Seventy Years or the QA's Past and Present." *Nurs Mirror*, 134 (7 Apr 1972), 13-16.

2330. "In Search of Unknown Nursing Literature. Nursing Literature Used in the Japanese Army and Navy." *Jap J Nurs Educ*, 16 (12) (Dec 1975), 754-758.

2331. Kiselev, A. "Participation of Feldshers and Midwives in the Secret and Partisan Activities During the Great Patriotic War." *Feldsher Akusl*, 40(9) (Sep 1975), 3-6. (Rus)

2332. Kroeze, R.C. "Information on the History of the Women's Military Medical Service." *Med Milit Geneesk T*, 17 (1964), 308-312. (Dut)

2333. Lady, A. [Martha Nicol]. *Ismeer (or Smyrna) and Its British Hospital in 1855*. London: Madden, 1856.

2334. Lapointe, G. "Souvenir from a War (Suzanne Giroux)." *Infirm Canad*, 14 (Nov 1972), 31-34. (Fr)

2335. Laws, M.E.S. "Before Florence Nightingale." *Nurs Times*, 44 (25 Dec 1948), 951.

2336. Lee, Y.B. "Historical Nursing Activities in National Emergencies." *Korean Nurs*, 14(5) (25 Oct 1975), 68-72. (Kor)

2337. Loch, C.G. "The Indian Army Nursing Service." *Nurs Rec* (12 Sep 1896), 204-205; (19 Sep 1896), 225-227; (26 Sep 1896), 244-245.

2338. Locke, E.I.J. *Post War Letters of a V.A.D. Nurse*. London: Stockwell, 1933.

2339. Longmore, T. *The Sanitary Contrasts of the British and French Armies During the Crimean War*. London: C. Griffin & Co., 1883.

2340. McCaul, Ethel. *Under the Care of the Japanese War Office*. London: Cassell, 1904.

2341. McLaren, Barbara. *Women of the War*. London: Hodder & Stoughton, 1917.

2342. McRae, C.J. "Honorary Nursing Sister to the Queen." *Aust Nurs J*, 56 (Apr 1958), 84.

2343. Marek, B. "Nurses in Silvery Helmets." *Pieleg Polozna*, 3 (Mar 1975), 22-23, 30. (Pol)

2343.1 Mary Aloysius, Sister. *Memories of the Crimea*. London:
        Burns, 1897.

2344.   Matron's Council. "Account of a Deputation to the War
        Office Before the Under Secretary of State for War, Sugges-
        tions of a Practical Nature in Reference to Army Nursing
        Reform." *Nurs Rec* (6 Apr 1901), 270; (27 Apr 1901), 331-
        335.

2345.   "Military and Naval Nursing; Scutari in Watercolours (2
        Sketches by Anne Morton, Who Worked in the Barrack Hospi-
        tal, Scutari from 1855-1856)." *Nurs Times*, 56 (1960), 108.

2346.   Mitchiner, P.H., and E.E.P. MacManus. *Nursing in Time of War*.
        London: Churchill, 1939; 2nd ed., 1943.

2347.   Morris, M. "Mum's Army." *Nurs Times*, 71(31) (31 Jul 1975),
        1228-1229.

2348.   Munroe, James Phinney. *Adventures of an Army Nurse in Two
        Wars*. Boston: Little, Brown & Co., 1903.

2349.   National Consul of Trained Nurses. "Resolution and Statement
        Sent to Secretary of State for War Expressing Dissatisfac-
        tion with Organization of Nursing Care of the Sick." *Brit
        J Nurs*, Supl. (30 Jan 1915).

2350.   Ndirangu, S. "Nursing Training and Practice During the World
        War II, 1939 to 1945 in Kenya." *Kenya Nurs J*, 3 (Jun 1974),
        13-14.

2351.   Nelson, R. "Nursing in the Royal Air Force." *Nurs Mirror*,
        121 (22 Oct 1965), 178-180; (29 Oct 1965), 207-210.

2352.   Nightingale, Florence. *Army Sanitary Administration and Its
        Reform Under Lord Herbert*. London: McCorquodale & Co.,
        1862. 11 pp.

2353.   ———. *Subsidiary Notes as to the Introduction of Female
        Nursing into Military Hospitals in Peace and War*. London:
        Privately printed by Harrison and Sons, 1858.

2354.   "The Nurse and the V.A.D. Members: Interesting Views for
        Military Matrons." *Nurs Times* (26 May 1917), 624-627.

2355.   "Nursing in the Zulu War, 1877-1879." *So Afr Nurs J*, 34
        (Oct 1967), 19-21; (Nov 1967), 34-35.

2355.1 "Nursing with the Navy." *Nurs Times* (19 Oct 1962), 1317-1319.

2356.   Odier, L. *Some Advice to Nurses and Other Members of the
        Medical Services of the Armed Forces*. Geneva: International
        Committee of the Red Cross, 1951.

2357.   Osborn, Sydney G. *Scutari and Its Hospitals*. London:
        Dickinson, 1855.

2358. Page, M. "Effect of War on Surgical Practice." Robert Jones Lecture. *Ann Assoc Coll Surg Eng*, 11 (Dec 1952), 335-349.

2359. Queen Alexandra's Imperial Military Nursing Service. *Reminiscent Sketches, 1914-1919.* London: Bale, 1922.

2360. ———. "A Qualification for Military Matrons. Examination of Sisters for the Rank of Matrons, Queen Alexandra's Imperial Military Nursing Service." *Brit J Nurs* (10 Mar 1906), 196-197.

2361. "Queen Alexandra's Imperial Military Nursing Service." *The Army Medical Service Administration.* Edited by F.A.E. Crew. Vol. 2. London: HMSO, 1955.

2362. "Queen Alexandra's Royal Naval Nursing Service: New Regulations." *Brit J Nurs* (9 Sep 1911), 207-208.

2363. Queen Alexandra's Royal Naval Nursing Service. *Nursing in the Navy: Queen Alexandra's Royal Naval Nursing Service Past and Present.* London: The Service, 1961.

2364. Number deleted.

2365. "Regulations for Queen Alexandra's Royal Naval Nursing Service." *Brit J Nurs* (29 Nov 1902), 437-439.

2366. "Regulations for Queen Alexandra's Royal Naval Nursing Reserve." *Brit J Nurs* (14 Jan 1911), 28-29.

2367. "Regulations for the Staff of Nursing Sisters in the Royal Naval Hospitals." *Nurs Rec* (2 Jul 1891), 7-9; (21 Jun 1902), 493-494.

2368. Rexford-Welch, S.C., ed. *The Royal Air Force Medical Services Volume I Administration.* London: HMSO, 1954.

2369. Richardson, Teresa Eden. *In Japanese Hospitals During Wartime; 15 Months with the Red Cross Society of Japan (April 1904 to July 1905).* London: Blackwood, 1905.

2370. Rogan, Rev. John. "Military Medical Services in the Reign of Elizabeth I." *Nurs Mirror* (1 May 1959), 349-350.

2371. Rosenbaum, S. "Report of the Royal Sanitary Commission (1858)." *J Royal Army Med Corps*, 106(1) (1960), 1-11.

2372. Ross, J.W. "Lessons Drawn from Practical Professional Experience with Trained Women Nurses in Military Service." *Brit J Nurs* (28 Feb 1903), 168-169; (7 Mar 1903), 187-188.

2373. Russell, W.H. *The British Expedition to the Crimea.* London: Routledge, 1858.

2374. St. John, C.F. "The Challenge Which Faced Florence Nightingale." *Med Bull US Army Europe*, 14(2) (Feb 1957), 28-29.

2375. Sandbach, Betsy, and Geraldine Edye. *Prison Life on a
       Pacific Raider: The Adventure of Nurse Escorts to the First
       500 Children Evacuated to Australia.* London: Hodder &
       Stoughton, 1941.

2376. Shimizu, A. "Nursing Described in Literature. From the
       Records by the Atomic Bomb Victims. (An Account by Miss
       Kiyoko Tanaka)." *Jap J Nurs Educ,* 16(11) (Nov 1975), 695-
       702.

2377. Simmons, Jessie E. *While History Passed: The Story of the
       Australian Nurses Who Were Prisoners of the Japanese for
       Three and Half Years.* London: Heineman, 1954.

2378. Smirnov, E.I. "The Nurse and Her Role in the War." *Med
       Sestra,* 34(5) (May 1975), 5-7. (Rus)

2379. Souttur, H.S. "Work of Our Doctors and Nurses in the Field
       of War." *Lond OR,* 124 (Jul 1915), 1-17.

2380. Soyer, Alexis. *Instructions to Military Hospital Cooks in
       the Preparation of Diets for Sick Soldiers.* London: Eyre &
       Spottiswoode, 1895.

2381. ———. *Soyer's Culinary Campaign: Being Historical Remini-
       scences of the Late War, with the Plain Art of Cookery for
       Military and Civil Institutions, The Army, Navy, Public
       etc.* London: Routledge, 1857.

2382. Speer, Theodore V. "Nursing on the Hospital Ship 'Solace.'"
       Nurs Rec (30 Dec 1899), 532-535.

2383. Stoney, A.H. *In the Days of Queen Victoria: Memories of a
       Hospital Nurse.* Bristol: Wright, 1931.

2384. Stratford, D.O. "Canadian Associations with the South Afri-
       can Military Nursing Service." *So Afr Nurs J* (Mar 1969),
       33-35.

2385. ———. "Women in Uniform. V. A History of Early Army
       Nursing Describing Nurses' Duties and Required Standards
       of Conduct." *So Afr Nurs J* (Mar 1961), 33-34.

2386. ———. "Women in Uniform. VI. Decorations, the Royal Red
       Cross; the Victoria Cross; the Florence Nightingale Medal."
       So Afr Nurs J (Sep 1961), 28-30.

2387. ———. "Women in Uniform. VII. Decorations Continued:
       Florence Nightingale Jewel." *So Afr Nurs J* (Oct 1961),
       24-36.

2388. ———. "Women in Uniform. VIII." *So Afr Nurs J* (Feb 1962),
       14-16; IX (Sep 1962), 33-35; X (Dec 1962) 33-35, 49.

2389. Terrot, S.A. "Reminiscences of Scutari Hospitals 1854-1855."
       Nurs Times (11 Sep 1909), 741-742; (18 Sep 1909), 761;
       (25 Sep 1909), 781-782.

2390. Thompson, A. "Military and Naval--Military Nursing Through the Ages." *J Roy Army Med Corps*, 89 (Oct 1947), 194-202.

2391. Thurston, Violetta. *Field Hospital and Flying Column: Being the Journal of an English Nursing Sister in Belgium and Russia.* New York: G.P. Putnam's Sons, 1915.

2392. Tinckler, L.F. "The Barracks of Scutari: Start of a Nursing Legend (F. Nightingale)." *Nurs Times*, 69 (2 Aug 1973), 1006-1007.

2393. "The Twenty-Fifth Anniversary of the Foundation of the KNA Branch Office--Army Nursing Corps." *Korean Nurs*, 12 (Sep-Oct 1972), 1-12. (Kor)

2394. Ward, I. *F.A.N.Y. Invicta.* London: Hutchinson, 1955.

2395. War Office. "Appointment to the Nursing Service of the Army." *Nurs Rec* (2 Jul 1891), 18-19.

2396. Watt, P.F. "The Work of the Indian Army Nursing Service." *Brit J Nurs* (13 Sep 1902), 214-215.

2397. Wenger, M.L., ed. "Army Nursing History (Opening of the QARANC Museum)." *Nurs Times*, 55 (1959), 623.

2398. Wizth, Alan. "Caring for the Sick and Wounded Sailors. An Account of the Development of Sickberth Staff in the Royal Navy." *Nurs Mirror* (14 Sep 1962), v-vi.

9.   NURSING SPECIALTIES

HOSPITAL NURSING

2399.   Abella, C.M.   "Tuberculosis in Nurses: Resume of Articles on
Investigations in Recent Years Especially in the United
States." *Hoja Tisiol*, 2 (Dec 1942), 283-294.

2400.   Armstrong, Dorothy Mary. *The First Fifty Years, A History
of Nursing at Royal Prince Alfred Hospital, Syndey from
1882-1932.* Sydney: Royal Prince Alfred Hospital Graduate
Nurses Assoc., 1965.

2401.   Aspinall, Archie. "Nursing Today and Yesterday." *Aust Nurs*,
31 (Jul 1933), 137-142.

2402.   Bauer, F. Deutsch. "Hospitals and the Nursing Profession in
Turkey." *Z Krankenpflege*, 11 (Dec 1967), 541-548.   (Ger)

2403.   Berwind, Anita. "The Nurse in the Coronary Care Unit."
The Law and the Expanding Nursing Role. Edited by Bonnie
Bullough. New York: Appleton-Century-Crofts, 1975. pp.
82-94.

2404.   Blackburn, Laura. "Meeting Local Hospital Needs." *Tr Nurs*,
98 (Feb 1937), 176-178.

2405.   Billings, J.S., and H.M. Hurd, eds. "Hospitals, Dispensaries,
and Nursing." *International Congress of Charities, Correction, and Philanthropy.* Sec. III. Baltimore: Johns Hopkins Press, 1894.

2406.   Blignault, A. "Keepers of the Flame; The History of Nursing
at Somerset Hospital." *So Afr Med J*, 36 (18 Aug 1962),
675-676.

2407.   Burdett, Henry Charles. *Hospitals and the State With an
Account of Nursing at London Hospitals and Statistical
Tables.* London: Churchill, 1881.

2408.   Cadbury, Mary. "Letters from a Nightingale Nurse." *Nurs
Times*, 36 (1940); 37 (1941); 27 times from Jun 1940 to Nov
1941.

2409.   Claridge, S.A. "A Nurse Remembers (50 Years Ago)." *Nurs
Times*, 45 (Jul 1949), 598-600.

2410.   Clarke, S.R. "Hospitals and Nursing in the Past." *Irish Nurs Hosp World*, 1 (15 Oct 1931), 9-10.

2411.   Cockayne, E. "The Nurse Within the National Health Service (Great Britain)." *Nurs Times*, 47 (8 Sep 1951), 883-884.

2412.   Cope, Zachary. *A Hundred Years of Nursing at St. Mary's Hospital*. London: Heinemann, 1955.

2413.   Coser, Rose L. *Life in the Ward*. New York: Atheneum, 1964.

2414.   DeLong, M.D., and W.L. Babcock. "Group Nursing--8 Years Experience." *Bull Am Hosp Assoc*, 9 (Oct 1935), 64-68.

2415.   Dilworth, Ava S. "Changes in Nursing from the 1930's to 1953" (abstr). *Nurs Res*, 5 (Oct 1956), 85-86.

2416.   Dock, Lavinia. "The Development of Nursing in Hospitals." *Nosokomeion*, 2 (Apr 1931), 265-275.

2417.   ————. "History of the Reform in Nursing in Bellevue Hospital." *Am J Nurs*, 1 (1901), 90.

2418.   Donnelley, P.G. "Royal Hobart Hospital Centenary of Nursing 1875-1975." *Aust Nurs J*, 5(4) (Oct 1975), 7-9.

2419.   ————. "History of Nursing at Royal Hobart Hospital. Our First 100 Years...." *Aust Nurs J*, 4(5) (Nov 1975), 10-11.

2420.   Dufton, Lena Irene. *History of Nursing at the New York Post-Graduate Medical School and Hospital*. New York: The Alumni Assoc., 1944.

2421.   "The Evolution of the Modern Nurse." *Hosp* (London), 35 (12 Dec 1903), 150-151.

2422.   "First Chairman, Private Duty Section, ANA Reminisces about Hospital Nursing." *Tr Nurs*, 107 (Aug 1941), 103-105.

2423.   "Florence Nightingale Planted the Seeds: A Commemorative Birthday Note in Honor of May 12, 1820." *Pub Hlth Nurs*, 38 (May 1946), 252.

2424.   Garrett, Elizabeth. *Volunteer Hospital Nursing*. London: Macmillan & Co., 1866. 8 pp.

2425.   Gelpin, Fanny. *Scenes from Hospital Life: Being the Letters of a Probationer Nurse*. London: Drane's Danegeld House, n.d.

2426.   Haldane, E.S. "Nursing in Scottish Poor Houses." *Brit J Nurs* (5 Jul 1902), 14-15.

2427.   "Have Times Changed? The Nursing Mirror, Sept. 22, 1906. Some Essentials of Sound Administration." *Nurs Mirror*, 141 (18) (30 Oct 1975), 76.

2428. "Have Times Changed? The Nursing Mirror, April 27, 1907. Hospitals and the Nursing of Out-Patients." *Nurs Mirror*, 141(21) (20 Nov 1975), 53.

2429. Henderson, V. "On Nursing Care Plans and Their History." *Nurs Out*, 21 (Jun 1973), 378-379.

2430. Hulburt, M. "The 19th Century Legacy for the Neurologic Nurse." *Nurs Clin No Am*, 4 (Jun 1969), 293-300.

2431. *Instructions pour les Fraters et les Infirmiers*. Berne: Imprimerie Huller, 1862. (Fr)

2432. Jacobs, G.B. "Keynote Address--American Association of Neurosurgical Nurses--April, 1976." *J Neurosurg Nurs*, 8(1) (Jul 1976), 2-7.

2433. Jari, K. "Hospital Nursing in Finland." *Bull Calif State Nurs Assoc* (Jan 1969), 6-7.

2434. Julian, E.E. "The Need of Nursing Reform in Workhouse Infirmaries." *Nurs Rec* (28 Jan 1899), 70-72.

2435. "Lady Nurses for the Sick Poor in Our London Workhouses." *Report of Proceedings at the Strands Union's Board of Guardians*. London: Board of Guardians, 1866.

2436. Lambertsen, Eleanor C. *Nursing Team Organization and Functioning*. New York: Teachers College, Columbia University, 1953.

2437. Landale, E.J.R. Nursing in a Workhouse Infirmary: Some of the Nurses' Difficulties. *Nurs Rec* (6 Jan 1894), 6-8.

2438. Lee, Florence. *Handbook for Hospital Sisters*. London: W. Isbister & Co., 1874.

2439. Logan, Laura R. "1936 ... Problems of the Staff Nurse from the Point of View of a Director of Nursing." *J NY State Nurs Assoc*, 7(1) (Mar 1976), 36-40.

2440. Luckes, Eva C.E. *Hospital Sisters and Their Duties*. London: The Scientific Press, Ltd., 1893.

2441. McIsaac, I. *Primary Nursing Technique*. New York: Macmillan Co., 1907.

2442. MacManus, Emily E.P. *Matron of Guys*. London: Andrew Melrose, 1956.

2443. Meltzer, L., and J. Roderick. "The Development and Current Status of Coronary Care." *Intensive Coronary Care*. Edited by L. Meltzer and A. Dunning. Philadelphia: Charles Press, 1970.

2444. Miller, Miriam C. *Through the Years with the Nurses at the
       Shadyside Hospital*. Pittsburgh: Miriam C. Miller, 1946.
       181 pp.

2445. Mollett, M. "On an Unpopular Branch of Our Profession (Work-
       house Infirmary Nursing)." *Nurs Rec* (20 Feb 1890), 90-93;
       (27 Feb 1890), 100-102.

2446. *Nursing of the Sick, 1893*. Edited by Isabel A. Hampton.
       Reprint. New York: McGraw-Hill Book Co., 1949.

2447. O'Neill, H.C., and Edith Barnett. *Our Nurses, and the Work
       They Have To Do*. London and New York: Ward, Lock & Co.,
       1888. 197 pp.

2448. "Pioneer Nursing." *Canad Nurs*, 44 (Feb 1948), 92, 126, 128.

2449. Regan, R.S. "Nursing Conditions in 1880 and After." *Hosp*
       (London), 31 (May 1935), 127-128.

2450. Reinkemeyer, Sister Agnes M. "It Won't Be Hospital Nursing."
       Am J Nurs, 68 (Sep 1968), 1936-1940.

2451. "Sheffield (Eng) Royal Infirmary in the Eighties." *Nurs
       Mirror* (Apr 1922), 17-18.

2452. Shmarov, A.A. "Nurses of a Kronstadt Hospital." *Med Sestra*,
       25 (Feb 1966), 50-51. (Rus)

2453. Show, Betty A. "History of Study of Tuberculosis Among
       Medical Students and Nurses." *Gray's Hosp Rep* (1952),
       302-312.

2454. Sleeper, Ruth, Dean A. Clark, Edward D. Churchill, Walter
       Bauer, and E. Lindemann. "Nursing's Contribution to a
       Famous Hospital." *Nurs Out*, 9 (May 1961), 276-280.

2455. Sloan, Raymond P. "Service Stripes for Hospital Women."
       Mod Hosp, 51 (Sep 1938), 56-59.

2456. Smith, Catherine. "1936 ... Problems of the Staff Nurse from
       the Point of a Staff Nurse." *J NY State Nurses Assoc*,
       7(1) (Mar 1976), 35.

2457. Snively, M.A. "A Nurse's Day in a Hospital." *Tr Nurs*, 13
       (1894), 8.

2458. Steele, J.C. "Account of the Nursing Arrangements Adopted in
       Guy's Hospital." *Guys Hosp Rep*, 120 (1971), 1067-1080.

2459. Thompson, C.J. "Nursing History. Nurses and Nursing at St.
       Bartholomew's Hospital (London, Eng.) in Olden Times."
       Brit J Nurs, 75 (Jun 1927), 137-138.

2460.   Twining, L. "The History of Workhouse Reform." In *Nursing
        of the Sick, 1893*. Ed. I.A. Hampton. Reprint. New York:
        McGraw-Hill, 1949.

2461.   ———. *Notes of Six Years' Work as Guardian of the Poor,
        1884-1890*. New York, 1893.

2462.   Whitney, J.S., and H.J. Stofer. *Tuberculosis Among Nurses*.
        New York: National Tuberculosis Association, 1941.

2463.   Whitney, Jessamine S. "Tuberculosis Among Young Women--With
        Special Reference to Tuberculosis Among Nurses." *Am J
        Nurs*, 28 (Aug 1928), 766-768.

2464.   Wilkie, C.B.S. "The Best Means of Providing and Training
        Nurses for the Indoor Poor." *Nurs Rec* (25 Feb 1899), 150-
        151; (4 Mar 1899), 170-172.

2465.   Wilson, T. *Nursing in Workhouses and Workhouse Infirmaries*.
        n.p.: University Press, 1890.

2466.   Wolf, Anna D. "Evolution in Nursing Service." *Nurs Out*, 4
        (Jan 1956), 47-49.

2467.   Wolf, L.K. "Development of Floor Nursing and Supervision."
        Hosp, 15 (Mar 1941), 53-56.

2468.   Woolsey, Jane Stuart. *Hospital Days*. New York: Privately
        printed, 1868. Reprint. New York: Van Nostrand, 1970.

2469.   Workhouse Infirmary Nursing Association. "Memorial to the
        Local Government Board, with Appendices on Suggested Rules
        for Nurses and Nursing in Workhouse Sick Wards." *Nurs Rec*
        (20 Jul 1893), 20-23.

INFECTIOUS DISEASE

2470.   Ackerknecht, Erwin Heinz. *History and Geography of the Most
        Important Diseases*. New York: Hafner Publishing Co., 1965.

2471.   Cipolla, Carlo M. *Cristofano and the Plague: A Study in the
        History of Public Health in the Age of Galileo*. Berkeley:
        University of California Press, 1973.

2472.   Davis, M.L. "Grendel Walks Again; Amateur Nurse in an Epi-
        demic." *Atlan*, 144 (Aug 1929), 173-185.

2473.   Defoe, Daniel. *A Journal of the Plague Year*. London: Falcon
        Press, 1957. Many editions.

2474.   Deming, Dorothy. "Influenza 1918." *Am J Nurs*, 57 (Oct 1957),
        1308-1309.

2475.   Fuller, Thomas. *Exantematologia: Or An Attempt to Give a
        Rational Account of Eruptive Fevers, Especially of the
        Small Pox*. London: Charles Rivington & Stephen Austen,
        1730.

2476.   Geister, Janet. "The Flue Epidemic of 1918." *Nurs Out*, 5
        (Oct 1957), 582-584.

2477.   Greenberg, D. "Influenza Statistics of the Visiting Nurse
        Association of New Haven." *Pub Hlth Nurs*, 12 (1920), 209.

2478.   Hanmer, G.A. "Tuberculosis Then and Now. 1." *Mid Hlth Visit*,
        10 (Jul 1974), 191-193.

2479.   ————. "Tuberculosis Then and Now. 2." *Mid Hlth Visit*, 10
        (Aug 1974), 233-236.

2480.   Harriss, Ethel Darrington. "Yellow Fever—History and
        Nursing." *Am J Nurs*, 16 (Jun 1916), 859.

2481.   Hoehling, A.A. *The Great Epidemic*. Boston: Little, Brown &
        Co., 1961.

2482.   Howard, John. *An Account of the Principal Lazarettoes in
        Europe: With Various Papers Relative to the Plague, Together
        with Further Observations on Some Foreign Prisons and Hos-
        pitals, and Additional Remarks on the Present State of
        Those in Great Britain and Ireland*. Warrington: William
        Eyres, 1789.

2483.   Ikeda, Yoshiko. "An Epidemic of Emotional Disturbance Among
        Leprosarium Nurses in a Setting of Low Morale and Social
        Change." *Psychiatry*, 29(2) (1966), 152-164.

2484.   La Motte, Ellen N. *Tuberculosis Nursing*. New York: G.P.
        Putnam's Sons, 1915.

2485.   Martin, Elsie, and Alice Taylor. "B.C.G. Vaccination Proce-
        dure and Results." *Nurs Mirror*, 107 (25 Jul 1958), 1281-
        1283.

2486.   Register, W.R. *Practical Fever Nursing*. Philadelphia:
        W.B. Saunders Co., 1907.

2487.   Rosenberg, Charles. *The Cholera Years*. Chicago: The Univer-
        sity of Chicago Press, 1962.

2488.   Sachs, Theodore B. "The Tuberculosis Nurse." *Am J Nurs*, 8
        (May 1908), 597-598.

2489.   Sieveking, E.H. "A Proposition to Supply the Labouring
        Classes with Nurses in the Time of Epidemic and Other Sick-
        ness." *Tr Epidemiol Soc Lond* (1856), 1-10.

2490.   Vaughan, Henry F., G.E. Harmon, and J.G. Molner. "Results of
        Mass Education for Tuberculosis Prevention in Detroit."
        Am J Pub Hlth, 27 (Nov 1937), 1116-1123.

MIDWIFERY AND OBSTETRICS

2491. Abbott, Grace. "The Midwife in Chicago." *Am J Soc*, 20 (Mar 1915), 684-699.

2492. Ackerknecht, Erwin H. "American Gynecology Around 1850." *Wisconsin Med J*, 51 (1952), 273-274.

2493. Adam, Shedden. "Obstetrics Through the Ages—An Historical Survey." *Aust Nurs J*, 37 (Dec 1939), 223-235; 38 (Jan 1940), 1-5.

2494. Addo, C. "The Midwife in Family Planning." *Nurs Mirror*, 133 (3 Dec 1971), 34-35.

2495. *An Appeal to the Medical Society of Rhode Island in Behalf of Woman to be Restored to Her Natural Rights as "Midwife" and Elevated by Education to be the Physician of Her Own Sex.* n.p.: Printed for the Author, 1851.

2496. *Aristotle's Compleat Midwife.* London: n.p., 1684 to well into the 19th century. Sometimes included with the sex and marriage manual known as *Aristotle's Masterpiece.*

2497. Arms, Suzanne. *Immaculate Deception: A New Look at Women and Childbirth in America.* Boston: Houghton Mifflin, 1975.

2498. Arthure, H. "Early English Midwifery." *Mid Hlth Visit Commun Nurs*, 11(6) (Jun 1975), 187-190.

2499. ————. "Midwifery Practice in the First Half of the 20th Century. Part 1." *Mid Hlth Visit Commun Nurs*, 11(10) (Oct 1975), 232-234.

2500. *Association for Childbirth at Home: Goals and Purposes.* Cerritos, CA: n.p., 1976.

2501. Atlee, H.B. "From Under the Blanket, 1908-1958." *Canad Nurs*, 54 (1958), 544-548.

2502. "Aunt Sarah: Tennessee's Champion Midwife." *Newsweek*, 48 (20 Aug 1956), 54.

2503. Aveling, J.H. *English Midwives, Their History and Prospects.* Reprint of 1872 edition. London: Elliot, Ltd., 1967.

2504. Azz, A. "Data Concerning the History of the School of Midwifery and Maternity Hospital of Sibiu. IV." *Ozv Szle*, 8 (1962), 213-216 (Magyar with Russian and English abstract).

2505. Bachu, A. "The Nurse's Role in Family Planning Services in India." *Int Nurs Rev*, 23(1) (1976), 25-28.

2506. Bagshaw, H.B. "What Ante-Natal Supervision Has Achieved." *Mid Chron & Nurs Notes*, 66 (Feb 1953), 28-29.

2507.   Bailey, Harold. "Control of Midwives." *Am J Obs Gyn*, 6
        (Sep 1923), 293-298.

2508.   Baker, S. Josephine. *Fighting for Life*. New York: Macmillan
        & Co., 1939.

2509.   —————. "Schools for Midwives." *Am J Obs & Dis Wom Child*,
        65 (1912), 256-270.

2510.   —————. "Why Do Our Mothers and Babies Die?" *Ladies Home J*,
        39 (Apr 1922), 39, 174.

2511.   Baldy, J.M. "Is the Midwife a Necessity?" *Am J Obs & Dis
        Wom Child*, 73 (Mar 1916), 399-407.

2512.   Bancroft, Livingston George. "Louise de la Vallieze and the
        Birth of the Man-midwife (Midwifery 17th Century)." *J
        Obstet Gyn Brit Eng*, 63 (1956), 261-267.

2513.   Bard, Samuel. *Compendium of the Theory and Practice of Mid-
        wifery*. New York: Collins, 1807.

2514.   Barnardo, Thomas J. "Dr. (Thomas J.) Barnardo's Homes."
        Mid Chron & Nurs Notes, 65 (Aug 1952), 219-222.

2515.   Barrett, Caroline V. "A Hundred Years of Maternity Nursing
        (Montreal Maternity Hospital)." *Canad Nurs*, 39 (1943),
        720-726.

2516.   Baughman, Greer. "A Preliminary Report Upon the Midwife
        Situation in Virginia." *Virg Med Monthly*, 54 (Mar 1928),
        749-750.

2517.   Beach, Wooster. *An Improved System of Midwifery Adopted to
        the Reformed Practice of Medicine*. New York: McAlister,
        1847; also New York: Scribner, 1851.

2518.   Bell, Arthur. "The Evolution of the Obstetric Service in
        Great Britain." *Nurs Mirror*, 115 (Oct 1962), 72-74.

2519.   Berkeley, Comyns. *A Handbook for Midwives and Maternity
        Nurses*. London: Cassell & Co., 1909.

2520.   Bigelow, Helen A. "Maternity Care in Rural Areas by Public
        Health Nurses." *Am J Pub Hlth*, 27 (Oct 1937), 975-980.

2521.   Biggar, J. "When Midwives Were Witches ... White Ones of
        Course. A Look at Maternity Care in the Middle Ages."
        Nurs Mirror, 134 (26 May 1972), 37-39.

2522.   Bowdoin, Joe P. "The Midwife Problem." *Transactions of the
        Section on Preventive Medicine and Public Health of the
        American Medical Association*. (1928), 90-95.

2523.   Breckinridge, Mary. "An Adventure in Midwifery." *Survey*,
        57 (Oct 1926), 25-27, 47.

2524.   ———. "Hard-Riding Nurses of Kentucky." *Lit Digest*, 96
        (Mar 1928), 29–30.

2525.   ———. "Maternity in the Mountains." *North Am Rev*, 226
        (Dec 1928), 765–768.

2526.   ———. "Midwifery in the Kentucky Mountains. An Investi-
        gation in 1923." *Q Bull Front Nurs Serv*, 17 (Spring 1942),
        29–53.

2527.   ———. "Nurse on Horseback." *Woman's J*, 13 (Feb 1928), 5–7.

2528.   ———. "Where the Frontier Lingers." *Rotarian*, 47 (Sep
        1935), 9–12, 50.

2529.   ———. *Wide Neighborhood: A Study of Frontier Nursing
        Service*. New York: Harper & Brothers, 1952.

2530.   Brockbank, W. "Mrs. Jane Sharp's Advice to Midwives." *Med
        Hist*, 2 (1958), 153–155.

2531.   Brocon, Charlotte B. "Obstetric Practice among the Chinese
        in San Francisco." *Pac Med Surg J*, 26 (Jul 1883), 15–21.

2532.   Brown, R. Chrisсie. "The History of Midwifery." *Mat & Child
        Wel*, 15 (Oct–Nov 1931), 243–245.

2533.   Browne, Helen E., and Gertrude Isaacs. "The Frontier Nursing
        Service: The Primary Care Nurse in the Community Hospital."
        Am J Obs Gyn, 124 (Jan 1976), 14–17.

2534.   Browne, J.C. "Ninth Dame Juliet Rhys Williams Memorial Lec-
        ture. "The Birthday Team." *Mid Chron*, 86 (Dec 1973),
        391–394.

2535.   Buchan, William. *Advice to Mothers*. London: T. Cadell and
        W. Davis, 1803.

2536.   Buchman, A.P. "Faulty Midwifery and Its Relations to Gyne-
        cology." *Obst Gaz*, 3 (1880), 62–66.

2537.   Buck, Dorothy F. "History of Midwifery." Master's Thesis,
        Teachers College, Columbia University, 1927.

2538.   Butler, Mary L. "Early History of Maternal Associations."
        Chautauguan, 31 (May 1900), 38–42.

2539.   Carter, Mary. "Fifty Years of Ante-Natal Care." *Mid Chron
        & Nurs Notes*, 64 (Nov 1951), 339–340.

2540.   Cartwright, F.F. "Robert Bentley Towd's Contributions to
        Medicine." *Proc R Soc Med*, 67(9) (Sep 1974), 893–897.

2541.   Chang, C.T. "Maternity Care in Free China." *Bull Am Coll
        Nurs-Mid*, 13 (1968), 139–142.

2542.   Channing, Walter. *Remarks on the Employment of Females as
         Practitioners in Midwifery.* Boston: Cummings & Hilliard,
         1820.

2543.   Chapin, Charles V. "The Control of Midwifery." *U.S. Depart-
         ment of Labor, Children's Bureau, Standards of Child Wel-
         fare: A Report of the Children's Bureau Conferences.*
         May and Jun 1919, White House Conference Series 1.
         Washington, D.C.: U.S. Government Printing Office, 1919.

2544.   ————. "The Control of Midwifery." *Med Prog*, 39 (Apr 1923),
         76-79.

2545.   Chisholm, Mary. "Paediatric After-Care." *Nurs Mirror*, 104
         (19 Oct 1956), vi-viii.

2546.   Chittick, R. "Our Anabases." *Aust Nurs J*, 67 (Mar 1964),
         58-67.

2547.   Cianfrani, Theodore. *A Short History of Obstetrics and
         Gynecology.* Springfield, IL: Charles C Thomas, 1960.

2548.   Cody, Edmund F. "The Registered Midwife: A Necessity."
         Bost Med Surg J, 168 (Mar 1913), 416-418.

2549.   Conant, Clarence M. *An Obstetric Mentor. A Handbook of
         Homeopathic Treatment Required During Pregnancy, Parturi-
         tion and the Puerperal Season.* New York: A.L. Chatterton,
         1884.

2550.   Corson, Hiram. "Thoughts on Midwifery." *Med Surg Rep*, 40
         (Jan 1879), 3-5.

2551.   Crowell, Elizabeth. "The Midwives of New York." *Charities*,
         17 (5 Jan 1907), 671-677.

2552.   Culikova, L. "History of Midwifery." *Zdrav Prac*, 19 (Apr
         1969), 218-224. (Cze)

2553.   ————. "History of Midwifery. 3." *Zdrav Prac*, 19 (Jun
         1969), 344-348. (Cze)

2554.   Culpeper, Nicolas. *Directory for Midwives.* London: n.p.,
         1653 and following years.

2555.   Cutter, Irving S., and Henry R. Viets. *A Short History of
         Midwifery.* Philadelphia: W.B. Saunders, 1964.

2556.   Darlington, Thomas. "The Present Status of the Midwife."
         Am J Obs Dis Wom Child, 63 (1911), 870-884.

2557.   Das, K. *Obstetric Forceps: Its History and Evolution.*
         St. Louis: C.W. Mobsy, 1929.

2558.   Davis, Dorothy Crane, and Lamar Middleton. "Rebirth of the
         Midwife." *Todays Hlth* (Feb 1968), 28-31, 70-71.

2559.   Deming, Dorothy. "General Summary of Findings of the Congress; Nursing Section." *Proc Am Cong Obs & Gyn*, 1 (1939), 881-883.

2560.   Dioneson, S.M. "The History of Midwifery Training at the Beginning of the XIXth Century in Russia." *Sovetsk Zdravoohr*, 20(6) (1961), 67-72. (Rus)

2561.   Donegan, Janet Bauer. "Midwifery in America, 1760-1860: A Study of Medicine and Morality." Ph.D. dissertation, Syracuse University, 1972.

2562.   Drogendijk, A.C. "De verloskundige voorziening te Gordrecht in de eerste helft van de 17e eeuw." *Ned T Geneesk*, 100 (1956), 928-935. (Dut)

2563.   Dublin, Louis I. *The First One Thousand Midwifery Cases of the Frontier Nursing Service.* New York: Metropolitan Life Ins. Co., 1932.

2564.   Eastman, Nicholsen J. "Whither American Obstetrics." *New England J Med*, 224 (1941), 89-93.

2565.   Edgar, J. Clifton. "The Remedy for the Midwife Problem." *Am J Obs Dis Wom Child*, 63 (1911), 881-884.

2566.   ————. "Why the Midwife." *Am J Obs Dis Wom Child*, 77 (1918), 242-255.

2567.   ————. "Why the Midwife?" *Trans Am Gyn Soc*, 43 (1918), 213-236.

2568.   *Education for Nurse-Midwifery: The Report of the Work Conference on Nurse-Midwifery.* New York: American College of Nurse-Midwifery, 1958.

2569.   *Education for Nurse-Midwifery: The Report of the Second Work Conference on Nurse-Midwifery Education.* New York: Maternity Center Assoc., 1967.

2570.   Ehrenreich, Barbara, and Diedre English. *Witches, Midwives and Nurses.* Old Westbury, NY: Feminist Press, 1973.

2571.   Elaut, L. "Voortgezet onderricht voor Vwedvzouwen in de Kastelenij van Aalst op het einde van de 18e eeux." *Het Land Van Aalst*, 8 (1956). (Dut)

2572.   Elfverson, K. "Uz Sophiahemmets Historie." *T Sver Sjukskoterskor NR, 10 Med Hist Azsh* (1959). (Swe)

2573.   Emmons, Arthur B., and James L. Huntington. "The Midwife: Her Future in the United States." *Am J Obs Dis Wom Child*, 65 (Mar 1912), 393-404.

2574.   ————. "A Review of the Midwife Situation." *Bost Med Surg J*, 164 (1911), 251-262.

2575.   Fedde, Helen Marie. "A Study of Midwifery with Special
         Reference to Its Historical Background, Its Present Status,
         and a Consideration of Its Future in the United States."
         Master's Thesis, University of Kentucky, 1950.

2576.   Fenwick, Ethel Gordon. "Nursing Homes. For Protest Action of
         National Council of Trained Nurses of Great Britain and
         Ireland led by Ethel Gordon Fenwick and Discussion of Bill
         Presented to Parliament." *Brit J Nurs*, 51 (20 Dec 1913),
         513-516; 52 (21 Mar 1914), 254; (25 Apr 1914), 364; 53
         (25 Jul 1914), 103-104; (1 Aug 1914), 110-111; (8 Aug
         1914), 132; 55 (15 Oct 1915), 322-324.

2577.   Ferguson, James H. "Mississippi Midwives." *J Hist Med*, 5
         (1950), 85-95.

2578.   Findley, Palmer. *Priests of Lucina: The Story of Obstetrics*.
         Boston: Little, Brown & Co., 1939. 42 pp.

2579.   ————. *The Story of Childbirth*. New York: Doubleday,
         Doran & Co., 1933.

2580.   Forbes, Thomas R. *The Midwife and the Witch*. New Haven:
         Yale University Press, 1966.

2581.   ————. "Midwifery and Witchcraft." *J Hist Med*, 17 (1962),
         264-283.

2582.   ————. "Perrette the Midwife--A 15th Century Witchcraft
         Case." *Bull Hist Med*, 36 (1962), 124-129.

2583.   ————. "The Regulation of English Midwives in the 16th and
         17th Centuries." *J Med Hist*, 8 (1964), 235-244.

2584.   Forman, Alice M. *Patterns of Legislation and the Practice of
         Nurse-Midwifery in the U.S.A.* New York: American College
         of Nurse-Midwives, 1974.

2585.   Fothergill, W.E. *Manual of Midwifery for the Use of Students
         and Practitioners*. New York: Macmillan & Co., 1896.

2586.   Foulkes, J.F. "Drugs Ancient and Modern in Obstetric Prac-
         tice." *Mid Chron & Nurs Notes*, 83 (Sep 1970), 288ff.

2587.   Fox, C.G. "Early Canadian Nursing." *Aust Nurs J*, 66 (Nov
         1968), 249-251.

2588.   ————. "Toward a Sound Historical Basis for Nurse-Midwifery."
         Bull Am Coll Nurs Mid, 14 (Aug 1969), 76ff.

2589.   "Frontier Nurse." *Lit Digest*, 124 (28 Aug 1937), 12.

2590.   Fullerton, Anna M. *A Handbook of Obstetrical Nursing for
         Nurses, Students, and Mothers*. Philadelphia: P. Blakiston,
         Son & Co., 1890.

2591. Galabin, Alfred L. *A Manual of Midwifery*. Philadelphia: P. Blakiston, Son & Co., 1886.

2592. Gardner, Augustus K. *A History of the Art of Midwifery*. New York: Stringer & Townsend, 1852.

2593. Garrigues, Henry J. *Practical Guide in Antiseptic Midwifery in Hospitals and Private Practice*. Detroit: G.S. Davis, 1886.

2594. Geffen, Dennis. *Public Health and Social Services: Elementary Text for Midwives*. London: Edward Arnold & Co., 1940.

2595. Gewin, W.C. "Careless and Unscientific Midwifery with Special References to Some Features of the Work of Midwives." *Alabama Med J*, 18 (1905-1906), 629-635.

2596. Gilliatt, Sir William. "Peel, John: The Life and Work of Sir William Gilliatt." *Nurs Mirror*, 106 (18 Oct 1957), 206-207; (25 Oct 1957), 283.

2597. Glisan, Rodney. *Textbook of Modern Midwifery*. Philadelphia: Presley Blakiston, 1881.

2598. Goldsmith, Seth B., John W.C. Johnson, and Monroe Lerner. "Obstetricians' Attitudes Toward Nurse-Midwives." *Am J Obs Gyn*, 111 (Sep 1971), 111-118.

2599. Goodell, William. "When and Why Were Male Physicians Employed as Accoucheurs?" *Am J Obs Dis Wom Child*, 9 (Aug 1876), 381-390.

2600. Gordon, J.E. "British Midwives Through the Centuries." *Mid Hlth Visit*, 3 (1967), 181-187, 237-240, 257-281.

2601. Graham, Harvey. *Eternal Eye: A History of Gynaecology and Obstetrics*. Garden City, NY: Doubleday, 1951.

2602. Gregory, Samuel. *Man-Midwifery Exposed and Corrected*. Boston: G. Gregory, 1848; New York: Fowleus and Wells, 1848.

2603. Guyonnett, G. "Le baptême administré par La Sage-femme." *Hist Med*, 8(8) (1958), 62-64.

2604. "Gynecological Nursing." *Int Nurs Rev*, 7 (Feb 1960), 3, supplement.

2605. Hanson, Henry, and Lucile S. Blackly. "Present Status of Midwifery in Florida." *So Med J*, 25 (Dec 1932), 1252-1258.

2606. Hardin, E.R. "The Midwife Problem." *So Med J*, 18(5) (1925), 349.

2607. Hartley, E.C., and Ruth E. Boynton. "A Survey of the Midwife Situation in Minnesota." *Minn Med*, 7 (Jun 1924), 439-446.

2608.   Haydon, M.O. "English Midwives in Three Centuries." *Mat Child Welf*, 3 (1919), 407-409.

2609.   Hellman, Louis, and Francis B. O'Brien, Jr. "Nurse-Midwifery --An Experiment in Maternity Care." *Obs Gyn*, 24 (Sep 1964), 343-349.

2610.   Hersey, Thomas. *The Midwife's Practical Directory: Or Woman's Confidential Friend*. Baltimore: n.p., 1836; Columbus, O: Clapp, Gillett & Co., 1834.

2611.   Hill, T.J. "Some Remarks on the Midwifery Question: Must the Midwife Perish?" *Med Rec*, 4 (Oct 1898), 474-475.

2612.   "History of Midwifery." *Nurs J India*, 60 (Dec 1969), 449ff.

2613.   Hitchcock, James. "A Sixteenth Century Midwife's License." *Bull Hist Med*, 41 (1967), 75.

2614.   Hollick, Frederick. *The Matron's Manual of Midwifery and the Diseases of Women During Pregnancy and in Child Bed*. 47th ed. New York: T.W. Strong, 1848.

2615.   Holmes, Rudolph W. "Midwife Practice: An Anachronism." *Ill Med J*, 37 (Jan 1920), 27-31.

2616.   Huard, P., and Z. Ohya. "L'obstetrique japonaise à la periode pre-meiji." *Aesculape*, 45 (1962), 41-46. (Fr)

2617.   Hudon, M. "Histoire de profesion Jean de Pieu." *Cah Nurs*, 38 (Dec 1965), 22-24. (Fr)

2618.   Hughes, Muriel Joy. *Women Healers in Medieval Life and Literature*. New York: King's Crown Press, 1943.

2619.   Huntington, James L. "The Regulation of Midwifery." *Bost Med Surg J*, 167 (1912), 84-87.

2620.   ————. "The Midwife in Massachusetts: Her Anomalous Position." *Bost Med Surg J*, 168 (Mar 1913), 418-421.

2621.   Jacobson, Paul H. "Hospital Care and the Vanishing Midwife." *Milbank Mem Fund O*, 34 (Jul 1956), 253-261.

2622.   Jameson, E. *Gynecology and Obstetrics*. New York: Hafner, 1962.

2623.   Jarrett, Elizabeth. "The Midwife or the Woman Doctor." *Med Rec*, 54 (Oct 1898), 610-611.

2624.   Jennings, Samuel K. *The Married Lady's Companion and Poor Man's Friend*. New York: n.p., 1908.

2625.   Jensen, Joan M. "Politics and the American Midwife Controversy." *Frontiers*, 1 (Spring 1976), 19-33.

2626.   King, Edward. "50 Years of Obstetrics in New Orleans."
        Obs Gyn, 19(6) (Jun 1962), 826-830.

2627.   King, Howard D. "The Evolution of the Male Midwife with
        Some Remarks on the Obstetrical Literature of Other Ages."
        Am J Obs Dis Wom Child, 77 (Feb 1918), 177-186.

2628.   Kobrin, Frances E. "The American Midwife Controversy: A
        Crisis of Professionalization." *Bull Hist Med*, 40 (Jul-
        Aug 1966), 350-363.

2629.   Kompert, G. "Midwives and Their Disregard for Antiseptics."
        Med Rec, 53 (Feb 1898), 331.

2630.   Kosmak, George W. "Certain Aspects of the Midwife Problem in
        Relation to the Medical Profession and Community." *Med
        Rec*, 85 (Jun 1914), 1013-1017.

2631.   Lader, Lawrence. *The Margaret Sanger Story*. Garden City,
        NY: Doubleday, 1955.

2632.   Laufe, Leonard. *Obstetrical Forceps*. New York: Harper &
        Row, 1968.

2633.   Lee, Florence Ellen, and Jay H. Glasser. "Role of Law Mid-
        wifery in Maternity Care in a Large Metropolitan Area."
        Pub Hlth Rep, 89 (Nov-Dec 1974), 537-544.

2634.   Leishman, William. *A System of Midwifery, Including the
        Diseases of Pregnancy and the Puerperal State*. 3rd Ameri-
        can ed. Philadelphia: H.C. Lea, 1879.

2635.   Leith, Mary Evelyn. *The Development of Midwife Education in
        South Carolina, 1919-1946*. M.A. thesis, Yale University,
        1948.

2636.   Levy, Barry S., Frederick S. Wilkinson, and William M.
        Marine. "Reducing Neonatal Mortality Rate with Nurse-
        Midwives." *J Obs Gyn*, 109 (Jan 1971), 50-58.

2637.   Levy, Julius. "The Maternal and Infant Mortality in Mid-
        wifery Practice in Newark, New Jersey." *Am J Obs*, 77
        (1918), 41-51.

2638.   Litoff, Judy Barrett. *American Midwives: 1860 to Present*.
        Westport, CT: Greenwood Press, 1978. 197 pp.

2639.   Lobenstine, Ralph W. "The Influence of the Midwife Upon
        Infant and Maternal Morbidity and Mortality." *Am J Obs
        Dis Wom Child*, 63 (1911), 876-880.

2640.   Lubic, Ruth W. "Myths About Nurse-Midwifery." *Am J Nurs*,
        74 (Feb 1974), 268-269.

2641.   Lusk, W.T. *The Science and Art of Midwifery*. New York:
        D. Appleton & Co., 1882.

2642.   McCoy, Samuel. "Ketchin' Babies: A Hundred Thousand Births
        that Need Safe Safeguarding." *Survey*, 54 (Aug 1925), 483-
        486.

2643.   Macy Foundation. *The Midwife in the United States*. New
        York: Josiah Macy, Jr. Foundation, 1968.

2644.   Maister, M. "The Control of Nursing Homes and Midwives:
        Legal Aspects and Education." *J Roy San Inst*, 59 (Jul
        1938), 118-128.

2645.   Mallon, Winifred. "Midwives in Relation to High Maternal
        Mortality." *Tr Nurs*, 82 (Jun 1929), 765-768.

2646.   Mango, M. "British Nurse-Midwife with WHO." *Nurs Mirror*, 99
        (26 Jun 1954), iv-v.

2647.   Manley, T.H. "Women as Midwives." *Trans NY State Med Assoc*,
        1 (1884), 370-375.

2648.   Marmol, Jose G., Alan L. Scriggins, and Rudolf F. Vollman.
        "History of the Maternal Mortality Study Committees in the
        United States." *Obs Gyn*, 34 (Jul 1969), 123-138.

2649.   Maternity Center Association. *Twenty Years of Nurse Mid-
        wifery, 1933-1953*. New York: Maternity Center Association,
        1955.

2650.   Mathews, W.S. "Why Were Physicians Employed as Accoucheurs
        Instead of Midwives?" *Toledo Med Surg J*, 3 (1879), 54-56.

2651.   Maygrier, Jacques Pierre. *Midwifery Illustrated*. Translated
        with notes by A. Sidney Doane. New York: J.K. Moore, 1833.

2652.   Meadows, Alfred. *A Manual of Midwifery*. Philadelphia:
        Lindsay & Blakiston, 1871.

2653.   Meglen, Marie C., and Helen V. Burst. "Nurse-Midwives Make a
        Difference." *Nurs Out*, 22 (Jun 1974), 386-389.

2654.   Mengert, William F. "The Origin of the Male Midwife." *Ann
        Med Hist*, 4 (Sep 1932), 453-465.

2655.   "The Midwife. Lying-in and Nursing Homes." *Brit J Nurs*, 51
        (1 Nov 1913), 366-368; (13 Dec 1913), 507-508.

2656.   "Midwife Mores--Some Sidelights on an Ancient Profession."
        MD Med News Mag, 2(11) (1958), 134-141.

2657.   "Midwifery in the Good Old Days." *Oest Hebammenzeitung*, 16
        (Jul 1969), 89-95.   (Ger)

2658.   "Midwives Dwindle Under Immigration Restrictions." *J Am Med
        Assoc*, 93(17) (26 Oct 1929), 1317.

2659.   Miles, D. "Heroines on Horseback." *Colliers*, 118 (31 Aug 1946), 24ff.

2660.   Monteiro, Lois. "Nursing's Acceptance of the Function of Family Planning Counselor." *Fam Cord*, 23(1) (Jan 1974), 67-72.

2661.   Mueller, Dietz H. "Der Whemütter-Eyd in Spandau zur geschichte der Hebammen-Ozdnungen." *Berl Med*, 14 (1963), 625-627. (Ger)

2662.   *Muller, Susanna, 1756-1785. An Old German Midwife's Record.* Edited by M.D. Learned and C.F. Bride. Philadelphia: Library of the College of Physicians of Philadelphia, n.d.

2663.   Mutton, M. "One Page, Two Pages, Three ... A History of Midwifery." *Aust Nurs J*, 63 (Nov 1965), 262ff.

2664.   Myers, Pauline. "Mountain Mothers of Kentucky." *Hygeia*, 7 (Apr 1929), 353-356.

2665.   Nash, Charles Elventon. *The History of Augusta, Including the Diary of Mrs. Martha Moore Ballard, 1785-1812.* Augusta, ME: Charles E. Nash & Son, 1904. pp. 229-464.

2666.   Newmayer, S.W. "The Status of Midwifery in Pennsylvania and a Study of the Midwives of Philadelphia." *Monthly Cyclopedia and Med Bull*, 4 (1911), 712-719.

2667.   Nicholson, William R. "The Midwife Situation." *Trans Am Gyn Soc*, 42 (1917), 623-631.

2668.   Nihell, Elizabeth. *A Treatise on the Art of Midwifery. Setting Forth Various Abuses Therein, Especially as to the Practice with Instruments: The Whole Serving to Put All Rational Inquirers in a Fair Way of Very Safely Forming Their Own Judgment Upon the Question: Which it is Best to Employ, in Cases of Pregnancy and Lying-In, A Man-Midwife or A Midwife.* London: Morley, 1760.

2669.   Noall, Claire. "Mormon Midwives." *Utah His Q*, 10 (1942), 84-144.

2670.   Olsen, L. "The Expanded Role of the Nurse in Maternity Practice." *Nurs Clin N Am*, 9 (1974), 459-466.

2671.   Olson, Ruth M. "A Home Delivery Service Based on a Study of Medical and Nursing Resources." *Am J Nurs*, 42 (Aug 1942), 877-878.

2672.   Paine, A.K. "The Midwife Problem." *Bost Med Surg J*, 173 (Nov 1915), 759-764.

2673.   Parvin, Theophilus. *Lectures on Obstetric Nursing.* Philadelphia: Blakiston, Son, 1889.

2674.   Paul, Lois. "Recruitment to a Ritual Role: The Midwife in a
         Maya Community." *Ethos*, 3(3) (Fall 1975), 449-467.

2675.   Peacock, Gladys Marcia. *I Wanted to Live in America.*
         Lexington, KY: Frontier Nursing Service, 1942.

2676.   Penman, W.R. "The Public Practice of Midwifery in Philadel-
         phia." *Trans Stud Coll Phys Phil*, 37 (Oct 1969), 124-132.

2677.   Playfair, W.S.A. *A Treatise on the Science and Practice of
         Midwifery.* 3rd Am. ed. Philadelphia: H.C. Lea, 1880.
         Many other editions, both in England and America.

2678.   Number deleted.

2679.   Plecker, W.A. "The First Move Toward Midwife Control in
         Virginia." *Virginia Med Monthly*, 45 (Apr 1918), 12-13.

2680.   ———. "The Midwife in Virginia." *Virginia Med Semi-
         Monthly*, 18 (Jan 1914), 474-477.

2681.   ———. "The Midwife Problem in Virginia." *Virginia Med
         Semi-Monthly*, 19 (Dec 1914), 456-458.

2682.   ———. "Virginia Makes Efforts to Solve Midwife Problem."
         Nat Hlth, 7 (Dec 1925), 809-811.

2683.   Poole, Ernest. "Nurse on Horseback: Frontier Nursing Ser-
         vice." *Good Housekeeping*, 94 (Jun 1932), 38-39, 203-210.

2684.   ———. *Nurses on Horseback.* New York: Macmillan Co.,
         1933.

2685.   Post, C.R. "De amsterdamse vroedvrouwen uit de 18e eeuw."
         Ned T Geneesk, 100 (1956), 167-174. (Dut)

2686.   Number deleted.

2687.   Pryor, J.H. "The Status of the Midwife in Buffalo." *New
         York Med J*, 11 (Aug 1884), 129-132.

2688.   Purrington, W.A. "The Midwifery Question." *Med Rec*, 53
         (Feb 1898), 286-287.

2689.   Puschel, E. "Die Hebamme ihr Stand und ihre Aufgabe un das
         Jahr 1600." *Dtsch Hekammer Z* (1957), part 7.

2690.   Radcliffe, Walter. *Milestones in Midwifery.* Bristol, Eng.:
         Wright, 1967.

2691.   Rayburn, O.E. "The 'Granny-Woman' in the Ozarks." *Mid
         Folklore*, 9 (1959), 145-148.

2692.   "Rebirth of the Midwife." *Life*, 71 (19 Nov 1971), 50-55.

2693.   Reed, Louis. *Midwives, Chiropodists, and Optometrists: Their Place in Medical Care*. Chicago: Univ. of Chicago Press, 1932. Committee on the Costs of Medical Care, Publication No. 15, 1932.

2694.   Reist, A. "Indication. Technic and Efficacy of Forceps in the Obstetric Department of Swiss Nursing School in Zurich from 1930 to 1949." *Scheweiz Med Wehnschr*, 82 (1 Mar 1952), 229-240.   (Ger)

2695.   *Remarks on the Employment of Females as Practitioners in Midwifery*. Boston: n.p., 1820.

2696.   Research Committee of the American College of Nurse-Midwives. *Descriptive Data: Nurse-Midwives--U.S.A.* New York: American College of Nurse-Midwives, 1972.

2697.   Roesslin, Eucharius. *Frauen Rosegarten*. Translated into English as *The Byrth of Mankind, Otherwyse Named the Womans Booke*. London: Thomas Raynalde, 1540. Reprinted until 17th century.

2698.   "Role of the Nurse-Midwife." *Am J Obs Gyn*, 124 (Mar 1976), 666.

2699.   Rolleston, Humphrey. "The Evolution of Nursing." *Nurs Times*, 32(11) (Apr 1936), 361-362.

2700.   Rosenberg, Charles, and Carroll Smith-Rosenberg, eds. *The Male Midwife and the Female Doctor: The Gynecology Controversy in Nineteenth Century America*. New York: Arno Press, 1974.

2701.   Ross, R.A. "Granny Gradiosity." *So Med Surg*, 96 (Feb 1934), 57-59.

2702.   Royer, B.F. "Midwives in Pennsylvania." *PA Med J*, 16 (Jan 1913), 289-294.

2703.   Rubin, R. "Maternity Nursing Stops Too Soon." *Am J Nurs*, 75(10) (Oct 1975), 1680-1684.

2704.   Sanger, Margaret. *An Autobiography*. New York: Dover Publications, 1971.

2705.   Sargent, C.A. "Midwifery in Delaware." *Del State Med J*, 5 (Aug 1933), 176-177.

2706.   Saur, Mrs. P.B. *Maternity: A Book for Every Wife and Mother*. Chicago: L.P. Miller & Co., 1899.

2707.   Scheffey. "The Early History and the Transition Period of Obstetrics and Gynecology in Philadelphia." *Ann Med Hist*, 3rd ser. (May 1940), 215-224.

2708.   Seaman, Valentine. *The Midwives' Monitor, and Mother's
        Mirror*. New York: Collins, 1800.

2709.   Shaver, Elizabeth. "Infant Mortality and the Midwife Prob-
        lem." *Louisville, KY Mont J Med Surg*, 19 (Jun 1912), 24-29.

2710.   Shoemaker, Sister M. Theophane. *History of Nurse-Midwifery
        in the United States*. Washington, D.C.: The Catholic
        University of America Press, 1947.

2711.   Skarica, M. "The Slovene, Andriji Mosetig and School for
        Midwives in Zador." *Zdrar Vestn*, 27 (1958), 462-463.
        (Serbo-Croat)

2712.   Slemons, Josiah Morris. "Progress in Obstetrics, 1890-1940."
        Am J Surg, 51 (1941), 79-96.

2713.   Slome, C.H., M. Daly Wetherbee, K. Christensen, M. Meglen,
        and H. Thiede. "Effectiveness of Certified Nurse-Midwives.
        A Prospective Evaluation Study." *Am J Obs Gyn*, 124 (Jan
        1976), 177-182.

2714.   Smith, Helena H. "Back to the Midwife?" *New Rep*, 79 (Jul
        1934), 207.

2715.   Smith, W.S. "Careless and Unscientific Midwifery, With
        Special Reference to Some Features of the Work of Midwives."
        Maryland Med J, 33 (1895-1896), 146-149.

2716.   Smythe, H.J. Drew. "Changes in Obstetric Technique." *Nurs
        Mirror*, 94 (16 Nov 1951), 149-150.

2717.   Snapper, I. "Midwifery, Past and Present." *Bull NY Acad Med*,
        39 (Aug 1963), 503-532.

2718.   Solenberger, Edith Reeves. "Nurses on Horseback: Frontier
        Nursing Service." *Hygeia*, 9 (Jul 1931), 633-638.

2719.   Soranus. *Gynecology*. Translated with introduction by Owsei
        Temkin. Baltimore: Johns Hopkins Press, 1956.

2720.   Speert, Harold. *Iconographia Gyniatrica: A Pictorial History
        of Gynecology and Obstetrics*. Philadelphia: F.A. Davis,
        1973.

2721.   ————. *Obstetric and Gynecologic Milestones: Essays in
        Eponymy*. New York: Macmillan Co., 1958.

2722.   Spencer, Herbert R. *The History of British Midwifery*.
        London: John Bale Sons & Danielson, 1927.

2723.   Sporlein, G., and H. Blanz. "Zur Geschichte des Hebammen-
        wesens in Suddeutschland." *Zbl Gyn*, 78 (1956), 478-482.
        (Ger)

2724.   Standlee, Mary W. *The Great Pulse: Japanese Midwifery and Obstetrics Through the Ages.* Rutland, VT: Charles E. Tuttle, 1959.

2725.   Stern, C.A. "Midwives, Male-Midwives, and Nurse-Midwives." *Obs & Gyn*, 39 (Feb 1972), 308-311.

2726.   Steudel, J. "Heilkundige Frauen des Abendlandes." *Zbl Gynak*, 81 (1959), 285-295. (Ger)

2727.   Stone, Ellen A. "The Midwives of Rhode Island." *Prov Med J*, 13 (1912), 57-60.

2728.   Stone, Sarah. *A Complete Practice of Midwifery.* London: T. Cooper, 1937.

2729.   Storer, Horatio R. *Criminal Abortion.* Boston: Little, Brown & Co., 1868.

2730.   Strachen, M. "History of Midwifery." *Front Nurs Serv Q Bull*, 49 (Summer 1973), 23-27.

2731.   Streshinsky, Shirley. "Are You Safer with a Midwife?" *MS*, 2 (Oct 1973), 24-27.

2732.   Stuerzbecher, M. "Der Stralsunder Hebammeneid Von 1717." *Zbl Gynak*, 79(2) (1957), 79-81. (Ger)

2733.   ———. "Zur Geschichte des Hebammen-wesens im Kreise Greifsweld." *Zbl Gynak*, 79 (1957), 1717-1724. (Ger)

2734.   Terry, Charles E. "Midwife Menace." *Delineator*, 91 (Oct 1917), 15-16.

2735.   ———. "The Mother, The Midwife and The Law." *Delineator*, 92 (Feb 1916), 12-13.

2736.   Thomas, Margaret W. *The Practice of Nurse-Midwifery in the United States, U.S. Department of Health, Education and Welfare, Children's Bureau Publication No. 436.* Washington, D.C.: U.S. Government Printing Office, 1965.

2737.   Thoms, Herbert. *Chapters in American Obstetrics.* Springfield, IL: Thomas, 1933

2738.   ———. *Classical Contributions to Obstetrics and Gynecology.* Springfield, IL: Thomas, 1935.

2739.   ———. *Our Obstetric Heritage.* Hamden, CT: Shoestring Press, 1960.

2740.   Tirpak, H. "Frontier Nursing Service: Fifty Years in the Mountains." *Nurs Out*, 23(5) (May 1975), 308-310.

2741.   Thornton, A. "The Past in Midwifery Services." *Aust Nurs J*, (1 Mar 1972), 19-23, *passim*.

2742.   *The Training and Responsibilities of the Midwife.* New York:
         Josiah Macy Foundation, 1967.

2743.   *200 Years of Nursing; The Story of Queen Charlotte's Mater-
         nity Hospital.* London: Churchill, 1952. 13 pp.

2744.   Tutzke, Dietrich. "Die Entwicklung des Hebammen-wessens in
         der Oberlausitz bis zum Beginn des 19 Jahrhunderts."
         Oberlausitzer Forsch (1961), 284-306. (Ger)

2745.   ————. "Uber Statistische Untersuchungen als Beitrag zur
         Geschichte der Hebammenwesens in Ausgehenden 18. Jahr-
         hundert." *Centaurus*, 4 (1956), 351-359. (Ger)

2746.   ————. "Zur materiellen Lage des Niederlausitzer Hebammen
         im 18. Jahrhundert." *Sudhoffs Arch Gesch Med*, 45 (1961),
         334-340. (Ger)

2747.   Underwood, Felix J. "The Development of Midwifery in
         Mississippi." *So Med J*, 19 (Sep 1926), 683-687.

2747.1   U.S. Congress, Senate. *Practice of Medicine and Midwifery
         in the District of Columbia.* Hearings on S.441, 69th Con-
         gress, 2d Session, 5 Jan 1927.

2748.   Van Blarcom, Carolyn C. "Has the Nursing Profession a
         Responsibility in Connection with Midwives?" *Brit J Nurs*,
         74 (Sep 1926), 212-214.

2749.   ————. *The Midwife in England: Being a Study in England of
         the Working of the English Midwives Act of 1902.* Phila-
         delphia: William F. Fell Co., 1913.

2750.   ————. "A Possible Solution of the Midwife Problem." *Proc
         Nat Conf Charities & Correction* (1910), 350-356.

2751.   ————. "Rat Pie: Among the Black Midwives of the South."
         Harpers, 160 (Feb 1930), 322-332.

2752.   Von Ramdohr, C.A. "Midwifery and Midwife." *Med Rec*, 3
         (Dec 1897), 882-883.

2753.   Waddel, W. "Obstetrics--From Prehistoric Times to the
         Present." *So Afr Nurs J*, 38 (Dec 1971), 14-18.

2754.   Wadsworth, L.C. "The Midwife and Midwifery." *Am Prac News*,
         26 (1898), 209-212.

2755.   Waite, Frederick C. *History of the New England Female Medi-
         cal College.* Boston: Boston University School of Medicine,
         1959.

2756.   Walker, Gretchen. "Nursing, Feminism and Maternity Care."
         Proceedings of the 1st International Childbirth Conference.
         Stamford, CT: New Moon Publications, 1973.

2757.   Wallace, Helen M., Curtis L. Mendelson, Leona Baumgartner,
        and Ruth Rothmayer. "The Practice of Midwives in New York
        City." *NY State J M*, 48 (Jan 1948), 67-71.

2758.   Weisl, Bernard A.G. "The Nurse-Midwife and the New York City
        Health Code." *W J Surg Obs Gyn*, 71 (Nov-Dec 1963), 266-269.

2759.   Welz, Walter E. "Michigan's Midwife Problem." *J Mich M Soc*,
        21 (Dec 1912), 788-793.

2760.   Wertz, Richard W., and Dorothy C. Wertz. *Lying-In; A History
        of Childbirth in America*. New York: Schocken Books, 1979.

2761.   *What Is A Nurse-Midwife?* New York: American College of Nurse-
        Midwives, 1973.

2762.   Wile, Ira S. "Immigration and Midwife Problems." *Bost Med
        Surg J*, 167 (1912), 113-115.

2763.   ————. "Immigration and the Midwife Problem." *Bull Am Acad
        Med*, 4 (1913), 197-202.

2764.   Williams, J. Whitridge. "Medical Education and the Midwife
        Problem in the United States." *J Am Med Assoc*, 58 (6 Jan
        1912), 4ff.

2765.   Williams, Linsly R. "Position of the New York State Depart-
        ment of Health Relative to Control of Midwives." *NY State
        J M*, 15 (Aug 1915), 296-301.

2766.   Williams, Philip F. "A Book Review of Samuel Bard's 'A Com-
        pendium of the Theory and Practice of Midwifery.'" *Am J
        Obs Gyn*, 70 (Oct 1955), 701-710.

2767.   Winslow, A. *Frontier Nursing Service*. Washington, D.C.: The
        Committee on the Costs of Medical Care, 1932.

2768.   Worden, H. "She Nurses Her Patients for a Dollar A Year:
        Frontier Nursing Service." *Am Med*, 112 (Dec 1931), 69ff.

2769.   Young, J. Van D. "The Midwife Problem in the State of New
        York." *NY State J M*, 15 (1915), 291-296.

2770.   Zeigler, Azelie. "The Midwife of the Past." *Q Bull Louisiana
        Dept Hlth*, 40 (Sep 1949), 5-10.

2771.   Ziegler, Charles Edward. "The Elimination of the Midwife."
        J Am Med Assoc, 60(1) (4 Jan 1913), 32-38.

NURSE ANESTHETISTS

2772.   Bankoff, G.A. *Conquest of Pain: The Story of Anesthesia.*
        London: MacDonald & Co., 1946.

2773.   Fife, Gertrude L. "The Nurse As Anesthetist." *Am J Nurs*,
        47 (May 1947), 308-309.

2774.   Keys, Thomas E. *The History of Surgical Anesthesia.* New
        York: Schuman, 1945.

2775.   Magaw, Alice. "Observations on 1092 Cases of Anesthesia from
        Jan. 1, 1899 to Jan. 1, 1900." *Tr Nurs & Hosp Rev*, 31
        (1903), 150.

2776.   ————. "A Review of Over 14,000 Surgical Anesthetics."
        Surg Gyn Obs, 3 (1906), 795-799.

2777.   Pougiales, J. "The First Anesthetizers at the Mayo Clinic."
        J Am Assoc Nurs Anes, 38 (Jun 1970), 235ff.

2778.   Thatcher, Virginia S. *A History of Anesthesia: With Emphasis
        on the Nurse Specialist.* Philadelphia: J.B. Lippincott,
        1952.

NURSE PRACTITIONERS AND CLINICAL SPECIALISTS

2779.   Abdellah, F. "Nursing Practitioners and Nursing Practice."
        Am J Pub Hlth, 66 (Mar 1976), 245-246.

2780.   Agree, Betty C. "Beginning an Independent Nursing Practice."
        Am J Nurs, 74 (Apr 1974), 636-642.

2781.   American Medical Association. Committee on Nursing. "Medi-
        cine and Nursing in the 1970s: A Position Statement." *J
        Am Med Assoc* (14 Sep 1970), 1881-1883.

2782.   American Nurses' Association. Health Nursing Practice Divi-
        sion and American Academy of Pediatrics. "Guidelines on
        Short-term Continuing Education Programs for Pediatric
        Nurse Associates." *Am J Nurs*, 71 (Mar 1971), 509-512.

2783.   Andrews, Priscilla, and Alfred Yankquer. "The Pediatric
        Nurse Practitioner; Growth of the Concept." *Am J Nurs*, 71
        (Mar 1971), 505-506.

2784.   Bates, Barbara. "Twelve Paradoxes: A Message for Nurse Prac-
        titioners." *Nurs Out*, 22 (Nov 1974), 686-688.

2785.   Bergman, Abraham, D. "Physicians' Assistants Belong in the
        Nursing Profession." *Am J Nurs*, 71 (May 1971), 975-977.

2786.   Berwind, Anita. "The Nurse in the Coronary Care Unit." *In
        the Law and the Expanding Nursing Role.* Edited by B. Bul-
        lough. New York: Appleton-Century-Crofts, 1975. pp. 82-95.

2787.   Browning, Mary H., and Edith Lewis. *Expanded Role of the
        Nurse.* New York: American Journal Nursing Co., 1973.

2788.   Bullough, Bonnie. "Barriers to the Nurse Practitioner Move-
        ment: Problems of Women in a Woman's Field." *Int J Hlth
        Serv,* 5(2) (1975), 225-233.

2789.   ————. "Influences on Role Expansion." *Am J Nurs,* 76
        (Sep 1976), 1476-1481.

2790.   Committee on Nursing. "Medicine and Nursing in the 1970s: A
        Position Statement." *J Am Med Assoc,* 21 (14 Sep 1970),
        1881-1883.

2791.   "Executive Board Initiates Child Health Manpower Training
        Program in a Major Effort to Improve Pediatric Care."
        Newsletter Am Acad Peds, 20 (1 Jul 1969), 1, 4.

2792.   "The Expanded Role of the Nurse: A Joint Statement of CNA/
        CMA." *Canad Nurs* (May 1973), 23-25.

2793.   *Extending the Scope of Nursing Practice: A Report of the
        Secretary's Committee to Study Extended Roles for Nurses,
        Nov. 1971.* Washington, D.C.: U.S. Government Printing
        Office, 1971. Dept. of HEW.

2794.   Farrisey, Ruth M. "How the Pediatric Nurse Associate Move-
        ment Began." *Child Health Care in the '70s: Eastern
        Regional Workshop on Pediatric Nurse Associate Programs.*
        New York: American Nurses Association and American Academy
        of Pediatrics, 1972.

2795.   Ferguson, Marion C. "Nursing at the Crossroads: Which Way to
        Turn, A Look at the Model of the Nurse Practitioner." *J
        Adv Nurs,* 1 (May 1976), 237-242.

2796.   Georgopoulas, Basil S., and Luther Christman. "The Clinical
        Nurse Specialist: A Role Model." *The Clinical Nurse
        Specialist; Interpretations.* Edited by Joan Riehl and Joan
        Wilcox McVay. New York: Appleton-Century-Crofts, 1973.

2797.   Hoekelman, Robert A. "Evaluating the Pediatric Nurse
        Associate." *Child Health Care in the '70s: Eastern
        Regional Workshop on Pediatric Nurse Associate Programs.*
        New York: American Nurses Association and American Academy
        of Pediatrics, 1972.

2798.   "An Interview with Dr. Loretta Ford." *Nurs Pract,* 1 (Sep
        Oct 1974), 9-12.

2799.   Kinlein, Lucille M. *Independent Nursing Practice with Clients*.
        Philadelphia: J.B. Lippincott, 1977.

2800.   ———. "Independent Nurse Practitioner." *Nurs Out*, 20
        (Jan 1972), 22-24.

2801.   Leininger, Madeleine. "An Open Health Care System Model."
        Nurs Out, 21 (Mar 1973), 171-174.

2802.   Longest, Virginia B. "Expanded Roles for Veterans Adminis-
        tration Nurses." *Am J Nurs*, 73 (Dec 1973), 2087-2089.

2803.   Lynaugh, Jean E., and Barbara Bates. "Physical Diagnosis a
        Skill for All Nurses?" *Am J Nurs*, 74 (Jan 1974), 58-59.

2804.   McGivern, Diane. "Baccalaureate Preparation of the Nurse
        Practitioner." *Nurs Out*, 22 (Feb 1974), 94-98.

2805.   Mauksch, Ingeborg C., and Martha Rogers. "Nursing is Coming
        of Age Through the Practitioner Movement." *Am J Nurs*, 75
        (Oct 1975), 1834-1843.

2806.   Morgan, D. "The Future Expanded Role of the Nurse." *Canad
        Hosp*, 75 (May 1972).

2807.   National Health and Welfare, Ministry of. National Conference
        on Assistance to the Physician. *The Complementary Roles of
        the Physician and the Nurse*. Ottawa: National Health and
        Welfare Ministry, 1972.

2808.   Noonan, Barbara R. "Eight Years in a Medical Nurse Clinic."
        Am J Nurs, 72 (Jun 1972), 1128-1130.

2809.   Riehl, Joan P., and Joan Wilcox McVay, eds. *The Clinical
        Nurse Specialist: Interpretations*. New York: Appleton-
        Century-Crofts, 1973.

2810.   Roemer, Ruth. "Nursing Functions and the Law: Some Perspec-
        tives from Australia and Canada." *The Law and The Expand-
        ing Nursing Role*. Edited by Bonnie Bullough. New York:
        Appleton-Century-Crofts, 1975.

2811.   Rogers, Martha E. "Nursing: To Be or Not To Be?" *Nurs Out*,
        20 (Jan 1972), 42-46.

2812.   Ross, W.F. "The Advanced Clinical Nurse and the Health Team."
        Cen Afr J Med, 21 (1975), 243-245.

2813.   Sackett, David L., et al. "The Burlington Randomized Trial
        of the Nurse Practitioner: Health Outcomes of Patients."
        Ann Int Med, 80 (Feb 1974), 137-142.

2814.   Schutt, Barbara G. "Frontier's Family Nurses." *Am J Nurs*,
        72 (May 1972), 903-909.

2815.   ———. "Spot Check on Primary Care Nursing." *Am J Nurs*, 72
        (Nov 1972), 1996-2003.

2816. Siegel, Earl, and Sylvia L. Bryson. "Redefinition of the Role of the Public Health Nurse in Child Health Supervision." *Am J Pub Hlth*, 53 (Jul 1963), 1015-1024.

2817. Silver, Henry, and Loretta Ford. "The Pediatric Nurse Practitioner at Colorado." *Am J Nurs*, 67 (Jul 1967), 1443-1444.

2818. Silver, Henry, Loretta Ford, and Susan Stearly. "A Program to Increase Health Care for Children: The Pediatric Nurse Practitioner Program." *Peds*, 39 (May 1967), 756-760.

2819. Smoyak, Shirley. "Specialization in Nursing: From Then to Now." *Nurs Out*, 24 (Nov 1976), 676-681.

2820. Stead, E.A., Jr. "Training and Use of Paramedical Personnel." *New England J Med*, 277 (12 Oct 1967), 800-801.

2821. Stoeckle, John D., Barbara Noonan, Ruth M. Farrisey, and Anne Sweatt. "Medical Nursing Clinic for the Chronically Ill." *Am J Nurs*, 63 (Jul 1963), 87-89.

2822. Sultz, Harry, Maria Zillezny, and Louis Kenyon. *Longitudinal Study of Nurse Practitioners: Phase I.* Washington, D.C.: U.S. Government Printing Office, 1976.

2823. Sultz, Harry A., O. Marie Henry, and Judith A. Sullivan. *Nurse Practitioner: USA.* Lexington, MA: D.C. Heath & Co., 1979.

2824. Weiler, P.G. "Health Manpower Dialectic--Physician, Nurse, Physician Assistant." *Am J Pub Hlth*, 65(8) (Aug 1975), 858-863.

2825. Willian, Mary Kay. "An Historical Perspective: The Pediatric Nurse Associate." *Ped Nurs*, 5 (Mar-Apr 1979), 2.

OCCUPATIONAL AND INDUSTRIAL NURSING

2826. Arms, F.C. "The First Industrial Nurse in the U.S. Was a Vermonter." *Am Assoc Ind Nurs J* (Oct 1962), 20.

2827. Bannister, Lucy A. "A New Field: The Nurse's Opportunity in Factory Work." *Fourteenth Annual Report of the American Society of Superintendents of Training Schools for Nurses.* New York, 1908. p. 104.

2828. Bauer, W.W. "The Nurse in Industry." *Am J Pub Hlth*, 22 (Aug 1932), 875-876.

2829. Bower, C. Ruth. "Caroline Pilcher." *Am J Nurs*, 35 (Mar 1935), 217-221.

2830. Bristol, Leverett Dale. "Industrial Nurses--Their Value to
       the Safety Movement." *Ind Med*, 4 (Jun 1935), 306-308.

2831. Charley, Irene H. *The Birth of Industrial Nursing*. London:
       Bailliere, 1954. 224 pp.

2832. ————. "Industrial Nursing." *Nurs Mirror*, 56 (19 Nov 1932),
       152; see also *Aust Nurs J*, 36 (Jan 1938), 17-20; *Cath Nurs*
       (London), 4 (Aug 1931), 269-271.

2833. ————. "The Place of the Nurse in Industry in Great Britain."
       *Section II of International Council of Nurses: Congress
       Papers. Eighth Quadrennial Congress, London, 1937*. London:
       The Council, 1937. 201 pp.

2834. Cross, M.B. "Remember Nursing Back When?" *Occup Hlth Nurs*
       (New York), 17 (Aug 1969), 21-22.

2835. "The Development of Industrial Nursing." *New Zeal Nurs J*, 41
       (Apr 1948), 55-58.

2836. "The First Factory Nurse." *Nurs Mirror*, 63 (11 Apr 1936),
       31.

2837. Hamilton, Alice. "Looking at Industrial Nursing." *Pub Hlth
       Nurs*, 38 (Feb 1946), 63-65.

2838. Holmes, Katherine M. *History of Industrial Nursing Up To
       Date*. Detroit, Mich.: n.p., 1931. 39 pp.

2839. "Industrial Nurses' Clubs." *Tr Nurs & Hosp Rev*, 107 (1941),
       191-192, 274-276.

2840. King, J.D. "The Industrial Nurse in Relation to Public
       Health." *Pub Hlth Nurs*, 11 (1919), 100.

2841. Lambie, Mary I. "The Development of Industrial Nursing."
       *International Council of Nurses: Congress Papers, Ninth
       Congress, Atlantic City, N.J., 1947*. London: The Council,
       1947. pp. 29-36.

2842. Lazenby, A.D. "The Place of the Nurse in Industry." *Pub
       Hlth Nurs*, 28 (Nov 1936), 713-718.

2843. Marino, R.A. "AAIN Salute to Bicentennial 1776-1976."
       Occup Hlth Nurs (New York), 23(9) (Sep 1975), 23.

2844. Markolf, Ada Stewart. "Industrial Nursing Begins in Vermont."
       Pub Hlth Nurs, 37 (Mar 1945), 125-129.

2845. McGrath, Bethel J. "Fifth Years of Industrial Nursing in
       the United States." *Pub Hlth Nurs*, 27 (Mar 1945), 119-123.

2846. ————. *Nursing in Commerce and Industry*. New York: Common-
       wealth Fund, 1946.

2847. Newquist, Melvin N. "Industrial Nursing--Past, Present and Future." *Pub Hlth Nurs*, 31 (Mar 1939), 162-166.

2848. Obuchowski, M., comp. *The Industrial Nurse in New England from the Horse and Buggy Days to the Atomic Age.* New England Association of Industrial Nurses, 1963.

2849. Owen, M.E. "Industrial Nursing During the First World War." *Nurs Mirror*, 115 (16 Nov 1962), xiff.

2850. Stricker, F. "Early Industrial Nursing in South Carolina." *Ind Nurs*, 7(7) (1948), 23.

2851. "A Study of Industrial Nursing Services." *Pub Hlth Nurs*, 32 (Oct 1940), 631-636.

2852. Thwing, Mary Dunning. "Factory Nursing." *Pub Hlth Nurs*, 5 (Apr 1913), 28-34.

2853. Waters, Yssabella. "Industrial Nursing." *Pub Hlth Nurs*, 11 (Sep 1919), 728-731.

2854. Watson, E. "Industrial Nursing." *Am Assoc Industr Nurs J*, 12 (Mar 1964), 16ff.

2855. Williams, M.M. "The Third Decade." *Occup Hlth* (London), 26 (Jan 1974), 10-15.

2856. Woodard, E. "Industrial Nursing in South Carolina: Its History and Growth." *Am Assoc Industr Nurs J*, 13 (Jun 1965), 29.

OPERATING ROOM NURSING

2857. Bullough, Vern, and Bonnie Bullough. "How Rough Red Hands Led to Rubber Gloves." *Am J Nurs*, 70 (Apr 1970), 777.

2858. James, T.G. "Surgical Nursing Through the Ages." *Nurs Mirror*, 94 (12 Oct 1951), vi-vii; (19 Oct 1951), 49-50.

2859. Laufman, Harold. "What's Happened to the Good Old OR Nurse." *AORN J*, 17 (Mar 1973), 61-70.

2860. Nicolo, S. "O.R. Nursing in Greece." *AORN J*, 19 (1974), 114-120.

2861. St. Mary's Hospital, Rochester, Minn. *The Operating Room: Instructions for Nurses and Assistants, St. Mary's Hospital.* Philadelphia: W.B. Saunders, 1924. 165 pp.

PEDIATRIC NURSING

2862.   "Activities of the 'Oeuvre Nationale de L'Enfance' (National
        Child Welfare Organization, Belgium)." *Queen's Nurs Mag*,
        25 (Dec 1932), 298-299.

2863.   Baker, S. Josephine. *Child Hygiene*. New York: Harper &
        Brothers, 1925.

2864.   ———. "Reduction of Infant Mortality in New York City."
        Am J Dis Child, 5 (Feb 1913), 151-161.

2865.   Evans, P.R. "A Hundred Years of Children's Hospitals: The
        Centenary of the Evelina Hospital for Sick Children."
        Proceedings Roy Soc Med, 63 (Jan 1970), 44-46.

2866.   Frankel, Lee K. *The Present Status of Maternal and Infant
        Hygiene in the United States*. New York: Metropolitan Life
        Insurance Co., 1927.

2867.   Goostray, Stella. "Pediatric Nursing at the Turn of the
        Century." *Am J Nurs*, 50 (Oct 1950), 624-625.

2868.   Hara, R. "20 Years of Pediatric Nursing at the Kiyose
        Children's Hospital Tokyo." *Jap J Nurs*, 31 (Jan 1967),
        34-37. (Jap)

2869.   "Have Times Changed? *The Nursing Mirror*; August 4, 1906.
        Training for Children's Nurses." *Nurs Mirror*, 141(14)
        (2 Oct 1975), 73.

2870.   Number deleted.

2871.   King-Hall, Magdalen. *The Story of the Nursery*. London:
        Routledge & Kegan Paul, 1958.

2872.   Moriyama, T.M. "Present Status of the Infant Mortality
        Problem in the United States." *Am J Pub Hlth*, 56 (Apr
        1966), 623-625.

2873.   Pearce, Evelyn Clare. "Nursing Care of Sick Children."
        Nurs Mirror, 77 (2 Oct 1943), 4.

2874.   Reese, D. Meredith. "Report on Infant Mortality in Large
        Cities, The Sources of Its Increase, and Means for Its
        Diminution." *Trans Am Med Assoc*, 10 (1857), 93-107.

2875.   Tsuneha, K. "Past and Present of Pediatric Nursing."
        Jap J Nurs, 39(9) (Sep 1975), 880-883. (Jap)

2876.   Van Ingen, Philip. "Child Health in the Past." *Am J Dis
        Child*, 34 (Jul 1927), 95-102.

2877.   West, Charles. *How to Nurse Sick Children*. London: Longman,
        Brown, Queen, & Longman, 1854. 79 pp. There was also a
        facsimile reprint, n.d.

2878.   *White House Conference on Child Health and Protection.*
        Washington, D.C.: U.S. Government Printing Office, 1930.

2879.   White House Conference on the Care of Dependent Children.
        Proceedings of the Conference Held at Washington, D.C.,
        January 25, 26, 1909. Washington, D.C.: U.S. Government
        Printing Office, 1909.

2880.   Wood, Catherine Jane. *A Handbook for Nursing Sick Children.*
        4th ed. London: Cassell, 1882; also London: Cassell, 1889.

PRIVATE DUTY NURSING

2881.   An American Woman. *Suggestions for the Sick-Room.* New York:
        Anson: D.F. Randolph & Co., 1876.

2882.   Boswall, Emily Oatway. "Development of Private Duty Nursing."
        Am J Nurs, 25 (Oct 1925), 848–850.

2883.   DeWitt, Katherine. *Private Duty Nursing.* Philadelphia:
        J.B. Lippincott Co., 1917.

2884.   Francis, Susan C. "The Private Duty Nurse in a New Era."
        Am J Nurs, 36 (Aug 1936), 773–777.

2885.   Geister, Janet M. "Hearsay and Facts in Private Duty."
        Am J Nurs, 26 (Jul 1926), 515–528.

2886.   ————. "More About General Duty." *Tr Nurs & Hosp Rev*,
        107 (1941), 346.

2887.   Maxwell, Anna C., and Mary L. Keith. "The Private Nurse and
        Twenty-four Hour Hospital Duty." *Am J Nurs*, 17 (1916), 191.

2888.   Ott, F.M. "Private Duty, Past and Present: Progress of 40
        Years." *Tr Nurs*, 80 (Jun 1928), 696–699.

2889.   Ross, Margaret. *Memoirs of a Private Nurse.* Glasgow:
        M'Naughton & Sinclair, 1928. 212 pp.

2890.   Stephen, Julia Prinsep (Mrs. Leslie). *Notes from Sick Rooms.*
        London: Smith, Elder & Co., 1883. 52 pp.

PSYCHIATRIC AND MENTAL HEALTH NURSING

2891.   Baird, Harriet H. "The Nursing and Care of the Insane."
        Tr Nurs, 36 (May 1906), 275–277.

2892.   Barrus, Clara. *Nursing the Insane.* New York: Macmillan Co.,
        1908.

2893.   Bennett, A.E., A.B. Purdy, and H.M. Jordan. "The History and
        Development of Modern Psychiatric Nursing." *Dis Nerv Syst*,
        1 (Sep 1940), 265-272.

2894.   Campbell, Robert Brown. "The Development of the Care of the
        Insane in Scotland." *J Ment Sci*, 78 (Oct 1932), 774-792.

2895.   Carini, Esta, Dorothy M. Douglas, Louis D. Heck, and Margue-
        rite Pearson. *The Mentally Ill in Connecticut: Changing
        Patterns of Care and the Evolution of Psychiatric Nursing:
        1936-1972.* Hartford, CT: Connecticut Dept. of Mental
        Health, 1974. 554 pp.

2896.   "A Century of Mental Nursing at Central Hospital (Hatton)
        Near Warwick (England)." *Nurs Mirror*, 95 (27 Jun 1952).

2897.   Clayton, Bonnie Clare Wilmot. *Historical Perspectives of
        Psychiatric Nursing in Higher Education.* Ph.D. disserta-
        tion, University of Utah, 1976.

2898.-
 2899. Numbers deleted.

2900.   Corcoran, M.E. "Review of Psychitric Progress: Psychiatric
        Nursing." *Am J Psychiat*, 105 (Jan 1949), 534-535.

2901.   Deutsch, Albert. "Life and Work of Dorothea Lynde Dix."
        Am J Nurs, 36 (Oct 1936), 987-997.

2902.   ————. *Mentally Ill in America: A History of Their Care and
        Treatment from Colonial Times.* New York: Doubleday, 1937.

2903.   Foote, John. "The Development of the Nursing Care of the
        Insane." *Tr Nurs*, 63 (Dec 1919), 401-403.

2904.   Frey, Lavonne M. "The Scope of Psychiatric Nursing Today."
        Nurs Out, 3 (Mar 1955), 152-155.

2905.   Goddard, D.L. "This History of Mental Nursing." *Brit J Nurs*,
        100 (Nov 1952), 106-107; 100 (19 Dec 1952), 121; 101 (Jun
        1953), 54-56; 77 (Jul 1953), 88-89; 77 (Oct 1953), 118-119;
        103 (Nov 1953), 130-131; 103 (May 1955), 46-48; 103 (Jun
        1955), 58-59.

2906.   ————. "Mental Nursing in U.S.A. and Russia." *Brit J Nurs*,
        102 (May 1954), 50-52.

2907.   Greene, B. "The Rise and Fall of the Asylum Workers' Assoc-
        iation." *Nurs Mirror*, 141 (26) (Dec 1975), 53-55.

2908.   Grob, G.N. *The State and the Mentally Ill: A History of the
        Worcester State Hospital in Massachusetts, 1830-1920.*
        Chapel Hill: University of North Carolina Press, 1966.

2909.   Harding, William. *Mental Nursing.* London: Scientific Press,
        1893. 131 pp.

2910. Hartman, C.R. "The Role Fusion of Psychiatric Nursing with Psychiatry." *Psychiat Opin*, 7 (Oct 1971), 7.

2911. Henry, George W. "The Care and Treatment of Mental Disease-- Yesterday and Today." *Mod Hosp*, 33 (Nov 1929), 49-54.

2912. Houliston, M. "Centenary of Mental Nurse Training." *Nurs Mirror*, 99 (17 Sep 1954), ii-iv.

2913. Hunter, P. "Community Psychiatric Nursing in Britain: An Historical Review." *Int J Nurs Studies*, 11(4) (Dec 1974), 223-233.

2914. Hunter, R.A. "In the Mental Hospital. The Rise and Fall of Mental Nursing." *Lancet* (14 Jan 1956), 98-99.

2915. Jones, K. *Lunacy, Law and Conscience, 1744-1845: The Social History of the Care of the Insane.* London: Routledge & Kegan Paul, 1955.

2916. Kiev, Ari, ed. *Magic, Faith and Healing: Studies in Primitive Psychiatry Today.* New York: The Free Press of Glencoe, 1964.

2917. Kukla, Rainer. "Zur Sozialisation von Krankenschwestern in der Psychiatrie" (On the Socialization of Nurses in Psychiatry). *Kölner Zeitschrift für Soziologie und Sozialpsychologie*, 25 (June), 484-498. (Ger)

2918. Laird, Donald A. "Psychopathic Nursing." *Am J Nurs*, 20 (Jun 1920), 85-89.

2919. Lee, L. "P.N.A.C.--Twenty-two Years of Progress." *Canad J Psychiatr Nurs*, 13 (Mar-Apr 1972), 8-11.

2920. Leninger, Model M. *Contemporary Issues in Mental Health Nursing.* Boston: Little, Brown & Co., 1973.

2921. MacAulay, Elizabeth L. "The Evolution of Mental Nursing." *Section II of International Council of Nurses: Congress Papers. Eighth Quadrennial Congress, London, 1937.* London: International Council of Nurses, 1937. 201 pp.

2922. McKinnon, Mary. "Psychiatric Nursing." *Tr Nurs*, 81 (Jul 1928), 80-82. Reprinted in *O J Chin Nurs*, 10 (Apr 1929), 6-11.

2923. Maier, S. "Psychiatric Nursing 70 Years Ago." *Z Krankepflege*, 11 (May 1967), 199-202. (Ger)

2924. "Mental Care Through Six Centuries." (Report Based on Document Issued by the Ministry of Health, 1949, London, HMSO). *Nurs Mirror*, 94 (7 Jul 1950), 261.

2925. "Mile Posts." *Tr Nurs & Hosp Rev*, 116 (May 1964), 353.

2926.   Mills, Charles K. *Nursing and Care of the Nervous and the Insane*. Philadelphia: J.B. Lippincott, 1887, 1904, 1915.

2927.   Mitchell, A. "Unique Mental Hospital in the Middle West." *Nurs Mirror*, 99 (23 Apr 1954), viii-ix.

2928.   Mitchell, W.T.B. "Mental Hygiene." *Canad Nurs*, 27 (Mar 1931), 120-124.

2928.1 National League for Nursing, Conference Proceedings (1957). *Concepts of the Behavioral Sciences in Basic Nursing Education*. New York: The League, 1958. 357 pp.

2928.2 National League for Nursing, Conference Proceedings (1959). *Psychiatric Nursing Concepts and Basic Nursing Education*. New York: The League, 1960. 151 pp.

2929.   Nelson, Jill K., and Dianne A. Schilke. "The Evolution of Psychiatric Liaison Nursing." *Perspectives in Psychiatric Care*, 4(2) (Apr-May-Jun 1976), 60-65.

2930.   Neuman-Rahn, Karin. *A Short Account of the Care of the Insane in Finland*. Helsingfor: Osakeyhtio Weilin & Goos Aktiebulag, 1925. 7 pp.

2931.   Patch, C.J. Lodge. "A Century of Psychiatry in the Punjab (India)." *J Ment Sci*, 85 (May 1939), 25-91.

2932.   Pinel, Philippe. *A Treatise on Insanity*. Translated by D.D. Davis. New York: Hafner, 1962.

2933.   Reilly, Grace L. "Psychiatry Through the Ages." *Tr Nurs*, 72 (Mar 1924), 229-233.

2934.   Rosen, George. *Madness in Society*. Chicago: University of Chicago Press, 1968.

2935.   Russell, William Logie. *The New York Hospital--A History of the Psychiatric Service, 1771-1936*. New York: Columbia University Press, 1945.

2936.   Santos, Elvin H., and Edward Stainbrook. "A History of Psychiatric Nursing in the Nineteenth Century." *J Hist Med*, 4 (Winter 1949), 48-74.

2937.   Smith, Philip. "Nursing Homes for Medical Patients." *Psychiat Q*, 7 (Oct 1933), 682-690.

2938.   Stevens, L.F., and D.D. Henrie. "A History of Psychiatric Nursing." *Bull Menninger Clin*, 30 (Jan 1966), 32-38.

2939.   Stills, Grayce M. "Historical Developments in Psychiatric and Mental Health Nursing." *Contemporary Issues in Mental Health Nursing*. Edited by Madelaine Leininger. Boston: Little, Brown & Co., 1973.

2940. Szasz, Thomas. *The Age of Madness*. New York: Jason Aronson, 1974.

2941. Tayona, S. "A Brief History of Psychiatric Nursing in the Philippines." *Phlp J Nurs* (Jan-Feb 1964), 12-22, 32.

2942. "Treatment of Mental Illness in the Middle Ages." *Nurs Mirror*, 98 (29 Jan 1954), v.

2943. Urano, S. "A Chronological Table of Psychiatric Nursing in Japan." *Kango*, 18 (1966), 99-110.

2944. Waek, A. "This History of Mental Nursing." *J Ment Sci*, 107 (Jan 1961), 1-17.

PUBLIC HEALTH NURSING

2945. Allen, M.H. "Victorian Order of Nurses for Canada." *Charities and the Commons*, 16 (7 Apr 1906), 19-21.

2946. Anderson, Genevieve. "An Experiment of the 1850's." *Am J Nurs*, 49 (Nov 1949), 717.

2947. ————. "An Oversight in Nursing History." *J Hist Med* (Summer 1948), 417-426.

2948. Andrews (nfn). "History and Development of the Ranyard Nurses, Nursing Branch of the London Biblewomen and Nurses Mission, 25 Russell Square, London, W.C." In *Report and Proceedings of the Jubilee Congress of District Nursing Held at Liverpool, 12-14 May 1909*. Liverpool: D. Marples & Co., 1898.

2949. Ashe, E. "Nurses' Settlements in San Francisco." *Charities and the Commons*, 16 (7 Apr 1906), 45-47.

2950. Axelsson, S., and U. Nicolausson. "Community Health Nursing --Farthest Outpost of the Health and Medical Service." *Cur Swed*, 144 (1977), 1-7.

2951. Barton, Eleanor C. "The Evolution of Poor Law Nursing." *Brit J Nurs* (23 Aug 1913), 149-151; (30 Aug 1913), 170-171.

2952. ————. *The History and Progress of Poor Law Nursing*. London: Law and Local Government Publications, Ltd., 1926.

2953. Bennett, Victoria. "Health Services of the London County Council." *Cath Nurs* (London), 5 (Aug 1937), 10.

2954. Bigelow, Helen A. "Maternity Care in Rural Areas by Public Health Nurses." *Am J Pub Hlth*, 27 (Oct 1937), 975-980.

2955.   Bodley (nfn). "State Aid for Poor Law Nurses." *Brit J Nurs*
        (Jan 1912), 25-26.

2956.   Boorer, D. "The District Nurse" (pictorial). *Nurs Times*, 61
        (14 May 1965), 669ff.

2957.   Bower, Irene M. *Public Health Nursing in Cleveland (Ohio),*
        1895-1928. Cleveland: Western Reserve University, 1930.
        120 pp.

2958.   Bowman, J. Beatrice. "Public Health Nursing in the Navy."
        Am J Pub Hlth, 17 (May 1927), 541-542.

2959.   Brainard, Annie M. *The Evolution of Public Health Nursing.*
        Philadelphia: W.B. Saunders, 1922. 454 pp.

2960.   "Brainard, Annie M." *Pub Hlth Nurs*, 34 (Jun 1942), 322-324.

2961.   "The British Nursing Sisters Institution." *Mid Chron & Nurs*
        Notes, 44 (Nov 1931), 170.

2962.   Butler, Elsa M. "The Polish Grey Samaritans." *Pub Hlth Nurs*
        (Cleveland), (1919), xi, 55-58.

2963.   Calder, J.M. "The Health Visitor--Past, Present and Future."
        Nurs Times, 43 (3 May 1947), 288-290.

2964.   Cardwell, V. "Public Health Nursing in Lebanon." *Pub Hlth*
        Nurs, 35 (1943), 430-434.

2965.   Carson, Agnes Douglas. "First District Nursing in Saint
        John, N.B. (Can.)." *Canad Nurs*, 27 (Jun 1931), 313-314.

2966.   Central Council for District Nursing in London. *History of*
        the Central Council for District Nursing in London 1914-
        1966. London: Central Council for District Nursing, 1966.
        15 pp.

2967.   "Childbed Fever." *Pub Hlth Nurs*, 35 (May 1943), 272.

2968.   Clement, F.F. "District Nurse in Rural Work." *National*
        Conference on Char. and Correc., Proceedings (1914), 279-
        288.

2969.   Codman, K.B. "District Nursing After the Chelsea Fire."
        Charities & the Commons, 32 (13 Feb 1909), 970-973.

2970.   Colton, Olive A. "This District Nurse of Yesterday and of
        Today." *Survey*, 32 (18 Jul 1914), 414-415.

2971.   Comstock, S. "Home Nurse Militant." *Good Housekeeping*, 61
        (Sep 1915), 280-288; 61 (Oct 1915), 421-429; 61 (Nov 1915),
        588-596.

2972.   Cope, Zachary. "Florence Nightingale and District Nursing."
        Dist Nurs (Nov 1958), 179-180.

2973. Cowen, E. "Algeria--Public Health Nursing in an Emergent State." *Nurs Mirror*, 136 (16 Mar 1973), 33-35.

2974. Crandall, Ella Philips. "An Historical Sketch of Public Health Nursing." *Am J Nurs*, 22 (May 1922), 641-645.

2975. Crockett, Bernice Norman. *The Origin and Development of Public Health in Oklahoma, 1830-1930*. Ph.D. dissertation, University of Oklahoma, 1953. 481 pp.

2976. Cullingworth, C.J. "Sick Nursing Amongst the Poor." *Hlth Lect* (London), (1880-1881), iv, 43-58.

2977. Davis, Maxine. "The Woman in Blue: The Public Health Nurse in Rural Areas." *Survey Graphic*, 27 (Oct 1938), 508-510.

2978. Deming, Dorothy. "Milestones of the Past 15 Years in Public Health Nursing." *Am J Pub Hlth*, 29 (Feb 1939), 128-134.

2979. Dening, F.C. "Another Jubilee/Public Health Nursing." *Nurs Times*, 73 (1977), 1384-1386.

2980. Depass, B. "Public Health Nursing." *J Pract Nurs*, 13 (May 1963), 24ff.

2981. "District Nursing." *Hosp* (London), 64 (8 Jun 1918), 209; 64 (22 Jun 1918), 255; 64 (29 Jun 1918), 285; 66 (31 May 1919), 228.

2982. "District Nursing in Westchester County, New York." *Vist Nurs Q*, 4 (Oct 1912), 55-57.

2983. Dock, Lavinia L. "The History of Public Health Nursing." *Pub Hlth Nurs*, 14 (Oct 1922), 522-526; (Nov 1922), 590-593.

2984. Donnan, S.G. "Looking Back. Early Experiences of a Health Visitor." *So Afr Nurs J* (Nov 1963), 13, 16.

2985. Dowling, W.C. "Health Visiting--Latter Days." *Hlth Visit*, 46(12) (Dec 1973), 410-413.

2986. Doyle, Ann. "Development of Federal Public Health Functions in the United States." *Pub Hlth Nurs*, 12 (Sep 1920), 723-727; (Oct 1920), 876-883.

2987. Drinker, Cecil K. "Problems and Progress in Public Health." *Pub Hlth Nurs*, 28 (Jan 1936), 10-14.

2988. Duffy, John. *A History of Public Health in New York City, 1866-1966*. New York: Russell Sage Foundation, 1974.

2989. Dunham, George C. "Community Public Health Nursing in the Philippine Islands." *Am J Pub Hlth*, 26 (Aug 1936), 771-777.

2990. Durgan, I. "Early Days in Nursing." *Pub Hlth Nurs*, 39 (Jun 1947), 289-293.

2991.   Eastwood, Cyril G. "The Public Health Service; Its History
        and Work." *Nurs Mirror*, 101 (10 Jun 1955), 721-722; 101
        (17 Jun 1955), 794-800; 101 (24 Jun 1955), xiii-xiv; 101
        (1 Jul 1955), v-vi; 101 (8 Jul 1955), vi-vii; 101 (15 Jul
        1955), x; 101 (22 Jul 1955), ii-iii, xii.

2992.   Ehrenfeld, Rose M. "The Evolution of the Public Health
        Nurse." *Am J Nurs*, 20 (Oct 1919), 14-18.

2993.   *Employment of Trained Nurses Among the Labouring Poor, Con-
        sidered in Relation to Sanitary Reform and the Arts of
        Life. By a Physician.* London: J. Churchill, 1860. 33 pp.

2994.   "The First Visiting Nurse in Boston." *Pub Hlth Nurs*, 43
        (May 1951), 294.

2995.   Fitzpatrick, M. Louise. *National Organization for Public
        Health Nursing 1912-1952: Development of a Practice Field.*
        Ph.D. dissertation, Columbia University, 1972; New York:
        National League for Nursing, 1975.

2996.   Fox, Elizabeth Gordon. "The Past Challenges the Future."
        Pub Hlth Nurs, 29 (May 1937), 275-279.

2997.   ————, et al. "Twenty Years of Red Cross Public Health
        Nursing." *Red Cr Courier*, 12 (Dec 1932), 173-177.

2998.   Fulmer, Harriet. "History of Visiting Nurse Work in America."
        Am J Nurs, 2 (Mar 1902), 411-425.

2999.   ————. "History of Visiting Nurses in America." Inter-
        national Council of Nurses. *Third International Congress
        of Nurses. (Buffalo, N.Y., Sept. 18-21, 1901).* Cleveland:
        J.B. Savage, 1901. 488 pp.

3000.   ————. "History of Visiting Nurses in America." *Nurs Rep*
        (21 Jun 1902), 496-498; (28 Jun 1902), 515.

3001.   ————. "Visiting Nurse in a Great City: A Short History of
        the Visiting Nurse Association of Chicago." *Charities*, 16
        (1906), 22.

3002.   Furman, B. *A Profile of the United States Public Health
        Service, 1798-1948.* Washington, D.C.: U.S. Government
        Printing Office, 1973.

3003.   Galdston, Iago. "Effects of Medical Advances on Nursing.
        Recent Advances in Medicine and the Development of Personal
        Preventive Medicine Imply Changes in Functions of the
        Public Health Nurse." *Pub Hlth Nurs*, 32 (1940), 352-359.

3004.   Gamble, L.A. "Should Public Health Nurses Give Much Bedside
        Care?" *Nation's Hlth*, 9 (1927), 11.

3005.   Gardner, Mary S. *Public Health Nursing.* 3rd ed. New York:
        Macmillan Co., 1936.

3006.   Green, Howard Whipple. *Time Study of the Cleveland Visiting Nurse Association.* Cleveland: Cleveland Health Council, 1938.

3007.   Greenwood, F.J.L. "The Evolution of the Health Visitor." *Nurs Times* (10 Feb 1917), 160-163; (17 Feb 1917), 186-188.

3008.   Haggard, Howard W. "Who Owns Health?" *Pub Hlth Nurs*, 28 (Apr 1936), 214-221.

3009.   Haig, Rena. *The Development of Nursing Under the California State Department of Public Health--A Short History.* New York: National League for Nursing, 1959.

3010.   Hardy, G., et al. "William Rathbone Staff College: Past, Present and Future." *Dist Nurs*, 15 (Sep 1972), 120-121.

3011.   Haupt, Alma C. "Forty Years of Teamwork in Public Health Nursing." *Am J Nurs*, 53 (Jan 1953), 81-84.

3012.   ————. "Thirty Years of Pioneering in Public Health Nursing." *Am J Nurs*, 39 (Jun 1939), 619-626.

3013.   Hawkyard, E.A. "On District Half-A-Century Ago." *Dist Nurs*, 13 (Mar 1971), 241.

3014.   "Health Visiting in the Early Days." *Nurs Mirror*, 66 (13 Nov 1937), 157-158.

3015.   Hentsch, Y. "The Student Nurse in the Community." *Canad Nurs*, 53 (Mar 1957), 205-207.

3016.   Hildreth, Peggy Bassett. "Early Red Cross: The Howard Association of New Orleans." *Louisiana Hist*, 20(1) (Winter 1979), 49-76.

3017.   Hill, Elma V. "Public Health Nursing." *Pac Cst J Nurs*, 22 (May 1926), 267-268.

3018.   Hodkinson, L.J. "A City's Progress in Public Health." *Nurs Mirror*, 102 (13 Jan 1956), iii.

3019.   *Hospital Nurse: Memories.* Bristol: John Wright, 1910.

3020.   Hubbard, Ruth W. "Public Health Nursing--1900-1950." *Am J Nurs*, 50 (Oct 1950), 608-611.

3021.   Hughes, Amy. "The Origin, Growth, and Present Status of District Nursing in England." *International Council of Nurses: Third International Congress of Nurses (Buffalo, N.Y., Sept. 18-21, 1901).* Cleveland: J.B. Savage, 1901. pp. 217-228. See also *Am J Nurs*, 2 (Jan 1902), 337-345; *Aust Nurs J*, 8 (Jun 1910), 201-202.

3022.   ————. "The Origin, Growth and Present Status of District Nursing in England." *Nurs Rec*, 28 (10 May 1902), 370-372; (17 May 1902), 391-393.

3023.   ————. "History of District Nursing in England and Other
          Countries." In *Report and Proceedings of the Jubilee Con-
          gress of District Nursing Held at Liverpool, 12-14 May 1909.*
          Liverpool: Marples and Co., 1909.

3024.   ————. "Rise of District Nursing in England." *Charities &
          the Commons*, 16 (7 Apr 1906), 13-16.

3025.   Jackson, E.M. "Future of District Nursing. Discussion."
          19th Cent, 102 (Oct 1927), 494-499; (Dec 1927), 865-870.

3026.   Johnson, Dorothy. "The Work of a District Nurse." *Nurs
          Notes*, 44 (May 1931), 70-72.

3027.   Jones, P.E. "Symposium on Community Nursing in Canada."
          Nurs Clin Nor Am, 10 (1975), 691-698.

3028.   Jubilee Congress of District Nursing. *Report and Proceedings
          of the Jubilee Congress of District Nursing Held at Liver-
          pool, 12-14 May 1909.* Liverpool: D. Marples & Co., 1909.

3029.   Junfrey, Marian. "The Monthly Nurse: Her Origin, Rise and
          Progress." *Nurs Rec* (21 May 1891), 267-272.

3030.   Kaneko, Mitsu. "Public Health Nursing in Japan." *Pub Hlth
          Nurs*, 42 (Feb 1950), 97-100.

3031.   Lent, Mary E. "This History and Development of Public Health
          Nursing." *Pac Cst J Nurs*, 13 (Mar 1917), 148-153.

3032.   ————. "Public Health Nursing and the War." Nat Conf Soc
          Work, *Proceedings* (1917), 214-218.

3033.   Lesson, Geoffrey. "District Nursing in Manchester Ninety
          Years Ago." *Nurs Times*, 53 (1957), 104-105.

3034.   Liverpool Queen Victoria District Nursing Association. *A
          Short History and Description of District Nursing in Liver-
          pool.* Liverpool: D. Marples & Co., 1898. 33 pp.

3035.   Livingston, M. Christine. "The Victorian Order of Nurses
          for Canada." *Nurs Out*, 6 (Jan 1958), 42-44.

3036.   London Biblewomen and Nurses Mission. "The District Nurses
          of the London Biblewomen and Nurses Mission." *Brit J Nurs*,
          (9 Jun 1906), 455-458.

3037.   McCloud, C. "District Nursing in Canada." *Am J Nurs*, 2
          (1901-1902), 503.

3038.   MacDougall, Eva. "Pioneering in Public Health Nursing in
          Italy." *Am J Pub Hlth*, 20 (Sep 1930), 1033-1034.

3039.   McIver, Pearl. "Analysis of the Present Qualifications of
          Public Health Nurses in the United States." *Am J Pub Hlth*,
          31 (Feb 1941), 151.

3040.　————. "Public Health Nursing Developments in the United States." *Int Nurs Rev*, 13 (Jul 1939), 217-225.

3041.　————. "Public Health Nursing in the United States Public Health Service." *Am J Nurs*, 40 (Sep 1940), 996-1000.

3042.　————. "Public Health Nursing Under the Social Security Act: Developments Under the U.S. Public Health Service." *Pub Hlth Nurs*, 28 (Sep 1936), 585-590.

3043.　————. "Trends in Public Health Nursing." *Am J Pub Hlth*, 25 (May 1935), 551-556.

3044.　McLure, R.E. "Education of Public Health Nursing Personnel." *Canad J Pub Hlth*, 57 (1966), 260-262.

3045.　MacMaster, Jennie. "Half a League Onward in Public Health Nursing." *Tr Nurs*, 100 (Apr 1938), 418-424.

3046.　Manchester District Nursing Service. "Centenary of District Nursing." *Manchester Nurs Times* (18 Dec 1964), 1667, 1670.

3047.　Martin, J. Middleton. "The District Nurse Grows Up." *Cath Nurs* (London), 1 (Jul 1933), 8-9.

3048.　Maternity Center Association. *Public Health Nurse in Obstetrics*. New York: Maternity Center Association, 1943.

3049.　"Metropolitan and National Association for Providing Trained Nurses for the Sick Poor." *Report of the Subcommittee of Reference and Enquiry*. London: Annual Report of the Metropolitan and Nat'l Assn., 1875.

3050.　Morris, Malcolm. *The Story of English Public Health*. London: Cassell, 1919. 165 pp.

3051.　National Organization for Public Health Nursing. *Manual of Public Health Nursing*. Prepared by NOPHN. New York: Macmillan Co., 1926.

3052.　Newsholme, Arthur. *Fifty Years in Public Health: A Personal Narrative with Comments*. London: G. Allen, 1935. 415 pp.

3053.　Nightingale, Florence. *Notes on Nursing for the Labouring Classes*. New ed. London: Harrison, 1876. 114 pp.

3054.　————. "Trained Nursing for the Sick Poor." *Int Nurs Rev*, 5 (Jul 1930), 426-433.

3055.　Norris, W. Perrin. "The Evolution of Hygiene and Public Health in Australia." *J Roy San Inst*, 36 (Jun 1915), 189-215.

3056.　"Notes on Nursing in Ireland." *Queen's Nurs Mag*, 25 (Sep 1932), 270.

3057.   "Nurse and Immigrant" (editorial). *Survey*, 35 (18 Dec 1915),
        334-335.

3058.   "Nursing and Community." *Korean Nurs*, 13 (Feb 1974), 9-15.

3059.   Parran, Thomas. "Public Health Nursing Marches On." *Pub
        Hlth Nurs*, 29 (Nov 1937), 617-622.

3060.   Paterson, Robert G. "Twenty Years of County Public Health
        Nursing in Ohio." *Pub Hlth Nurs*, 25 (Jun 1933), 329-332.

3061.   ————. "The Development of State Public Health Nursing."
        Pub Hlth Nurs Q, 8 (1916), 69.

3062.   Peterkin, A.M. "The Scope of Conditions of District Nursing."
        Pub Hlth Nurs, 25 (May 1931), 128-132.

3063.   Petry, Lucile. "One Hundred Fifty Years of Service." *Am J
        Nurs*, 48 (Jul 1948), 435.

3064.   Pierson, M.H. "Orange Visiting Nurses' Settlement."
        Charities & the Commons, 16 (7 Apr 1906), 48-51.

3065.   Porter, Charles. "Presidential Address." *J Roy San Inst*, 59
        (Jan 1939), 529-535.

3066.   "Public Health Nursing in California." *Pac Cst J Nurs*, 32
        (Jun 1936), 360-362, 365.

3067.   "Public Health Nurse--Or Health Visitor? Some Thoughts Aris-
        ing from Important Decisions in Eire." *Nurs Mirror*, 97
        (17 Apr 1953), 164.

3068.   "Queen Victoria's Jubilee Institute for Nurses Regulations
        as to the Training and Engagement of District Nurses for
        Sick Poor." *Nurs Rec* (24 Jul 1890), 44-45.

3069.   "Queen Victoria's Jubilee Institute for Nurses Statement as
        to the Past and Present Position of Queen Victoria's Jubilee
        Institute for Nurses." *Nurs Rec* (17 Jul 1890), 34-35.

3070.   Queen's Institute of District Nursing Survey of District
        Nursing in England and Wales. *Information Obtained and
        Compiled by the Queen's Institute of District Nursing.*
        London: The Institute, 1939.

3071.   Ramaiah, K. "Development of Public Health Nursing in India."
        Nurs J India, 57 (Aug 1966), 233-235, *passim*.

3072.   Randall, M.G. "Public Health Nursing Service for Rural
        Children." *Milbank Mem Fund Q*, 10 (1932), 276.

3073.   Rathbone, William. *Sketch of the History and Progress of
        District Nursing from Its Commencement in the Year 1859 to
        the Present Date.* New York: Macmillan Co., 1890.

3074. Ravenel, Mazych R., ed. *Half Century of Public Health.* New York: American Public Health Association, 1921.

3075. Rayfield, Stanley. "A Study of Negro Public Health Nursing." *Pub Hlth Nurs,* 22 (Oct 1930), 525-536.

3076. Rivers, F., S.H. Schuman, L. Simpson, and S. Olansky. "20 Years of Follow-up Experience in Long Range Medical Study (Emphasizing the Part of the Public Health Nurse) in a Continued Study of Untreated Syphillis in Male Negros." *Pub Hlth Rep,* 68 (Apr 1953), 391-395.

3077. Roach, W.W. "Origins of District Nursing." *Aust Nurs J,* 2 (Jul 1973), 18.

3078. Rosen, George A. *History of Public Health.* New York: M.D. Publications, 1958.

3079. Rosenberg, Charles E., and Carroll S. Rosenberg. "Pietism and the Origins of the American Public Health Movement." *Hist Med,* 23 (1968), 16-35.

3080. Rosnagle, Laura. "Nursing School Aids Fight on Disease (Cincinnati, Ohio)." *Phi Chi Q,* 39 (1942), 47-48.

3081. Sanavitis, A. "Historical Dates in the Development of Public Health and Public Health Nursing in Puerto Rico." *P Rico Enferm,* 44 (Sep 1969), 7-15. (Spa)

3082. Sayles, M.B. "Visiting Nurse and the Nurses' Settlement." *Nurs Out,* 81 (21 Oct 1905), 419-424.

3083. Scamman, Clarence L., ed. *Papers of Charles V. Chapin, M.D.* New York: Commonwealth, 1934. 244 pp.

3084. ————. "The Voluntary Nursing Agency." *Pub Hlth Nurs,* 38 (Nov 1946), 608-614.

3085. "Scenes from the Early History of District Nursing." *Nurs Mirror,* 100 (15 Oct 1954), viii-ix.

3086. Scharlibe, M. "The Health Visitor 1919." *Hlth Visit,* 46 (May 1973), 163-165.

3087. Sedgwick, M.K.R. "Instructive District Nursing." *Forum,* 22 (1896), 297.

3088. Shafer, Donald M. "Improving the Health of the Worker." *Pub Hlth Nurs,* 31 (Dec 1939), 677-681.

3089. Shatz, Rebecca, and Bessie S. LeLaucheur. "The General Visiting Nurse." *Pub Hlth Nurs Q,* 7 (Jan 1915), 23-28.

3090. Shaw, Flora Madeline. "The Visiting Nurse." *Canad Nurs,* 5 (Jan 1909), 11-20.

3091.   Shepard, William P., and George M. Wheatley. "Visiting
        Nurse Service." *J Am Med Assoc*, 149 (7 Jun 1952), 554-557.

3092.   Shimizu, T., et al. "History of Public Health Nursing in
        Niigata Prefecture." *Jap J Pub Hlth Nurs*, 26 (Feb 1970),
        11-27. (Jap)

3093.   Siegel, Earl, and Sylvia Bryson. "Redefinition of the Role
        of the Public Health Nurse in Child Health Supervision."
        Am J Pub Hlth, 53 (Jul 1963), 1015-1024.

3094.   Silcock, Josephine. "District Nursing: A Brief History."
        Nurs Times, 66 (24 Sep 1970), 1244.

3095.   "Sixty Years of Nursing Service (Visiting Nurse Association
        of Boston)." *New England J Med*, 234 (1946), 680-681.

3096.   Skaife, W.F. "Some Aspects of District Nursing." *So Afr
        Nurs Rec*, 20 (Nov 1932), 30.

3097.   Smillie, Wilson G. *Public Health; Its Promise for the
        Future, 1607-1914.* New York: Macmillan Co., 1955. 449 pp.
        Reviewed in *Am J Nurs*, 56 (Aug 1956), 1047.

3098.   Smith, Elizabeth. "From Toboggan to Aeroplane in Public
        Health Nursing." *Canad Nurs*, 51 (Mar 1955), 220-222.

3099.   Smith, M. "American Public Health Methods in the Near East."
        Am J Nurs, 28 (1928), 463-465.

3100.   "Spread of Visiting Nursing." *Charities & the Commons*, 16
        (7 Apr 1906), 1-6.

3101.   Stewart, M.P. "Public Health Nursing in Rural Districts."
        Am City, 21 (Nov 1919), 421-424.

3102.   Stockler, Rebecca Adams. *Development of Public Health
        Nursing Practice as Related to the Health Needs of the
        Jewish Population of Palestine, 1913-1948.* Ed.D. disser-
        tation, Teachers College, Columbia University, 1975.
        176 pp.

3103.   Subhadra, V. "An Evaluation of Public Health Services at an
        Urban Health Center." *Int J Nurs Studies*, 7 (1970), 257-
        265.

3104.   Sumner, A.B., and R.A. David. "Public Health Nursing Amongst
        the Maori People in New Zealand." *Int Nurs Rev News*, 3
        (Oct 1956), 21-25.

3105.   Sumner, Mary R. "When We Were Very Young." *Pub Hlth Nurs*,
        33 (Jul 1941), 422-423.

3106.   Talcott, Agnes G. "First Municipal Nurse in United States."
        Pac Cst J Nurs, 35 (Jun 1939), 340-341.

3107. Temple, Sara L. "The Origin and Growth of District Visiting Nursing." *Canad Nurs*, 10 (Jan 1914), 21-23.

3108. Tinkham, Catherine, and Eleanor Voorhees. *Community Health Nursing--Evolution and Process*. New York: Appleton-Century-Crofts, 1972.

3109. Townsend, J.G. "Public Health Nursing." *Pub Hlth Rep*, 40 (6 Nov 1925), 2471-2478; 41 (1926), 651.

3110. ————. "Town and Country Nursing." *Hosp* (London), 38 (30 Sep 1905), 416-417.

3111. Trujillo, Berta Arango. "Brief History of Public Health Nursing in Columbia." *Int Nurs Rev*, 11 (Nov-Dec 1964), 64-66.

3112. Turner, Ethel. "Six Decades of Service (Instructive Visiting Nurse Association of Baltimore)." *Maryland Med J*, 4 (1955), 666-667.

3113. "Twenty Years of It In the Henry Street Nurses' Settlement." *Survey*, 31 (14 Feb 1914), 606-608.

3114. "Two Unpublished Letters." *Pub Hlth Nurs*, 29 (May 1937), 307.

3115. Valkonen, I. "First Course in Public Health Nursing is 50 Years Ago." *Sairaanhoitaja*, 50 (11 Dec 1974), 18-20. (Fin)

3116. Van Kooy, Nelly. "Development of Public Health Nursing in Wisconsin." *Pub Hlth Nurs*, 14 (Feb 1922), 87-89.

3117. Wald, Lillian D. "Development of Public Health Nursing in the United States." *Tr Nurs*, 80 (Jun 1928), 689-692.

3118. ————. "Henry Street Settlement, New York." *Charities & the Commons*, 16 (7 Apr 1906), 35-38.

3119. ————. *The House on Henry Street*. New York: Holt, 1943. Other editions.

3120. ————. "Nurse and the Community." *Survey*, 30 (19 Jul 1913), 516-517.

3121. ————. "Nursing." *Survey*, 31 (27 Dec 1913), 355-356.

3122. ————. "What Keeps the Nurses Going?" *Survey*, 68 (15 Nov 1932), 590-591.

3123. Waters, Ysabella. "Rise, Progress and Extent of Visiting Nursing in the United States." *Charities & the Commons*, 16 (7 Apr 1906), 16-19.

3124. ————. *Visiting Nursing in the United States*. New York: Charities Publication Committee, 1909.

3125. Welsh, Mabelle S. "What is Public Health Nursing?" *Am J Nurs*, 36 (May 1936), 452-456.

3126. "Whence the Term 'Public Health Nursing'? An Authority Speaks." *Pub Hlth Nurs*,29 (Dec 1937), 712-714.

3127. White, R. "Development of Poor-Law Nursing-Service." *Int J Nurs Studies*, 14(1) (1977), 19-27.

3128. Williams, J. Harley. *A Century of Public Health in Britain 1832-1929*. London: A. & C. Black, 1932. 314 pp.

3129. Wilson, Russell H., and Lila Anderson. "A Wartime Public Health Program." *Pub Hlth Nurs*, 36 (Apr 1944), 160-163.

3130. Winslow, Charles-Edward A. "Has Public Health Nursing Reached Its Destination?" *Pub Hlth Nurs*, 36 (Dec 1944), 609-616.

3131. ————. "National Health Challenges: How the Public Health Nurse is Meeting Them." *Pub Hlth Nurs*, 27 (Feb 1935), 120-124.

3132. ————. "Public Health Nursing." *Forum*, 78 (Nov 1927), 726-732.

3133. ————. "The Role of the Visiting Nurse in the Campaign for Public Health." *Am J Nurs*, 11 (Aug 1911), 909-920.

3134. Wood, C.J. "The Present Position of Poor Law Nursing." *Nurs Times* (10 Jun 1905), 91-95.

3135. Worcester, Alfred. *Nurses for Our Neighbors*. Boston: Houghton Mifflin, 1914.

SCHOOL NURSING

3136. Brown, Jefferson. "School Nursing Aims and Development." *Ariz Pub Hlth News* (1940), 1-4.

3137. Campbell, Katherine. "School Nursing in Edmonton." *Canad Nurs*, 16 (Apr 1920), 197-199.

3138. Chayer, Marry Ella. *School Nursing*. New York: G.P. Putnam's Sons, 1937.

3139. Doster, Mildred. "The Role of the Schools in Primary Health Care." *J Sch Hlth*, 49 (Feb 1979), 2.

3140. Grittinger, E.C. "Work of the School Nurse." Natl Educ Assn. *Addresses and Proceedings* (1917), 513-515.

3141. Jordan, Ora Gertrude. "The School Nurse in Relation to the Child and Its Future." *Tr Nurs*, 63 (Dec 1919), 421-423.

3142.   Keene, Charles H. "Development of School Health Services."
         J Sch Hlth, 23 (Jan 1953), 23-33; 23 (Feb 1953), 51-59;
         23 (Mar 1953), 88-96.

3143.   National Commission for the Study of Nursing and Nursing
         Education. *Bell, Book and Candle: The National Commission
         and the School Nurse*. New York: The Commission, 1972.

3144.   Phelps, Orra A. "School Health Service in the First Super-
         visory School District, Montgomery County, New York."
         Sch Phys Bull, 2 (May 1932), 5-8.

3145.   Power, P. "School Nurse: Her Duties and Methods." *Am City*,
         25 (Sep 1921), 190-192.

3146.   Regan, Patricia Ann. *A Historical Study of the Nurse's Role
         in School Health Programs from 1902 to 1973*. Ed.D. disser-
         tation, Boston University School of Nursing, 1974. 183 pp.

3147.   Rogers, Lina L. "Another Age in School Nursing." *Visit
         Nurs Q* (Apr 1910). Reprinted in *Pub Hlth Nurs*, 29
         (Sep 1937), 540-542.

3148.   "School Nurses Successfully Used in Massachusetts." *Sch
         Life*, 10 (Mar 1925), 139.

3149.   "School Health Program Dates Back to Early Greeks." *Hygeia*
         (Sep 1931).

3150.   Schwab, Ernestine. "Eliabeth Ashe--First School Nurse in
         California." *Pac Cst J Nurs*, 35 (Jun 1939), 336-339.

3151.   Short, Beatrice. "Weather Vanes." *Pub Hlth Nurs*, 19 (Sep
         1927), 427-429.

3152.   "Silver Anniversary of School Nurses in Boston." *Sch Phys
         Bull*, 2 (Dec 1932), 11.

3153.   Struthers, Lina Rogers. *School Nurse*. New York: G.P.
         Putnam's Sons, 1917.

OTHER

3154.   Coppes, M.A. "I've Been Nursing on the Railroad ..." *RN*,
         39 (Jul 1976), 34-37.

3155.   Davis, B.A. "Geriatric Nursing Through the Looking Glass."
         J NY State Nurs Assoc, 2 (Winter 1971), 7-12.

3156.   Ornstein, S. "Establishing A Therapeutic Climate for
         Geriatric Care." *J NY State Nurs Assoc*, 3 (Nov 1972),
         21-29.

3157.   Stroup, Leora B. "A New Service in an Old Cause (Aerial
        Nurse Corps of America--Its Development)." *Tr Nurs & Hosp
        Rev*, 105 (1940), 184-188.

GENERAL

3158.   Adler, S.P. "Swedish Student Nurses: A Descriptive Study."
        Nurs Res, 18 (1969), 363-365.

3159.   Ahad, M.A. "Nursing Education in India." *Int Nurs Rev*, 17
        (3) (1970), 224-237.

3160.   Aikens, C.A. *Hospital Training--School Methods and the Head
        Nurse*. Philadelphia: W.B. Saunders Co., 1907.

3161.   Allemang, Margaret May. *Nursing Education in the United
        States and Canada 1873-1950: Leading Figures, Forces, Views
        on Education*. Ph.D. dissertation, University of Washington,
        1974.

3162.   Allen, Dotaline E. "Nursing Education at Indiana University
        1931-1945." *Monthly Bull Ind Board Hlth*, 49 (1946), 105-
        114, 116.

3163.   American Nurses Association. *Educational Preparation for
        Nurse Practitioners and Assistants to Nurses: A Position
        Paper*. New York: A.N.A., 1965. Reprinted in *Am J Nurs*,
        66 (Mar 1966), 515-517.

3164.   ————. *The Study of Credentialing in Nursing: A New
        Approach*. Kansas City, MO: A.N.A., 1979.

3165.   Anderson, Bernice E. *Nursing Education in Community Junior
        Colleges*. Philadelphia: J.B. Lippincott, 1966.

3166.   Andreoli, A. "Nursing Education Today." *Professioni Infer-
        mieristiche*, 28(4) (1976), 121-124. (Ital)

3167.   Antrobus, Susan. "Nursing Forty Years Ago." *Nurs Times*, 3
        (12 Jan 1907), 34.

3168.   Bachu, A. "Problems of Nursing Education in India in an Age
        of Technology." *Int Nurs Rev*, 18 (1971), 85-95.

3169.   Baggallay, Olive. "The Wider Influence of the Nightingale
        Training School." *Nurs Times*, 56 (13 May 1960), 604-607.

3170.   Bankoff, G.A. "The Social, Economic, and Educational Status
        of the Nurse." *Am J Nurs*, 20 (1919-1920), 955-962.

3171.   Barber, Calvin F.   "The Trained Nurse--Her Education."   *Tr Nurs*, 25 (Aug 1900), 108-114.

3172.   Barritt, Evelyn R.   "Florence Nightingale's Values and Modern Nursing Education."   *Nurs Forum*, 12 (1973), 7-47.

3173.   ———.   "Florence Nightingale's Values and Modern Nursing Education. 1."   *Compr Nurs Q* (Spring 1974), 75-91.   (Jap)

3174.   ———.   "Florence Nightingale's Values and Modern Nursing Education. 2."   *Compr Nurs Q*, 9(4) (Nov 1974), 80-98. (Jap)

3175.   Bauman, M.B.   "Baccalaureate Nursing in a Selected Number of English Speaking Countries."   *Int Nurs Rev*, 9(1) (1972), 12-38.

3176.   Bayldon, Margaret C., ed.   "Diploma Schools: The First Century. The Long Road of Today."   *RN*, 36 (Feb 1973), 33-44, 67-68, 83-86, 90-92.

3177.   Beard, Richard Olding.   "Fair Play for the Trained Nurse."   *Pict Rev* (Feb 1922), 28, 95-96.

3178.   Bertrand, Alvin Lee.   *A Study of Practical Nurse Education and Practical Nursing in Louisiana 1950-1959*.   Baton Rouge: State Department of Education, 1956.

3179.   "The Birth of the American Trained Nurse."   *Nurs Mirror*, 119 (30 Oct 1964), xii.

3180.   Bogue, Jessie Parker.   *The Community College*.   New York: McGraw-Hill, 1950.

3181.   Boyd, E.   "Postbasic Nursing Education in New Zealand."   *Int Nurs Rev*, 17(1) (1970), 43-52.

3182.   Bridgman, Margaret.   *Collegiate Education for Nursing*.   New York: Russell Sage Foundation, 1953.

3183.   ———.   "The Status of Nursing Education in Institutions of Higher Education."   *The Nursing Program in the General College*.   Edited by Olivia Gowan.   Washington, D.C.: Catholic University Press, 1954.

3184.   Bristowe, J.S.   "How Far Should Our Hospitals Be Training Schools for Nurses?"   *J Hosp Assoc* (London) (1884), 26-36.

3185.   Brooks, M.M.   "Contribution of Methodist Hospitals to Nursing During Last 40 Years."   *Tr Nurs*, 80 (Jun 1928), 709-711.

3186.   Brown, Katharine.   "Evolution of the Training-School."   *Nurs J Pac Cst*, 1 (Jun 1905), 164-168.

3187.   Buckinghamshire County Council. North Bucks Technical Educa-
        tion Committee. *Health at Home: Report of the Training of
        the Rural Health Missioners and of Their Village Lecturing
        and Visiting.* Winslow: Bucks County Council, 1892. Re-
        printed in *Reproduction of a Printed Report Containing
        Letters from Miss Florence Nightingale on Health Visiting.*
        1911.

3188.   Bullough, Bonnie. "Public Legal and Social Pressures for a
        Career Ladder in Nursing." In *Proceedings: Council of
        Baccalaureate and Higher Degree Programs*, Mar 22-24, 1972.

3189.   ————. "You Can't Get There from Here." *J Nurs Educ*
        (Nov 1972), 4-10.

3190.   Bullough, Bonnie, and Vern Bullough. "A Career Ladder in
        Nursing: Problems and Prospects." *Am J Nurs*, 71 (1971),
        1938-1943.

3191.   ————. "Collegiate Nursing in the United States—A His-
        torical Review." *Int Nurs Rev*, 10 (1963), 41-47.

3192.   Burgess, Elizabeth C. "Eight Years of the Grading Committee."
        Am J Nurs, 34 (Oct 1934), 937-945.

3193.   ————. "What are Nurses Going to Do About It?" *Am J Nurs*,
        32 (May 1932), 553-556.

3194.   Burgess, May Ayres. *Nursing Schools Today and Tomorrow.*
        New York: National League of Nursing Education, 1934.

3194.1 Canadian Nurses Association. *A Proposed Curriculum for
        Schools of Nursing in Canada.* Montreal: Canadian Nurses
        Assoc., 1936.

3194.2 ————. *A Supplement to a Proposed Curriculum.* Montreal:
        Canadian Nurses Assoc., 1940.

3195.   Chance, K. "A History of the Emerging Discipline of Nursing
        into American Higher Education: Some Philosophical and
        Social Considerations." *Georgia Nurs*, 37 (1977), 4-5.

3196.   Chittick, Rae. "Nursing Comes to the Last Frontier." *Canad
        Nurs*, 36 (Apr 1940), 201-205.

3197.   Christy, T.E. "An Appraisal of an Abstract for Action."
        Am J Nurs, 71 (Aug 1971), 1574-1581.

3198.   Clayton, Bonnie Clare Wilmot. "Historical Perspectives of
        Psychiatric Nursing in Higher Education: 1946 to 1975."
        Ph.D. dissertation, University of Utah, 1976.

3199.   Clemence, B.A. "Baccalaureate Nursing Education in Nigeria."
        Int Nurs Rev, 18(1) (1971), 40-48.

3200.   Committee for the Study of Nursing Education (Josephine C.
        Goldmark). *Nursing and Nursing Education in the United
        States*. New York: Macmillan Co., 1923.

3201.   Committee on the Grading of Nursing Schools. *Nurses: Produc-
        tion, Education, Distribution, and Pay*. New York: National
        League of Nursing Education, 1930.

3202.   —————. *Nursing Schools Today and Tomorrow: Final Report*.
        New York: National League of Nursing Education, 1934.

3203.   —————. *Results of the First Grading of Nursing Schools*.
        3 vols. New York: National League of Nursing Education,
        1931.

3204.   —————. *The Second Grading of Nursing Schools*. New York:
        National League of Nursing Education, 1932.

3205.   "Contribution to Nursing Education Made by Sisters of Mercy
        (1843-1928)." *Tr Nurs*, 80 (Jun 1928), 706.

3206.   Cooper, Singe S. "A Brief History of Continuing Education in
        Nursing in the United States." *Cont Educ Nurs*, 4 (May-Jun
        1973), 5-14.

3207.   —————. "A Century of Nursing Education." *Cont Educ Nurs*, 3
        (Sep-Oct 1972), 3-4.

3208.   Cope, Zachary, Sr. "Evolution of the Sister Tutor." *Nurs
        Times* (9 Dec 1955), 1388-1391.

3209.   "Credentialing in Nursing: A New Approach; Report of the Com-
        mittee for the Study of Credentialing in Nursing." *Am J
        Nurs*, 79 (Apr 1979), 674-683.

3210.   Cunningham, Elizabeth V. "Education for Leadership in Nurs-
        ing 1899-1959." *Nurs Out*, 7 (May 1959), 268-272.

3211.   —————. *Today's Diploma Schools of Nursing*. New York:
        National League for Nursing, 1963.

3212.   *A Curriculum for Schools of Nursing*. New York: National
        League of Nursing Education, 1927.

3213.   *A Curriculum Guide for Schools of Nursing*. New York:
        National League of Nursing Education, 1937.

3214.   Davies, C. "Four Events in Nursing History: A New Look--2.
        Case 4, Education and Management: Options for Change."
        Nurs Times, 74(26) (1978), 69-70.

3215.   Davis, Fred. "Problems and Issues in Collegiate Nursing
        Education." *The Nursing Profession: Five Sociological
        Essays*. New York: John Wiley, 1966.

3216.   Davis, Graham Lee. "33,000 Loss in 12 Hospitals Due to
        Nursing Schools." *Hosp Mgmt* (Aug 1931).

3217.   Davis, Mary D. "I Was a Student Over Fifty Years Ago."
        Nurs Out, 9 (Apr 1961), 221-222.

3218.   DeHaan, M.C. "The Student of the Intermediate Professional
        Nursing Education in Training and Practice." *Tejdschreft
        voor Ziekenverplegeng*, 29(9) (1976), 408-417. (Dutch)

3219.   Denny, F.P. "The Need of an Institution for the Education of
        Nurses Independent of the Hospitals." *Bost Med Surg J*, 148
        (1903), 657.

3220.   Diekmann, J.A. "Nursing Schools in Hospitals Under 100 Beds
        Should Close." *Hosp Mgmt*, 37 (1934), 29.

3221.   Dock, L.L. "Nursing Education." *Charities & the Commons*,
        17 (3 Jan 1907), 743-744.

3222.   Donnie, C. "SNA Conference: The Theme: 'Nursing Students of
        the 70's'." *Nurs of India*, 64 (Dec 1973), 410-411.

3223.   Downing, L.C. "Early Negro Hospitals with Special Reference
        to Nurse's Training Schools." *J Nat Med Assoc*, 33 (1941),
        13-18.

3224.   Drage, Martha. "Core Courses and a Career Ladder." *Am J
        Nurs*, 71 (Jun 1977), 1356-1358.

3225.   *Education for Nursing: Past, Present, and Future*. New York:
        National League for Nursing, Division of Nursing Education,
        1959.

3226.   "Educational Preparation for Nursing." *Nurs Out*, 18 (Sep
        1970), 53-57; 19 (Sep 1971), 604-607; 20 (Sep 1972), 599-
        602; 21 (Sep 1973), 586-593.

3227.   Eichhorn, S. "Trends in the Professional Education of
        Doctors, Nurses, and Other Paramedical Staff in the German
        Federal Republic." *World Hosp*, 5 (1969), 77.

3228.   Eldredge, A. "How Many Girls of 15 Years are Enrolled in
        Nurse Schools?" *Hosp Mgmt*, 25 (1928), 49.

3229.   Emblin, R. "Degree Courses in Nursing." *Nurs Times*, 72
        (7 Oct 1972), 141-143; 72 (14 Oct 1972), 145-146.

3230.   "Examination Questions for R.N., Given Dec 5, 1914 (Cali-
        fornia)." *Pac Cst J Nurs*, 10 (1914), appendix.

3231.   Fagen, Claire, Margaret McClure, and Rozelle Schlotfeldt.
        "Can We Bring Order Out of the Chaos of Nursing Education?"
        Am J Nurs, 76 (Jan 1976), 98-107.

3232.   ————. "Baccalaureate Preparation for Primary Care." *Nurs
        Out*, 20 (Apr 1972), 240.

3233.   Fenwick, E.G.   "Evolution of the Trained Nurse." *Outlook*,
        64 (6 Jan 1900), 56-67.

3234.   Fillmore, Anna M.   "Scene--U.S.A., 1900." *Am J Nurs*, 41
        (Aug 1941), 913-915.

3235.   Fitzpatrick, M.L.   "Nursing Education and Change." *Alum Mag*,
        (Baltimore), 76 (1977), 2-7.

3236.   Forbes, Mary.   "The Small General Hospital: Its Advantages
        and Difficulties as a Field for Training." *Am J Nurs*, 3
        (Feb 1903), 341-344.

3237.   Frey, Don C.   "Futurism and Health Occupations Education:
        The Implications of Changes in the Delivery System, Address
        to Health Occupations Section at the Annual Meeting of the
        American Vocational Association." *Proceedings*.   Atlanta,
        GA: American Vocational Association, 1973.

3238.   Fulmer, Harriet.   "Does Public Health Nursing Belong in the
        Curriculum of the School of Nursing?" *Tr Nurs & Hosp Rev*,
        95 (1935), 539.

3239.   Gilpin, Fanny.   *Scenes from Hospital Life: Being the Letters
        of a Probationer Nurse*.   London: Drane's Danegeld House,
        1923.

3240.   Gipe, Florence Meda.   *The Development of Nursing Education in
        in Maryland*.   Ed.D. dissertation, University of Maryland,
        College Park, 1952.

3241.   Good, Harry G.   *A History of American Education*.   New York:
        The Macmillan Co., 1956.

3242.   Goodrich, Annie Warburton.   "The Gift of Dr. Richard Olding
        Beard to Nursing Education." *Am J Nurs*, 35 (Mar 1935),
        251-259.

3243.   ————.   "The Nurse as an Interpreter of Life." *Am J Nurs*,
        29 (Apr 1929), 427-428.

3244.   Gowan, Sister M. Olivia, ed.   *The Nursing Program in the
        General College*.   Washington, D.C.:   The Catholic Univer-
        sity of America Press, 1954.

3245.   Grace, Helen K.   "The Development of Doctoral Education in
        Nursing: A Historical Perspective."   In *The Nursing Pro-
        fession: Views Through the Mist*.   Edited by Norma L.
        Chaska.   New York: Blakiston, 1978.

3246.   Grady, Thomas E.   "Nurse Training and Education--History and
        Hopes." *Nurs Times*, 68 (11 May 1972), 585-586.

3247.   Grey, Grace G.   "The Past, Present, and Future of Nursing
        Education." *Mod Hosp*, 36 (Feb 1931), 124, 126, 128.

3248.   Grippando, Gloria. *Nursing Perspectives and Issues*. Albany, NY: Delmar, 1977.

3249.   Grobellaan, A. "South African Experiments with the Basic Collegiate Program." *Am J Nurs*, 58 (1958), 1401-1402.

3250.   Grunau, D.L. "Are Nurses Over-Educated?" *Tr Nurs & Hosp Rev*, 122 (1949), 210.

3251.   Guanes, H. "Nursing Education in Brazil." *Int Nurs Rev*, 5 (1958), 32-33.

3252.   Gunter, Laurie M. "The Effects of Segregation on Nursing Students." *Nurs Out*, 9 (Feb 1961), 74-76.

3253.   Hadley, Ernest C. "A Review of the Training of Nurses in the Light of Modern History." *Brit J Nurs*, 94 (Jan 1946), 6-7.

3254.   Harmer, H.M. "Nurses Old and New." *Nurs Times*, 25 (5 Jan 1929), 6.

3255.   Harris, Susan S. "Evolution of Nursing in Colorado Springs." *Tr Nurs*, 39 (Dec 1907), 359-362.

3256.   Hassenplug, Lulu Wolf. "Nursing Education in Universities." *Nurs Out*, 8 (1960), 92-95, 154-155.

3257.   ———. "Preparation of the Nurse Practitioner." *J Nurs Educ*, 4 (Jan 1965), 29-42.

3258.   "Have Times Changed? The *Nursing Mirror*; September 7, 1907. How to Prepare for Becoming a Probationer." *Nurs Mirror*, 141(23) (4 Dec 1975), 76.

3259.   "Have Times Changed? The *Nursing Mirror*: June 1, 1907. Training, Discipline and Courtesy." *Nurs Mirror*, 141(22) (27 Nov 1975), 81.

3260.   Herdmann, W.J. "Evolution of the Trained Nurse." *Tr Nurs* (1896), xvi, 389-395.

3261.   Hintz, Anna A. "The Probationary Term." In *How to Become a Trained Nurse*. Edited by Jane Hodson. New York: William Abbott, 1898. pp. 15-19.

3262.   ———. "The Training Term." In *How to Become a Trained Nurse*. Edited by Jane Hodson. New York: William Abbott, 1898. pp. 20-24.

3263.   Hodson, Jane, ed. *How to Become a Trained Nurse*. New York: William Abbott, 1898.

3264.   Holland, Howard Owen. *Historical Survey of Attendant-Nurses Training in Michigan*. Ph.D. dissertation, Michigan State University, 1974.

3265.   "Impressions of Pacific Coast Training Schools." *Nurs J Pac
        Cst,* 2 (Mar 1906), 19-20.

3266.   Ingles, Thelma. "The University Medical Center as a Setting
        for Nursing Education." *J Med Educ,* 37 (1962), 411-420.

3267.   International Council of Nurses. *Constitution and Regula-
        tions. International Directory of Nurses with Doctoral
        Degrees.* New York: American Nurses Foundation, 1973.

3268.   Jamme, Anna C. "Changing Aspects of Nursing." *Pac Cst J
        Nurs,* 24 (Sep 1928), 521-526.

3269.   Johnson, Dorothy. "Competence in Practice: Technical and
        Professional." *Nurs Out,* 14 (Oct 1966), 30-33.

3270.   Johnson, Walter. "Educational Preparation for Nursing."
        Nurs Out, 23 (Sep 1975), 578-582; 24 (Sep 1976), 568-573;
        25 (Sep 1977), 587-592; 26 (Sep 1978), 568-573.

3271.   Johnston, M.F., et al. "Question of Modern Trained Nurse."
        19th Cent, 51 (Jun 1902), 966-979.

3272.   Kalisch, B.J., and P.A. Kalisch. "Slaves, Servants, or
        Saints? An Administrative Analysis of the System of Nurse
        Training in the United States, 1873-1948." *Nurs Forum,*
        14(3) (1975), 222-263; *Sogo Kango,* 12 (1977), 23-55. (Jap)

3273.   Katscher, C. "Current Status of Nursing Education." *Deutsche
        Krankenpflegzeitschrift,* 29 (1976), 250-253. (Ger)

3274.   Kelly, Lucie Young. "Open Curriculum--What and Why." *Am J
        Nurs,* 74 (Dec 1974), 2232-2238.

3275.   Kelly, M.A. "Beliefs of Iranian Nurses and Nursing Students
        about Nurses and Nursing Education." *Int Nurs Rev,* 20
        (Jul-Aug 1973), 108-111.

3276.   Krekeler, Kathleen. "Continuing Education--Why?" *Cont Educ
        Nurs,* 6 (Mar-Apr 1975), 2, 12-16.

3277.   Krishnan, S. "Planning Nursing Education for the 70s in
        India." *Int Nurs Rev,* 18(1) (1971), 181-191.

3278.   Lambertsen, Eleanor C. *Education for Nursing Leadership.*
        Philadelphia: J.B. Lippincott, 1958.

3279.   Ledakis, S. "Nursing Education in Greece." *Int Nurs Rev,* 4
        (Jan 1957), 49-54.

3280.   Lenburg, Carrie B. *Open Learning and Career Mobility in
        Nursing.* St. Louis: C.V. Mosby, 1975.

3281.   Lenburg, Carrie B., Walter Johnson, and JoAnn T. Vahey.
        Directory of Career Opportunities in Nursing. New York:
        National League for Nursing, 1973.

3282. Logan, Laura R. *National League of Nursing Education: Annual Report, 1923 and Proceedings of 29th Convention.* Baltimore: Williams & Wilkins, 1923. 282 pp.

3283. ————. "The National League of Nursing Education." *Sch & Soc*, 18 (14 Jul 1923), 51-52.

3284. ————. "A Review of the Progress of Nursing and Nursing Education in 1924." *Mod Hosp*, 24 (1925), 18-22.

3285. Longway, Ina Madge. "Curriculum Concepts—An Historical Analysis." *Nurs Out*, 20 (Feb 1972), 116-120; see also *IM Kango*, 24 (Jul 1972), 20-25. (Jap)

3286. Loyer, M.A. "Should Nursing Education Be Under the Domain of Hospitals?" *Canad Nurs*, 62 (1966), 25-26.

3287. Lückes, Eva C.E. "How Far Should Our Hospitals Be Training Schools for Nurses?" *J Hosp Assoc* (London), (1884), 36-44.

3288. Ludlam, G.F. "The Organization and Control of Training Schools." *NY Med J*, 83 (1906), 850.

3289. Number deleted.

3290. MacBride, O. "An Overview of the Health Professions Education Assistance Act, 1963-1971." *Health Manpower Policy Discussion Paper Series Number D. I.* Ann Arbor: University of Michigan Press, 1973.

3291. MacDonald, Gwendoline. *Development of Standards and Accreditation in Collegiate Nursing Education.* New York: Teachers College Press, Columbia University, 1965.

3292. MacEachern, Malcolm T. "Which Shall We Choose—Graduate or Student Service?" *Mod Hosp*, 38 (1932), 97-104.

3293. McGivern, Diane. "Baccalaureate Preparation of the Nurse Practitioner." *Nurs Out*, 22 (Feb 1974), 94-98.

3294. McKay, R. "A Comparative Approach to the Development of Nursing Education." *Nurs Sci*, 2 (Apr 1964), 125.

3295. McQuarrie, Frances. "The Evolution of Nursing Education." *Canad Nurs*, 51 (Mar 1955), 194-199.

3296. Martel, Gabrielle D., and Marilyn Winterton Edmunds. "Nurse-Internship in Chicago." *Am J Nurs*, 72 (May 1972), 940-943.

3297. Matarazzo, Joseph D. "Perspective." In *Future Directions of Doctoral Education for Nurses.* Report of a Conference. Bethesda, MD: U.S. Government Printing Office, 1971. pp. 64-67. DHEW Pub. #78-82.

3297.1 ————, and F. Abdellah. "Doctoral Education for Nurses in the United States." *Nurs Res*, 20 (Sep-Oct 1971), 404-414.

3298.   Meyers, M.A. "Three Year Study of Student Nurses, 1935-1937
        (Result of Tuberculin Testing)." *J Indiana MA*, 30 (Dec
        1937), 638-639.

3299.   Moghadassy, M. "Progress: Postbasic Nursing Education in
        Iran." *Int Nurs Rev*, 19(1) (1972), 3-11.

3300.   Montag, Mildred, and L.C. Gotkin. *Community College Educa-
        tion for Nursing: Technical Education for Nursing.* New
        York: McGraw-Hill Book Co., 1959.

3301.   Montag, Mildred. *The Education of Nursing Technicians.* New
        York: G.P. Putnam's Sons, 1951.

3302.   ———. *Evaluation of Graduates of Associate Degree Nursing
        Programs.* New York: Columbia University, Teachers College
        Press, 1972.

3303.   Morgan, James Dudley. "Are the Trained Nurses Over-
        Educated?" *Am J Nurs*, 6 (Sep 1906), 858-860.

3304.   Moss, M. "Evolution of the Trained Nurse." *Atlan*, 91 (May
        1903), 587-599.

3305.   Nagayoshi, T. "Historical Aspects of Nursing Education."
        Jap J Nurs Educ, 15(9) (Sep 1974), 577-580.   (Jap)

3306.   Nakazato, R. "Early History of Nursing Education in Japan."
        Kango, 26(6) (June 1974), 97-102.   (Jap)

3307.   ———. "History of Establishing Nursing Education in Modern
        Japan." *Kango*, 26 (Jan 1974), 88-93; (Feb 1974), 59-64;
        (Mar 1974), 89-90; (Apr 1974), 103-108.   (Jap)

3308.   National Commission for the Study of Nursing and Nursing
        Education, Jerome P. Lysaught, Director. *An Abstract for
        Action.* New York: McGraw-Hill Book Co., 1970.

3309.   ———. *Action in Nursing: Progress in Professional Purpose.*
        New York: McGraw-Hill Book Co., 1974.

3309.1 National Committee for the Improvement of Nursing Services.
        Final Report. Battle Creek, MI: Kellogg Foundation, 1953.

3310.   ———. *Interim Classification of Schools of Nursing Offer-
        ing Basic Programs.* New York: The Authors, 1949.

3311.   ———. *Nursing Schools at the Mid-Century.* New York: The
        Authors, 1950.

3312.   National League for Nursing. *The Nursing Data Book: Statis-
        tical Information on Nursing Education and Newly Licensed
        Schools.* New York: The League, 1978.

3313.   ———. *Nurse Faculty Census, 1972.* New York: The League,
        1972.

3313.1 ———. The Open Curriculum in Nursing Education: Final
        Report of the NLN Open Curriculum Study. Lucille E. Natter,
        Project Director. New York: The League, 1972.

3314.   ————. *Report on the Associate Degree Programs in Nursing*.
         New York: The League, 1961.

3314.1   ————. Selected Readings from Open Curriculum Literature:
         An Annotated Bibliography. 2nd ed. Walter Johnson,
         Division of Research, NLN. New York: The League, 1977.

3315.   National League of Nursing Education. *A Curriculum Guide for
         Schools of Nursing*. New York: The League, 1927.

3316.   ————. *A Curriculum Guide for Schools of Nursing*. New
         York: The League, 1937.

3317.   ————. *Essentials of a Good School of Nursing*. New York:
         The League, 1936. Rev. Ed. 1942.

3318.   ————. *Standard Curriculum for Schools of Nursing*. New
         York: The League, 1917.

3319.   Newman, Margaret A. "Nursing's Theoretical Evolution."
         Nurs Out (Jul 1972), 53.

3320.   Nightingale, Florence. *On Trained Nursing for the Sick Poor*.
         London: Metropolitan and National Nursing Association,
         1876.

3321.   ————. "The Reform of Sick Nursing and the Late Mrs. Ward-
         roper, the Extinction of Mrs. Gamp." *Brit Med J* (21 Dec
         1892), 1448.

3322.   ————. "Trained Nurses." *Cent*, 81 (Nov 1910), 159-160.

3323.   ————. "The Training of Nurses." *Nurs Mirror*, 99 (7 May
         1954), iv-vi.

3324.   ————, ed. "To the Probationer Nurses in the Nightingale
         Fund School at St. Thomas' Hospital." *Int Nurs Rev*, 18
         (1971), 3-5.

3325.   Noall, Sandra Hawkes. *A History of Nursing Education in
         Utah*. Ph.D. dissertation, University of Utah, 1970.

3326.   Notter, Lucille, ed. *Proceedings: Open Curriculum Conference
         I*. New York: National League for Nursing, 1974.

3327.   "Nursing in the Nineties." *Nurs Times*, 31 (20 Apr 1935),
         410, 412.

3328.   Nutting, Mary Adelaide. "Developments in Teaching Since
         1873." *National League of Nursing Education: Annual Report,
         1923, and Proceedings of 29th Convention*. Baltimore:
         Williams & Wilkins, 1923. pp. 231-237.

3329.   ————. *The Education and Professional Position of Nurses,
         United States Bureau of Education*. Washington, D.C.:
         U.S. Government Printing Office, 1907.

3330.   ————. *Educational Status of Nursing, United States Bureau
         of Education*. Washington, D.C.: U.S. Government Printing
         Office, 1912.

3331. ———. "Historical Summary of the Relations of Nursing Education to Universities." *Proceedings of Conference on Nursing Schools Connected with Colleges and Universities, January 21-25, 1928.* New York: National League of Nursing Education, 1928. pp. 5-12.

3332. ———. "Miss Nutting's Report." *Am J Nurs*, 3 (Jan 1903), 272-273.

3333. ———. *A Sound Economic Basis for Schools of Nursing and Other Addresses.* New York: G.P. Putnam's Sons, 1926.

3334. ———. "Thirty Years of Progress in Nursing." *Am J Nurs*, 23 (1923), 1027.

3335. Nutting, Mary Adelaide, and Lavinia L. Dock. *A History of Nursing.* 4 vols. New York: G.P. Putnam's Sons, 1907-1912.

3336. "On Accreditation. Faculty, Curriculum, Philosophy." *Am J Nurs*, 60 (1960), 1475-1478.

3337. Osgood, Robert Bayley. "Hazards and Hopes in the Education of Trained Nurses." *New England J Med*, 204 (25 Jun 1931), 1369-1373.

3338. Papamicrouli, S. "Hellenic Red Cross School of Nursing: A Combined Program in General and Public Health Nursing." *Int J Nurs Studies*, 6 (1969), 27-35.

3339. Paylor, Mary Margaret. *A History of Nursing Education in Florida from 1893 to 1970.* Ph.D. dissertation, Florida State University, 1975.

3340. Peck, E.S. *Nurses in Time Developments in Nursing Education, 1898-1963.* Berea, KY: Berea College Press, 1964.

3341. Petry, L., and E.M. Vreeland. "Nursing Education." *Higher Educ*, 8 (1952), 181.

3342. Prangley, P.R., and L. DeYoung. "Nursing Education Changes to Meet Service Needs of Patient Care." *Rocky Mountain Med J*, 56(1) (Jan 1959), 48-52.

3343. "The Preliminary Education of Nurses." *Am J Nurs* (Jan 1903), 272-273.

3344. Rafuse, Ella M. "Nursing Education--What is the Challenge?" *Tr Nurs*, 100 (Apr 1938), 425-431.

3345. Rawnsley, M.M. "The Goldmark Report: Midpoint in Nursing History." *Nurs Out*, 21 (Jun 1973), 380-383.

3346. Reinkemeyer, Sister Mary Hubert. "An Inherited Pathology." *Nurs Out*, 15 (Nov 1967), 51-53.

3347. ———. "It Won't Be Hospital Nursing." *Am J Nurs*, 68
(Sep 1968), 1936-1940.

3348. "Report of the Nursing Consultant Group to the Surgeon-
General." *Toward Quality on Nursing Needs and Goals*.
Washington, D.C.: U.S. Government Printing Office, 1963.

3349. "Report on Committee on Nursing Education." *Nations Hlth*, 4
(1922), 408.

3350. "Report of Committee on the Training of Nurses." *Trans Am
Med Assoc* (1869), 161-174.

3351. Riahi, A. "Nursing Education in Iran." *Int J Nurs Studies*,
5 (1968), 267-271.

3352. Richards, Linda. "Early Days in the First Training School for
Nurses." *Am J Nurs*, 26 (Nov 1915), 174-179; 73 (Sep 1973),
1574-1575.

3353. ———. "How Trained Nursing Began in America--At the New
England Hospital." *Am J Nurs*, 2 (1901), 88-89.

3354. ———. "Nagat." *Jap J Nurs Educ*, 10 (May 1969), 60-63;
(Jun 1969), 49-51. (Jap)

3355. Rines, Alice R. "Associate Degree Education: History,
Development, and Rationale." *Nurs Out*, 25 (Aug 1977),
496-501.

3356. Robb, Isabel Hampton. "The Affiliation of Training Schools
for Nurses for Educational Purposes." *Am J Nurs*, 5 (Jul
1905), 666-677.

3357. ———. "The Three Years' Course of Training in Connection
with the Eight Hours System." *First and Second Annual
Reports of the American Society of the Superintendents of
Training Schools for Nurses*. New York, 1897.

3358. Rogers, Martha E. *Educational Revolution in Nursing*. New
York: Macmillan Co., 1961.

3359. ———. *Reveille in Nursing*. Philadelphia: F.A. Davis, 1964.

3360. Rottman, E. "Why Should a Hospital Close Its Nursing School?"
Mod Hosp, 39 (Aug 1932), 77.

3361. Rowsell, G.S. "University Nursing Education--Facts and
Trends." *Canad Nurs*, 62 (1966), 31-33.

3362. Sand, Annie. "Nurses--Their Education and Their Role in
Health Programmes." *Phlp J Nurs*, 24 (Jul-Sep 1954), 101-
105, 128-131.

3363.   Scanlan, P.P. *Nursing Education in Ireland: Background,*
         Present Status, and Future, 1964. Ph.D. dissertation,
         Catholic University of America, 1966.

3364.   ————. "Nursing Education in Ireland." *Int Nurs Rev*, 16
         (Apr 1969), 153.

3365.   Schwier, Mildred E., Lena R. Paskewita, Frances K. Peterson,
         and Florence E. Elliot. *Ten Thousand Nurse Faculty Members*
         in Basic Professional Schools of Nursing. New York:
         National League for Nursing, 1953.

3366.   Scott, Jessie M. "Federal Support for Nursing Education
         1964-1972." *Am J Nurs*, 72 (Oct 1972), 1855-1861.

3367.   Searle, Charlotte, "Developments in Nursing Education in
         South African Universities." *Int J Nurs Studies*, 6 (1969),
         107-113.

3368.   ————. "Nursing Education in South Africa." *Int Nurs Rev*,
         41 (1959), 49-62.

3369.   Setzler, L. "Nursing and Nursing Education in Germany."
         Am J Nurs, 45 (1945), 993-995.

3370.   Shadbolt, Y.T. "Nursing Education in New Zealand." *New*
         Zeal Nurs J, 68(1) (1975), 19-22.

3371.   Sharp, Bonita H. "The Beginning of Nursing Education in the
         United States: An Analysis of the Times." *J Nurs Educ*, 12
         (Apr 1973), 26-32.

3372.   Shulamith, L.A. "A Nursing School in Palestine." *Am J Nurs*,
         40 (1960), 880-884.

3373.   Simpson, T.H. "College Women as Nurses." *Rev of Reviews*,
         57 (May 1918), 527-528.

3374.   Slater, P.V. "The Future Development of the College of
         Nursing, Australia and the Proposed Basic Nursing Course."
         Aust Nurs J, 2 (Mar 1973), 26-30.

3375.   Sleeper, Ruth. "Nursing Education in Evolution." *New*
         England J Med, 271 (1964), 27.

3376.   ————. "A Reaffirmation of Belief in the Diploma School."
         Nurs Out, 6 (1958), 616-618.

3377.   ————. "The Two Inseparables--Nursing Services and
         Nursing Education." *Am J Nurs*, 48 (Nov 1948), 478-481.

3378.   Smith, Lesley. *Four Years Out of Life.* Glasgow: Philip
         Allan, 1931.

3379.   Sotejo, J.V. "Nursing Education in the Philippines, 1907-
         1967." *S Tomas Nurs J*, 5 (Mar 1967), 284-295.

3380. Spector, Audrey F. *Regional Planning for Nursing Education in the South, 1972-1975: A Study in Transition*. Atlanta: Southern Regional Education Board, 1975.

3381. Spingarn, Natalie Davis. "Biggest of the Health Professions, Nursing is Beset with Paradoxes." *Chron High Educ* (4 Feb 1974).

3382. Stankova, M. "Fifteen Years of Nurses' High School Education." *Zdrav Prac*, 25(4) (Apr 1975), 198-199. (Cze)

3383. Steed, M.E. "Trends in Diploma Nursing Education." *Canad Nurs*, 64 (1968), 40-41.

3384. Stephenson, Gladys E. "Nursing School Curricula. The Value of History of Nursing." *Q J Chin Nurs*, 10 (Jan 1929), 19-22.

3385. Stevenson, Deva. "Curriculum Development in Practical Nurse Education." *Am J Nurs*, 64 (1974), 81-86.

3386. Stewart, Isabel Maitland. "Developments in Nursing Education Since 1918." *US Bur Educ Bull*, 20 (1921), 1.

3387. ———. *The Education of Nurses: Historical Foundation and Modern Trends*. New York: Macmillan Co., 1945.

3388. ———. "A Half-Century of Nursing Education." *Am J Nurs*, 50 (Oct 1950), 617-621.

3389. ———. "The Movement for Shorter Hours in Nurses' Training Schools." *Am J Nurs*, 19 (Mar 1919), 439-443.

3390. ———. "Problems of Nursing Education." *Teach Coll Rec*, 11 (May 1910), 7-26.

3391. ———. "Readjustments in the Training School Curriculum to Meet the New Demands in Public Health Nursing." *Am J Nurs*, 20 (Nov 1919), 102-109.

3392. ———. "Trends in Nursing Education." *Am J Nurs*, 31 (1931), 601.

3393. Strangford, Viscountess. *Hospital Training for Ladies, An Appeal to the Hospital Boards in England*. London: Harrison & Sons, 1874.

3394. Suhrie, Eleanor Brady. *Evidences of the Influence of Ruth Perkes Kuehn on Nursing and Nursing Education*. Ph.D. dissertation, University of Pittsburgh, 1975.

3395. Suleiman, Louise Wailus. *A Critical Analysis of the Nurse Training Act of 1964*. Ed.D. dissertation, Boston University School of Education, 1974.

3396.   Suzuki, S. "Re-evaluation of Nursing Education in History.
        3. A Study on the Organization of Nursing Training Follow-
        ing the End of World War II." *Jap J Nurs Art*, 22(4) (Mar
        1976), 139-147. (Jap)

3397.   Swanson, R. "Nursing Education--What It Costs the Hospital."
        Hosp, 27 (1953), 68.

3398.   Taylor, Henry L. *Professional Education in the United
        States*. Albany: University Press of the State of New York,
        1900.

3399.   "Then and Now." *Tr Nurs & Hosp Rev*, 102 (Feb 1939), 140-143.

3400.   Thoms, A.B., and C.E. Bullock. "Developments of Facilities
        for Colored Nurse Education." *Tr Nurs & Hosp Rev*, 80
        (1928), 722.

3401.   Thomson, M. "Change in Nursing Education." *New Zeal Nurs J*,
        68 (1975), 22-23.

3402.   "Training Camps for Nurses." *Outlook*, 119 (1918), 94.

3403.   U.S. Public Health Service. *The U.S. Cadet Nurse Corps and
        Other Federal Nurse Training Programs, 1943-1948*.
        Washington, D.C.: U.S. Government Printing Office, 1950.

3404.   Urch, Daisy D. "The Blooming. What Shall the Fruitage Be?"
        Pac Cst J Nurs, 22 (Nov 1926), 654-655.

3405.   "Vassar Preparatory Course: A New Experiment in Nursing
        Education." *Am J Nurs*, 18 (Sep 1918), 1155-1159.

3405.1 Vaughn, John C., and Walter Johnson. "Educational Prepara-
        tion for Nursing." *Nurs Out*, 27 (Sep 1979), 608-614.

3406.   Walters, Verle H., Shirley S. Chater, Mary Louise Vivier,
        Judith H. Urrea, and Holly Skodel Wilson. "Technical and
        Professional Nursing: An Exploratory Study." *Nurs Res*, 21
        (Mar-Apr 1972), 124-131.

3407.   Washburn, Frederic A. "The Development of Nursing Education."
        Hosp, 11 (Feb 1937), 15-20.

3408.   Waters, Charles Edward. "The Professional Nurse and the
        Schools for the Training of Professional Nurses." *Tr
        Nurs*, 41 (Jul 1908), 8-10.

3409.   Watson, J. "The Evolution of Nursing Education in the United
        States: 100 Years of a Profession for Women." *J Nurs Educ*,
        16 (1977), 31-38.

3410.   Weir, George M. *Survey of Nursing Education in Canada*.
        Toronto: University of Toronto Press, 1932.

3411.   West, Margaret, and Christy Hawkins. *Nursing Schools at the
        Mid-Century*. New York: National Committee for the Improve-
        ment of Nursing Services, 1950.

3412.   Whitaker, Judith. "The Issue of Mandatory Continuing Educa-
         tion." *Nurs Clin No Am*, 9 (Sep 1974), 475-483.

3413.   Williams, H.J. "The Importance of Intelligent Nursing and
         the Training of Nurses." *Atlanta Med Surg J* (1885-1886),
         ii, 257-268.

3414.   Winslow, Charles Edward A. "Nursing Education--Its Past and
         Its Future." *Mod Hosp*, 25 (Sep 1925), 237-240.

3415.   Woolley, Alma S. "The Long and Tortured History of Clinical
         Evaluation." *Nurs Out*, 25(5) (May 1977), 308-315.

3416.   Worcester, Alfred. "The Training of Nurses in Private Prac-
         tice." *Med Comm Mas Med Soc* (1887), xiv, 89-100; see also
         Bost Med Surg J (1887), cxvii, 193-195.

3417.   ————. *A New Way of Training Nurses*. Boston: Cupples and
         Hurd, 1888.

3418.   Yukinaga, M. "Historical Observation on Nursing Education
         and Clinical Training." *Jap J Nurs Art*, 19 (Jan 1973),
         1-7. (Jap)

3419.   Zorn, Joan M., and Robert L. Zorn. *The Phenomenal Growth of
         the Associate Degree Program in Nursing*. ERIC Data Retrie-
         val Service, unpublished paper. 8 pp.

MIDWIFERY EDUCATION

3420.   Calder, A.B. *Lectures on Midwifery for Midwives*. New York:
         William Wood & Co., 1905.

3421.   Campbell, Janet M. "Training of Midwives." *Pub Hlth Rep*, 39
         (Feb 1924), 341-348.

3422.   Clark, Taliaferro. "Training of Midwives." *Chicago Med
         Recorder*, 46 (1924), 297-304.

3423.   Clifton, Edgar J. "The Education, Licensing and Supervision
         of the Midwife." *Am J Obs Dis Wom Child*, 73 (Mar 1916),
         385-398.

3424.   Jones, Anita M. *Manual for Teaching Midwives*. United States
         Department of Labor, Children's Bureau Publication No. 260.
         Washington, D.C.: U.S. Government Printing Office, 1941.

3425.   McCord, James R. "The Education of Midwives." *Am J Obs Gyn*,
         21 (1931), 837-852.

3426.   Macy Foundation. *The Training and Responsibilities of the
         Midwife*. New York: Josiah Macy, Jr. Foundation, 1967.

3427.   Maternity Center Association. *Twenty Years of Nurse Mid-
         wifery 1933-1953*. New York: The Maternity Center Associa-
         tion, 1955.

3428.   Monroe, Robert F. "Historical Development of Obstetric Edu-
         cation in the South." *So Med J*, 52 (1959), 1142-1148.

3429.   Nightingale, Florence. *Introductory Notes on Lying-In
         Institutions; Together with a Proposal for Organizing an
         Institution for Training Midwives and Midwifery Nurses*.
         London: Longmans, 1871.

3430.   Noyes, Clara D. "The Training of Midwives in Relation to the
         Prevention of Infant Mortality." *Am J Obs Dis Wom Child*,
         66 (1912), 1051-1059.

3431.   Wile, Ira S. "Schools for Midwives." *Med Rec*, 81 (Mar 1912),
         517-518.

                        PUBLIC HEALTH NURSING EDUCATION

3432.   Connor, M.C. "Education 1940-1947 in Retrospect." *Pub Hlth
         Nurs*, 40 (Mar 1948), 123-127.

3433.   Davies, M.O. "Trends in Nursing Education and Public Health
         Nursing Education." *Am J Pub Hlth*, 43 (1953), 1289.

3434.   Fulmer, Harriet. "Does Public Health Nursing Belong in the
         Curriculum of the School of Nursing?" *Tr Nurs & Hosp Rev*,
         95 (1935), 539.

3435.   National Organization for Public Health Nursing. *Courses in
         Public Health Nursing for Graduate Nurses. 1*. New York:
         The Organization, 1924, 1926, 1927.

3436.   ————. *The Public Health Nursing Curriculum Guide*. New
         York: The Organization, 1942.

                        OTHER SPECIALTY EDUCATION

3437.   Clemons, B. "Diploma Schools: The Operating Room, Nursing's
         First Specialty." *RN*, 36 (Feb 1973), 1-9.

3438.   Daley, Mary Anselm. "Historical Development of the Medical-
         Surgical Nursing Course in the United States from 1873 to
         1950." Ph.D. dissertation, St. Louis University, 1963.

3439.   Pittman, Jacquelyn. "The Development of Graduate Programs in
         Psychiatric Nursing, 1932-1968, and the Relationship to
         Congressional Legislation." Ed.D. dissertation, Columbia
         University, 1974.

3440.   Schubert, Florence Marguerite. "The Emergence of Preparation
         for Psychiatric Nursing in Professional Nursing Education
         Programs in the United States, 1873-1918." Ed.D. disser-
         tation, Columbia University, 1972.

3441.   Smith, A.A. *Operating Room: A Primer for Public Nurses*.
         Philadelphia: W.B. Saunders Co., 1924.

                    SCHOOLS OF NURSING: AMERICAN--GENERAL

3342.   American Nurses' Association. *Schools of Nursing Accredited
         by the State Boards of Nurse Examiners, 1918-1928*. 5 vols.
         New York: The Association, 1918-1929.

3443.   Bayldon, Margaret C. "Diploma Schools: First Century."
         RN, 36 (Feb 1973), 33.

3444.   "Beginnings of Some Famous Schools." *Tr Nurs & Hosp Rev*, 101
         (Aug 1938), 115-122.

3445.   Campbell, A.F. "Two Chicago Hospitals and Training Schools."
         Tr Nurs & Hosp Rev, 23 (1899), 130.

3446.   Clinton, Fred S. "The First Hospital and Training School for
         Nurses in the Indian Territory, Now Oklahoma." *Chron
         Oklahoma*, 25 (1947), 218-228.

3447.   "Diploma Schools: The Long Road to Today." *RN*, 36 (Feb 1973),
         34-48.

3448.   "Diploma Schools: for Negro Schools, Nearly a Century." *RN*,
         36 (Feb 1973), 67-68.

3449.   "Diploma Schools: Famous Graduates: 'A Notable Company, Long
         Remembered.'" *RN*, 36 (Feb 1973), 83-86.

3450.   "Diploma Schools: Massachusetts General, Yesterday and
         Today." *RN*, 36 (Feb 1973), 75-80.

3451.   Dolan, Josephine A. "Nurses in American History: Three
         Schools--1873." *Am J Nurs*, 75(6) (Jun 1975), 989-992.

3452.   Labecki, Geraldine. "Baccalaureate Programs in Nursing in
         the Southern Region, 1925-1960." Ed.D. dissertation,
         George Peabody College for Teachers, 1967.

3453.   May, Mary Elizabeth. "Nurse Training Schools of the New York
         State Hospitals." *Am J Nurs*, 8 (Oct 1907), 18-24.

3454.   National League of Nursing Education, Publication Committee.
         Calendar, 1925. Early Schools of Nursing in America. New
         York: The League, 1924.

3455.   New York (City). Department of Health. "New York City's
         Facilities for the Training of Nurses." *Weekly Bull Dept
         Hlth C NY* (22 Apr 1916).

3456.   The New York Inspector Editor. "Announcement of and Comment
         on Appointment of Annie W. Goodrich as Inspector of Schools
         of Nursing Under Department of Education New York State."
         NY Inspector, 10 (Jul 1910), 32-33.

3457.   "Nurses' Schools and Illegal Practice of Medicine." *J Am
         Med Assoc*, 47 (1906), 1835.

3458.   Putnam, Charles Pickering. *Training Schools for Nurses in
         America*. New York, 1874. Read at the annual meeting of
         the American Social Science Assn., October 14, 1874.

3459.   Sutlittle, Irene. "History of American Training Schools
         Hospital, Dispensary and Nursing." *Int Cong Char 1893*
         Baltimore and London, 1894.

3460.   Thompson, William Gilman. *Training Schools for Nurses with
         Notes on Twenty-two Schools*. New York: G.P. Putnam's Sons,
         1883.

3461.   Titus, Shirley. "Factors Determining the Development of
         Nursing and Schools of Nursing (with Special Reference to
         Vanderbilt University School of Nursing)." *Methods and
         Problems of Medical Education*. New York: The Rockefeller
         Foundation, 1932.

3462.   "Two Early American Schools of Nursing." *Am J Nurs*, 48
         (Oct 1948), 612-615.

3463.   U.S. Bureau of Education. *Nurse Training Schools 1917-1919*.
         Washington, D.C.: U.S. Government Printing Office, 1920.

3464.   Woolsey, Abby Howland. *Hospitals and Training Schools Report
         of the Standing Committee on Hospitals of the State
         Charities Aid Association*. New York: G.P. Putnam's Sons,
         1950.

SCHOOLS OF NURSING: AMERICAN--SPECIFIC

ARMY SCHOOL OF NURSING

3465.   Goodrich, Annie W. "The Plan for the Army School of Nursing."
         *Twenty-fifth Annual Report of the National League of Nurs-
         ing Education*. New York: National League of Nursing Edu-
         cation, 1918.

3466.   Jamme, Anna C. "The Army School of Nursing." *Pub Hlth Mich*,
         7 (1919), 97.

BELLEVUE

3467. Cooper, Page. *The Bellevue Story*. New York: Thomas Y. Crowell, 1948.

3468. Crosby, Alice B. "The First Training School for Nurses in America." *Am J Nurs*, 16 (Dec 1915), 236-237.

3469. Dock, Lavinia L. "How Trained Nursing Began in America. History of the Reform Nursing in Bellevue Hospital." *Am J Nurs*, 2 (Nov 1901), 89-98.

3470. Giles, Dorothy. *A Candle in Her Hand*. New York: G.P. Putnam's Sons, 1949.

3471. Hobson, Elizabeth Christophers. *Founding of the Bellevue Training School for Nurses*. New York: G.P. Putnam's Sons, 1916. Reprinted, *A Century of Nursing*. New York: G.P. Putnam's Sons, 1950.

3472. "Professional Education in the Seventies." *Tr Nurs & Hosp Rev*, 90 (Jan 1933), 24-25.

3473. Woolsey, Abby Howland. *A Century of Nursing with Hints Toward the Organization of Training Schools, and Florence Nightingale's Historic Letter on the Bellevue School*. New York: G.P. Putnam's Sons, 1950. Originally published anonymously in 1876 as Publication No. 11 of State Charities Aid Association, New York.

BOLTON

3474. Faddis, Margene O. *The History of the Frances Payne Bolton School of Nursing*. Cleveland: Alumni Association of the Frances Payne Bolton School of Nursing, 1948.

3475. ————. *A School of Nursing Comes of Age: A History of the Frances Payne Bolton School of Nursing, Case Western University*. Cleveland: Alumnae of the Frances Payne Bolton School of Nursing, 1973.

BOSTON

3476. Curtis, Mrs., and Miss Denny. "Early History of the Boston Training School." *Am J Nurs*, 2 (Feb 1902), 331-335.

3477. Riddle, Mary M. *Boston City Hospital Training School for Nurses*. Boston: n.p., 1928. 203 pp.

CALEDONIAN

3478. "Nursing--Past and Present ... Caledonian Hospital School of Practical Nursing in Brooklyn, New York." *Nurs Care*, 8 (Mar 1975), 18-19.

CAPITAL CITY

3479.   Youtz, Dorothy, with Irene B. Page and Mary Goodreau. *The*
        Capital City School of Nursing: Formerly the Washington
        Training School for Nurses 1877-1972. Washington, D.C.:
        Capital City School of Nursing Alumnae Association, 1975.

CHILDREN'S HOSPITAL: BOSTON

3480.   Goostray, Stella. *Fifty Years: A History of the School of*
        Nursing, the Children's Hospital, Boston. Boston: The
        Alumnae Association of the Children's Hospital School of
        Nursing, 1940.

COLORADO

3481.   Boyd, L.C. "Colorado School for Nurses 1887-1924: A Bit of
        Western Nursing History." *Tr Nurs & Hosp Rev*, 72 (1924),
        433.

COLORADO TRAINING SCHOOL

3482.   Mumey, Nolie. *Cap, Pin and Diploma; A History of the Colorado*
        Training School. Boulder, CO: Johnson Publishing Co.,
        1968.

CONNECTICUT TRAINING SCHOOL

3483.   Bacon, F. "Founding of the Connecticut Training School for
        Nurses." *Tr Nurs*, 15 (1895), 187-193.

3484.   Stack, Margaret K. "Resumé of the History of the Connecticut
        Training School for Nurses." *Am J Nurs*, 23 (Jul 1923),
        825, 829.

CORNELL UNIVERSITY--SEE NEW YORK HOSPITAL

FARRAND

3485.   Deans, Agnes G., and Anne L. Austin. *The History of the*
        Farrand Training School for Nurses. Detroit: Alumnae
        Association of the Farrand School for Nurses, 1936.

FLOWER MISSION

3486.   Wishard, W.N. "Early Days of Flower Mission Training
        School." *J Ind Med Assoc*, 27 (Jan 1934), 21-25.

HARRIS COLLEGE

3487.   Harris, L. *Harris College of Nursing: Five Decades of*
        Struggle for a Cause. Fort Worth: Texas Christian Univer-
        sity Press, 1973.

ILLINOIS

3488.   McIsaac, D. "Illinois School for Nurses, Chicago, U.S.A."
        Nurs Mirror, 27 (1900), 261.

3489.   Schryver, Grace Fay. *History of the Illinois Training School
        for Nurses 1880-1929*. Chicago: Board of Directors of the
        Illinois Training School for Nurses, 1930.

JOHNS HOPKINS

3490.   Johns, Ethel, and Blanche Pfefferkorn. *The Johns Hopkins
        Hospital School of Nursing 1889-1949*. Baltimore: The Johns
        Hopkins Press, 1954.

3491.   Leone, L.P. "Closing Ceremony the Johns Hopkins Hospital
        School of Nursing." *Alum Mag*, 72 (Jul 1973), 35-44.

3492.   Osler, William. "Address at Commencement of the Nurses'
        Training School." *Johns Hop Nurs Alum Mag* (Jul 1913),
        72-81.

LOMA LINDA UNIVERSITY

3493.   Atteberry, Maxine. *From Pinafores to Pantsuites: The Story
        of Loma Linda University School of Nursing*. Whittier, CA:
        Fenn Lithographics, 1975.

MARION COUNTY

3494.   Wishard, W., Jr. "The Genesis of Marion County General Hos-
        pital and Its Training School for Nurses." *J Ind Med Assoc*,
        59 (Mar 1966), 264-274.

MARY HITCHCOCK MEMORIAL HOSPITAL

3494.1 Land, Loretta Churney. *Hiram Hitchcock's Legacy: The History
        of the Mary Hitchcock Memorial Hospital School of Nursing*.
        Canaan, NH: Phoenix Publishing, 1980.

MASSACHUSETTS GENERAL

3495.   Parsons, Sara E. *History of the Massachusetts General Hos-
        pital Training School of Nursing*. Boston: Whitcomb and
        Barrows, 1922.

3496.   Perkins, Sylvia. *A Centennial Review: The Massachusetts
        General Hospital School of Nursing 1873-1973*. Boston:
        Alumnae Association of the Massachusetts General Hospital
        School of Nursing, 1975.

MEDICAL COLLEGE OF SOUTH CAROLINA

3497.   Chamberlin, Ruth. *The School of Nursing of the Medical
        College of South Carolina: Its Story*. Columbia, SC: 1970.

MONTANA STATE UNIVERSITY

3498.   Sherrick, Anna Pearl, with Jeanne M. Claus and John P. Parker.
         Montana State University School of Nursing. Bozeman, MT:
         Big Sky Books, 1976.

NEW YORK HOSPITAL--CORNELL UNIVERSITY

3499.   Dufton, Lena, ed. *History of Nursing at the New York Post-*
         graduate Medical School and Hospital. New York: Alumnae
         Association of New York Hospital School of Nursing, 1944.

3500.   Jones, Cadwalader, Mrs. "Looking Back Through Fifty Years."
         Alum J NYC Hosp Sch Nurs, Golden Anniversary Number, 1875-
         1929 (Jul 1925), 11.

3501.   Number deleted.

3502.   Jordan, Helen Jamieson. *Cornell University--New York Hos-*
         pital School of Nursing 1877-1952. New York: New York
         Hospital, 1952.

PENNSYLVANIA HOSPITAL

3503.   Tomes, N. "Little World of Our Own; The Pennsylvania Hospi-
         tal Training School for Nurses, 1895-1907." *J Hist Med*, 33
         (1978), 507-530.

3503.1   Stachniewicz, Stephanie A., and Jean K. Axelrod. *The Double*
         Frill: A History of the Philadelphia General Hospital
         School of Nursing. Philadelphia: George F. Stickley, 1978.

PRESBYTERIAN HOSPITAL AND COLUMBIA UNIVERSITY

3504.   Lamb, Albert R. *The Presbyterian Hospital and the Columbia-*
         Presbyterian Medical Center 1868-1943. New York: Columbia
         University Press, 1955.

3505.   Lee, Eleanor. *History of the School of Nursing of the Pres-*
         byterian Hospital, New York, 1892-1942. New York: G.P.
         Putnam's Sons, 1942.

3506.   ————. *Neighbors 1892-1967: A History of the Department of*
         Nursing, Faculty of Medicine, Columbia University 1937-1967
         and Its Predecessor, the School of Nursing of the Presby-
         terian Hospital New York, 1892-1935. New York: Columbia
         University, Presbyterian Hospital School of Nursing Alumnae
         Association, 1967.

PURDUE UNIVERSITY

3507.   Johnson, Helen R. *A History of Purdue University's Nursing*
         Education Programs. Ed.D. dissertation, Purdue University,
         1975. 195 pp.

ST. LOUIS CITY HOSPITAL

3508.   Green, E. *History of the St. Louis City Hospital Training
        School for Nurses Which Later Became the St. Louis City
        Hospital Training School for Nurses.* St. Louis: n.p.,
        1941. 12 pp.

ST. LUKE'S HOSPITAL

3509.   Keller, Malvina W. *History of the St. Luke's Hospital
        Training School for Nurses.* New York: St. Luke's Hospital,
        1938.

ST. VINCENT'S HOSPITAL

3510.   "Fifty Years of Nursing Education at St. Vincent's Hospital."
        Hosp (Oct 1942), 16, 50-51.

3511.   Loftus, Maria D. Andrea. *A History of St. Vincent's Hospital
        School of Nursing, Indianapolis, Indiana: 1896-1970.*
        Indianapolis: Litho Press, 1972.

TEACHERS COLLEGE--COLUMBIA UNIVERSITY

3512.   Number deleted.

3513.   "A Century of Progress in Nursing." *Nurs Mirror*, 99 (11 Jun
        1954), 697.

3514.   Christy, Teresa E. *Cornerstone for Nursing Education: A
        History of the Division of Nursing Education of Teachers
        College, Columbia University, 1899-1947.* New York:
        Teachers College Press, 1969.

3515.   Nursing Education of Teachers College, Department of and the
        Committee on University Relations of the National League
        of Nursing Education. *Proceedings of Conference on Nurs-
        ing Schools Connected with Colleges and Universities.* New
        York: National League of Nursing Education, 1928.

3516.   "Proceedings, Alumnae Celebration of the Fortieth Anniversary
        of Nursing Education in Teachers College, 1939." *Nurs Educ
        Bull* (Feb 1940), 1-84.

UNIVERSITY OF MICHIGAN

3517.   Kirkconnell, Norma E., and R. Faye McCain. "The Development
        of the Degree Program of Nursing at the University of
        Michigan." *Mich Med Bull* (1956).

UNIVERSITY OF MINNESOTA

3518.   Gray, James. *Education for Nursing: History of the Univer-
        sity of Minnesota School of Nursing.* Minneapolis: Univer-
        sity of Minnesota Press, 1960.

UNIVERSITY OF MISSOURI

3519.   Potter, R., and J. Hofmann. "The School of Nursing at the
        University of Missouri." *Missouri Med* (1960).

UNIVERSITY OF PENNSYLVANIA

3520.   Stephenson, M.V. *The First Fifty Years of the Training
        School for Nurses of the Hospital of the University of
        Pennsylvania*. Philadelphia: J.B. Lippincott Co., 1940.

UNIVERSITY OF TEXAS

3521.   Brown, Billye Jean. *The Historical Development of the Univer-
        sity of Texas System School of Nursing, 1890-1973*.
        Ed.D. dissertation, Baylor University, 1975.

UNIVERSITY OF WASHINGTON

3522.   Lawrence, Cora Jane. *University Education for Nursing in
        Seattle, 1920-1950: An Inside Story of the University of
        Washington School*. Ph.D. dissertation, University of
        Washington, 1972.

VINELAND, NEW JERSEY

3523.   Vernon, Mary L. "Notes on the Early Days of the Training
        School." *Tr Sch Bull* (1942), 22-25.

WALTHAM TRAINING SCHOOL

3524.   Parker, Martha P. "Preparatory Work at the Waltham Training
        School." *Am J Nurs*, 3 (Jan 1903), 264-266.

WARSAW SCHOOL OF NURSING

3525.   Pohlman, Helen Bridye. *Warsaw School of Nursing, 1921-1928*.
        Moskogee, OK: Donald Kilgour Sharlte, 1966.

YALE

3526.   "Great University to Train Nurses." *World's Work*, 47 (1923),
        142-143.

3527.   "Twenty-fifth Anniversary Exercises, Yale School of Nursing."
        Yale J Biol Med, 21 (1949), 263-292.

3528.   "Undergraduate School of Nursing of Yale University." *Sch
        & Soc*, (28 Apr 1923), 460.

SCHOOLS OF NURSING: BRITISH

3529.   "Alfred Hospital, 1871-1971, The Training School." *UNA Nurs J*, 69 (Jun 1971), 14-20.

3530.   "The Committee or the Council of the Nightingale Fund Desire to Make the Following Report of Their Proceedings to the Council." *Canad Nurs*, 8 (Feb 1912), 71-73, 96. Reprint of the Committee's First Report by J. Jebb, Chairman, 1861.

3531.   "Extract from the First Report of the Bristol Nurses' Training Institute and Home 1862." *Queen's Nurs J*, 17 (Feb 1975), 238.

3532.   "The First Nursing School in the World--St. Thomas' Hospital School in London." *Munca Sanit*, 17 (Aug 1969), 449-454. (Rum)

3533.   Gould, Marion E. "Growth of the Nightingale School." *Nurs Times*, 56 (13 May 1960), 590-592.

3534.   Hallowes, Ruth M. "The Nightingale Training School of St. Thomas' Hospital, London." *Int Nurs Rev*, 7 (Jun 1960), 11-16.

3535.   Hillyers, G.V. "Nightingale Training School of St. Thomas Hospital." *St Thom Hosp Gaz*, 36 (Oct 1938), 490-495.

3536.   McInnes, E.M. "The History of Nursing in St. Thomas' Hospital." *Nurs Mirror*, 114 (31 Aug 1962), 2893.

3537.   Nightingale, Florence. "Letter to the Nurses of the Nightingale School." *Caridad Cienc Arte*, 8 (Jan-Mar 1971), 3-4. (Spa)

3538.   *The Nightingale Training School: St. Thomas' Hospital, 1860-1910*. London: Privately printed for the Nightingale Nursing School for Nurses, 1960.

3539.   *Organization of Nursing; An Account of the Liverpool Nurses' Training School, Its Foundation, Progress, and Operation in Hospital, District, and Private Nursing*. Liverpool and London: A. Holden, 1865.

3540.   Turner, T. "The Nightingale Training School 1860-1960." *St. Thom Hosp Gaz*, 58 (1960), 65-67.

SCHOOLS OF NURSING: CANADIAN

3541.   Cavers, Anne S. *Our School of Nursing 1899 to 1949*. Vancouver: Vancouver General Hospital, n.d.

3542.   Greene, C.H. "Canadian Training Schools for Nurses." *Canad Nurs*, 4 (Dec 1908), 596-601.

3543.   Johns, Ethel. *The Winnipeg General Hospital School of Nursing, 1887-1953*. Winnipeg: Alumnae Association, 1957. 85 pp.

3544.   MacDermot, H.E. *History of the School for Nurses of the Montreal General Hospital*. Montreal: Alumnae Association of the School for Nurses of the Montreal General Hospital, 1940.

3545.   "Miss Harmer Goes to McGill School for Graduate Nurses." *Am J Nurs*, 28 (Apr 1928), 465.

3546.   Tunis, B.L. *In Caps and Gowns; The Story of the School for Graduate Nurses, McGill University 1920-1964*. Montreal: McGill University Press, 1966.

SCHOOLS OF NURSING: OTHER COUNTRIES

3547.   Almeida, Prado E.N. de. "Study ... of Nursing School of Sao Paulo." *Gaz Clin*, 40 (Mar 1942), 79-82.

3548.   Armstrong, D.M., and E.A. Cottee. *The First Fifty Years--A History of Nursing at the Royal Prince Alfred Hospital, Sydney, from 1882 to 1952*. Sydney: Alfred Hospital Graduate Nurses Association, 1965.

3549.   Balunsat, Rosa, et al. "Histories of Nursing Schools in Philippine Islands." *Filipino Nurs*, 3 (Apr 1929), 32-43.

3550.   Cusak, Frank. *Lister House: the Story of the North District School of Nursing*. Melbourne: Hawthorne Press, 1976.

3551.   De Carvalho, A.C. "Historico da Escola de Enfermagem 'Lauriston Job Lone.'" *Rev Brasil Enferm*, 18 (Apr-Jun 1965), 151-156. (Por)

3552.   Disselhoff, D. "The Deaconesses of Kaiserwerth; A Hundred Years' War." *Int Nurs Rev*, 9 (1934), 19-28.

3553.   "Early History of the 80 Year Old Tokyo University School of Nursing." *Nakazata R Kango*, 22 (Jan 1970), 71-78. (Jap)

3554.   Garfield, Richard. "Nursing Education in China." *Nurs Out*, 26 (May 1978), 312-315.

3555.   Ghini, Laura. "Ineamenti Della Organizzazione Strutturale Della Scuola Per Infermiere Professionali (Outlines of the Structural Organization of the School for Professional Nurses)." *Annali Di Sociologia*, 7 (1970), 136-150. (Ital)

3556.   Goffe, G. "Jamaica's First School of Nursing." *Jamaica Nurs*,
        5 (Aug 1965), 11.

3557.   Guzman, C. "History of a School." *P Rico Enferm*, 48 (Jun
        1972), 15-20. (Spa)

3558.   Harnar, Ruth May. *The Place of Church Related Schools of
        Nursing in the Health Care Systems of India*. Ed.D. disser-
        tation, Columbia University Teachers College, 1975.

3559.   Hibbard, M. Eugenie. "The Establishment of Schools for
        Nurses in Cuba." *Am J Nurs*, 2 (Sep 1902), 985-989.

3560.   "History of Two Philippine Schools of Nursing." *Filipino
        Nurs*, 17 (Oct 1947), 83-84.

3561.   Knudsen, H. "Preparatory Education in the Testrup College
        Will End at the Turn of the Year. A Chapter in Nursing
        Will Soon Be Over." *Sygeplejersken*, 74(50) (18 Dec 1974),
        4, 5, 17. (Dan)

3562.   Kockx, A. "The Higher Institute for Nursing: Past, Present
        and Future." *FNIB*, 56(3) (1978), 11-22. (Dut)

3563.   Lourens, S.G. "History of the Pretoria College of Nursing."
        So Afr Nurs J, 31 (Jun 1974), 7-12.

3464.   Nightingale, Florence. *The Institute of Kaiserwerth on the
        Rhine, for the Practical Training of Deaconesses*. London:
        Inmates of the Ragged Colonial Training School, 1851.

3565.   "Norwegian Nursing College, 50 Years." *Sykepleien*, 62(18)
        (20 Sep 1975), 836-841. (Nor)

3566.   Reinhart, A. *A Memorial: The Kaiserswerth Deaconesses at
        Alexandria*. Alexandria: Kaiserswerth Deaconesses' Hospital,
        1932.

3567.   "Sao Paulo's Women in White, Sao Paulo's School of Nursing."
        Americas, 1 (Dec 1949), 28-31.

3568.   Shala, Sarah G. "Nursing in Syria (American University Hos-
        pital School of Nursing)." *Am J Nurs*, 30 (Dec 1930), 1515-
        1518.

3569.   "Thirtieth Anniversary of Helsinki's Swedish Nursing Insti-
        tute." *Sairaanhoitaja*, 54(8) (1978), 29. (Fin)

3570.   Tsuboi, Y. "History of Nursing Education at Kikei Hospital."
        Kango Kyoiku, 19 (1978), 255-259, 317-323, 385-391, 447-
        453. (Jap)

3571.   "Ulleval's Nursing School: 75th Anniversary." *Sykepleien*,
        62(9) (5 May 1975), 376-377. (Nor)

3572.   Vanegas, L.W. "Historical Development of the Nursing Career
        in the National University of Columbia." *ANEC*, 7(17) (Jan-
        Apr 1976), 51-55. (Spa)

3573.   "Victoria House Nurse Training School, Friedrichshain Kranken-
        haus, Berlin." *Nurs Rec* (25 Jan 1902), 69-70.

3574.   Zepps, K. "The Role of the N.S.W. College of Nursing Regard-
        ing the Educational and Professional Development of Nursing
        in N.S.W." *Lamp*, 23(2) (Dec 1975), 3, 5, 7.

                TEXTBOOKS WITH HISTORICAL SIGNIFICANCE

            See also Nursing Specialties and Education for addi-
            tional listings of texts.

3575.   An American Woman. *Suggestions for the Sick Room.* New York:
        Anson D.F. Randolph, 1876.

3576.   Barwell, Richard. *The Care of the Sick: A Course of Practi-
        cal Lectures Delivered at the Working Women's College.* 1st
        ed. London: Chapman, 1857. 2nd ed. London: n.p., 1857.
        171 pp.

3577.   Chayer, Mary Ella. "The Trail of the Nursing Textbook."
        Am J Nurs, 50 (Oct 1950), 606-607.

3578.   Connecticut Training School for Nurses. *Handbook of Nursing
        for Family and General Use.* Philadelphia: J.B. Lippincott
        Co., 1878.

3579.   Dock, Lavinia L. *Textbook of Materia Medica for Nurses.*
        4th ed. New York: G.P. Putnam's Sons, 1905. 330 pp.

3579.1 Donahoe, Mary Frances. *A Manual of Nursing.* New York:
        D. Appleton & Co., 1910.

3580.   G.P. *Home-Nursing: A Manual for the Use of All Who Would
        Nurse the Sick in a Private House.* London: George Rout-
        ledge & Sons, 1867.

3581.   Hill, S.C. *A Cook Book for Nurses.* Boston: Whitcomb &
        Barrows, 1906.

3582.   Hodson, Jane. *How to Become a Trained Nurse.* New York:
        William Abbott, 1898.

3583.   *How to Nurse Sick Children--Intended Especially as a Help to
        the Nurses at the Hospital for Sick Children.* London:
        Longman, Brown, Green and Longmans, 1854.

3584.   *Instruction Pour Les Fraters et Les Infirmiers de l'Armee
        Federale.* Berne: Imprimerie Haller, 1862.

3585. Kimber, D.C., and C.E. Gray. *Anatomy and Physiology for Nurses*. New York: Macmillan Co., 1893.

3586. Ladies' Sanitary Association. *"The Black Hole" in Our Own Bedroom*. London: Jarrold and Sons, after 1857.

3587. ————. *The Cheap Doctor: A Word About Fresh Air*. London: Jarrold & Sons, after 1857.

3588. ————. *Health Rules*. 3rd ed. London: Jarrold & Sons, after 1857.

3589. Lees, Florence. *Handbook for Hospital Sisters*. London: W. Ibister & Co., 1874.

3590. Nightingale, Florence. *Notes on Nursing: What It Is, and What It is Not*. New York: D. Appleton & Co., 1860.

3591. *Plain Words About Sickness, Addressed to the Mothers and Wives of Working Men. By a Doctor's Wife*. London: Seeley, Jackson, and Halliday, 1861. 156 pp.

3592. *The Sick Room Attendant: Containing Directions for the Young or Inexperienced Nurse. By a Lady*. London: n.p., 1844; new edition, 1859.

3593. Warrington, Joseph. *The Nurses' Guide. Containing a Series of Instructions to Females Who Wish to Engage in the Important Business of Nursing Mother and Child in the Lying-in-Chamber*. Philadelphia: T. Cowperthwait & Co., 1839. Excerpted in *History of Nursing Source Book*, Anne L. Austin. New York: G.P. Putnam's Sons, 1957. pp. 255-256.

3594. Number deleted.

3595. Weeks-Shaw, C.S. *A Textbook of Nursing for the Use of Training Schools, Families and Private Students*. New York: D. Appleton, 1885. Rev. ed., 1897.

3596. Wilcox, R.W. *A Manual of Fever Nursing*. 2nd ed. Philadelphia: P. Blakiston's Sons & Co., 1904.

3597. Wilson, J.C. *Fever Nursing*. Philadelphia: J.B. Lippincott, 1888.

3598. Zabriskie, L. *Nurses Handbook of Obstetrics*. Philadelphia: J.B. Lippincott Co., 1929.

11. NURSING LICENSURE AND THE LAW
AS IT RELATES TO NURSING

3599.   Agree, Betty C. "The Threat of Institutional Licensure."
        Am J Nurs, 73 (Oct 1973), 1758-1763.

3600.   "All Those Who Nurse for Hire!" (editorial). *Am J Nurs*, 39
        (Mar 1939), 275-277.

3601.   Amberg, Emil. "State Registration of Nurses." *Brit J Nurs*
        (18 Jun 1904), 494-496.

3602.   "Amendment of the Arizona Nursing Practice Law Broadens
        Definition of Professional Nursing." *Am J Nurs*, 72 (Jul
        1972), 1203.

3603.   American Hospital Association. "Statement on Licensure of
        Health Care Personnel." *Hosp*, 45 (16 Mar 1971).

3604.   American Nurses Association. *Legal Aspects of Nursing*.
        Reprints of articles by Nathan Hershey. New York: ANA,
        1962.

3605.   ————. "Resolution on Institutional Licensure." *Am J Nurs*,
        72 (Jun 1972), 1106.

3606.   Amthill, Lord. "State Registration of Nurses." *Nineteenth
        Cent*, 68 (Aug 1910), 303-306.

3607.   "A.N.A. Board Approves a Definition of Nursing Practice."
        Am J Nurs, 55 (1955), 1474.

3608.   Anderson, Bernice E. *Facilitation of the Interstate Movement
        of Nurses*. Philadelphia: J.B. Lippincott Co., 1950.

3609.   Barbee, Grace. "When is the Nurse Held Liable?" *Am J Nurs*,
        54 (1954), 1343-1346.

3610.   ————. "Special Procedures: I.V.s, Blood Transfusions, and
        Skin Testing." *Proceedings: Institute on Medico-Legal
        Aspects of Nursing Practice*. Santa Monica, CA: California
        Nurses' Association, 1961. pp. 41-44.

3611.   Barnett, R.P. "Speech Made When Moving the 2nd Reading of
        the Nurses Registration Bill in the House of Commons
        March 28th." *Brit J Nurs* (5 Apr 1919), 217-229.

3612.   Bonham-Carter, H. "Is a General Register for Nurses Desir-
          able?" *Nurs Rec* (6 Sep 1888), 301-304.

3613.   Booth, Audrey. "Legal Accommodation of the Nurse Practitioner
          Concept--The Process in North Carolina." *Nurs Pract*, 2
          (Nov-Dec 1977), 13-15, 27.

3614.   Boyd, Louie C. *State Registration for Nurses*. 2nd ed.
          Philadelphia: W.B. Saunders Co., 1915.

3615.   "Brief History and Current Provisions of the Law to Regulate
          the Practice of Nursing in Maine, October 18, 1972."
          Maine Nurs, 4 (Jul 1973), 10-13.

3616.   British Medical Association. "Memorandum on the Bills for
          State Registration of Nurses Prepared Respectively by the
          Association for the State Registration of Trained Nurses
          and the Royal British Nurses Association." *Brit J Nurs*
          (11 Jun 1904), 472-473.

3617.   ———. "Circular Sent to the Chairmen of the Committees of
          Management of Hospitals Throughout the UK Having Nurse
          Training Schools Attached Suggesting the Foundation of a
          Registration Council." *Nurs Rec* (21 Nov 1889), 284-285.

3618.   Bullough, Bonnie. "The Law and the Expanding Nursing Role."
          Am J Pub Hlth, 66 (Mar 1976), 249-254; see also Bonnie
          Bullough, *The Law and the Expanding Nursing Role*. New
          York: Appleton-Century-Crofts, 1975. 2nd ed. 1980.

3619.   ———. "The Medicare-Medicaid Amendments." *Am J Nurs*, 73
          (Nov 1973), 1927-1929.

3620.   Cazalas, Mary W. *Nursing and the Law*. Germantown, MD: Aspen
          Systems Corp., 1978.

3621.   Central Committee for the State Registration of Nurses.
          "Correspondence Between Committee and the College of Nurs-
          ing on the Nurses Registration Bill." *Brit J Nurs* (2 Dec
          1916), 447-454.

3622.   ———. "Deputation to the Home Secretary." *Brit J Nurs*
          (8 Aug 1914), 115-122.

3623.   ———. "State Legislation and the College of Nursing
          (Negotiations Between the Commission and the College of
          Nursing to Join a Bill)." *Brit J Nurs* (16 Sep 1916),
          238-240.

3624.   Clarke, Alice R. "Legislation--News and Views" (editorial).
          RN, 12 (Apr 1949), 39-41, 55.

3625.   Cohen, H.S., and L.K. Milike. *Developments in Health Man-
          power Licensure: A Follow Up to the 1971 Report on Licen-
          sure and Related Health Personnel Credentialing*.

Washington, D.C.: Department of H.E.W. Publication, HRA 74-3101, 1973.

3626. College of Nursing. "College of Nursing Opposes the Nurses Petition to the Prime Minister." *Brit J Nurs* (9 Jun 1917), 398-399.

3627. ————. "Conference on State Registration." *Brit J Nurs* (1 Apr 1916), 292-300.

3628. ————. "The Reasons for the State Registration of Trained Nurses." *Nurs Rec* (25 Aug 1900), 149-150.

3629. Conference on State Registration of Nurses. "Conference Between Representatives of Various Nursing Bodies and the Parliamentary Bills Committee of the B.M.A. Held on 14th January 1896; Report of Proceedings." *Nurs Rec* (18 Jan 1896), 55-57.

3630. Corning, Peter A. *The Evolution of Medicare; From Idea to Law.* U.S. Department of Health, Education and Welfare, Social Security Administration, Research Report 19. Washington, D.C.: U.S. Government Printing Office, 1969.

3631. Crawford, J.A. "The Reasons for the State Registration of Trained Nurses." *Nurs Rec* (25 Aug 1900), 149-150.

3632. Creighton, Helen. *Law Every Nurse Should Know.* 2nd ed. Philadelphia: W.B. Saunders, 1970. 3rd ed., 1975.

3633. Davis, Anne J., and Mila A. Aroskar. *Ethical Dilemmas and Nursing Practice.* New York: Appleton-Century-Crofts, 1978.

3634. Dean, W.J. "State Legislation for Physician's Assistant: A Review and Analysis." *Hlth Serv Rep*, 88 (Jan 1973), 3-12.

3635. Dent, V. *United States Reports: Cases Adjudged in the Supreme Court.* (1888), pp. 114-128.

3636. "Deputation of Anti-Registrationists at the Privy Council Office." *Brit J Nurs* (23 Jun 1905), 499-501.

3637. Derbyshire, Robert C. *Medical Licensure and Discipline in the United States.* Baltimore: The Johns Hopkins Press, 1969.

3638. DeSilva, E.B. "Jurisprudence for Nurses." *Hosp Prog*, 14 (Jan 1933), 23-26.

3639. deTornyay, R. "State Board Member." *Am J Nurs*, 69 (Mar 1969), 570-572.

3640. Dietrich, Clay. "The Nurse and the Law." *Hosp*, 10 (Feb 1936), 34-39.

3641.   "Discussion on Proposed Legislation Against Midwives." *Med Rec*, 53 (Feb 1898), 210-211.

3642.   Dock, Lavinia. "The Progress of Registration in Holland and Australia." *Am J Nurs*, 5 (1905), 318-319.

3643.   ———. "State Registration." *Brit J Nurs* (Feb 1905), 148-151.

3644.   ———. "What We May Expect from the Law." *Am J Nurs*, 1 (Oct 1900), 8-12.

3645.   Doubleday, E.M. "Journal of Midwifery. Nursing Homes (Registration) Bill." *Nurs Times*, 23 (15 Oct 1927), 1236.

3646.   Driscoll, V.M. "Reflections on the Birth of an Idea." *J NY State Nurs Assoc*, 2 (Winter 1971), 5.

3647.   Eccard, Walter T. "Revolution in White: New Approaches in Training Nurses as Professionals." *Vanderbilt Law Rev*, 30 (May 1977), 839-879.

3648.   Eve, Robert C. "Licensing of Midwives." *Charlotte Med J*, 6 (1895), 990-995.

3649.   "The Expanded Role of the Nurse: A Joint Statement of CNA/CMA." *Canad Nurs* (May 1973), 23-25.

3650.   Fenwick, Ethel Gordon. "The Nurses' Registration Act." *Brit J Nurs* (10 Jan 1920), 20-22.

3651.   ———. "The Nursing Profession and the Board of Trade." *Brit J Nurs* (22 Jan 1916), 73-75; (29 Jan 1916), 94-99.

3652.   ———. "The Organization and Registration of Nurses." *Nurs Rec* (12 Apr 1902), 284-287.

3653.   ———. "State Registration of Trained Nurses." *19th Cent*, 67 (Jun 1910), 1049-1060.

3654.   Ferguson, H.M. "State Registration of Nurses." *19th Cent*, 55 (Feb 1904), 310-317.

3655.   Fogotson, Edward, Ruth Roemer, Roger W. Newman, and John L. Cook. "Licensure of Other Medical Personnel." *Report of the National Advisory Commission on Health, Manpower*. Vol. 2. Washington, D.C.: U.S. Government Printing Office, 1967. pp. 407-492.

3656.   ———. "Legal Regulation of Health Personnel in the United States." *Report of the National Advisory Commission on Health Manpower*. Vol. 2. Washington, D.C.: U.S. Government Printing Office, 1967. pp. 416-418.

3657.   Forman, Alice M. *Patterns of Legislation and the Practice of Nurse Midwifery in the U.S.A.* New York: American College of Nurse-Midwives, 1974.

3658.   Forman, A.M., and E.M. Cooper. "Legislation and Nurse-Midwifery Practice in U.S.A." *J Nurs Mid* (American College of Nurse-Midwives), 21(2) (Summer 1976).

3659.   Friedmann, W.G. *Law in a Changing Society.* New York: Columbia University Press, 1964.

3659.1 Green, Karen. *Occupational Licensing and the Supply of Non-professional Manpower.* U.S. Department of Labor, Manpower Research Monograph No. 11. Washington, D.C.: U.S. Government Printing Office, 1969.

3660.   Hall, Virginia. *Statutory Regulation of the Scope of Nursing Practice: A Critical Survey.* Chicago: National Joint Practice Commission, 1975.

3661.   Harrison, G., and J.H. Harrison. *The Nurse and the Law.* Philadelphia: F.A. Davis, 1945.

3662.   Health Care Financing Administration, HEW. "Rural Health Clinics: Conditions for Certification." *Fed Reg,* 43 (8 Feb 1978), 5373-5377.

3663.   Health Law Center. *Nursing and the Law.* Edited by Eric W. Springer. Pittsburgh: Aspen Systems Corp., 1970.

3664.   Hemelt, M.D., and M.E. Mackert. *Dynamics of Law in Nursing and Health Care.* Reston, Va.: Reston, 1978.

3665.   Hershey, Nathan. "Alternative to Mandatory Licensure of Health Professionals." *Hosp Prog,* 50 (Mar 1969).

3666.   ————. "Legal Issues in Nursing Practice." *Professional Nursing: Foundations, Perspectives and Relationships.* Edited by Eugenia K. Spalding and Lucile E. Notter. Philadelphia: J.B. Lippincott, 1970. pp. 110-127.

3667.   ————. "Nurses' Medical Practice Problems, Part I." *Am J Nurs,* 62 (Jul 1962), 82-83.

3668.   ————. "Nursing Practice Acts and Professional Delusion." *J Nurs Admin* (Jul-Aug 1974), 36-39.

3669.   Hershey, Nathan, and W. Wheeler. *Health Personnel Regulation in the Public Interest, Questions and Answers on Institutional Licensure.* Sacramento: California Hospital Association, 1973. pp. 13-14.

3670.   Hicks, E.J. "New Nurse Practice Act: Close Up and Its Workings; What the New Law Will Mean to Physician Hospital Administrator and Nurse." *NY State J Med,* 38 (1 Aug 1938), 1098-1102.

3671.   "History and Development of Official Examination of Nurses
        and Social Hygiene Workers." *Rev Philanthrop*, 50 (15 Feb
        1930), 81-90.

3672.   Holland, Sydney. "Manifesto Against State Registration."
        Brit J Nurs (Mar 1904), 246-248.

3673.   ———. "State Registration of Nurses." *19th Cent*, 68 (Jul
        1910), 143-147.

3674.   Hutchison, Dorothy. "Certification: New Impetus to Continu-
        ing Education." *Cont Educ Nurs* (Sep-Oct 1973), 3-4.

3675.   "The Impact of Title VI on Health Facilities." *George
        Washington Law Rev*, 36 (May 1968), 980-993.

3676.   "Institutional Licensure Opposed by NCSNNE." *Am J Nurs*, 72
        (Apr 1973), 701.

3677.   International Council of Nurses: Florence Nightingale Inter-
        national Foundation. *Report of an International Seminar on
        Nursing Legislation, Warsaw, 1970*. Basel: S. Karger, 1971.

3678.   Iverson, M. "Our Nursing Laws." *Tr Nurs & Hosp Rev*, 9
        (1918), 78.

3679.   Kelly, Lucie Young. "Credentialing of Health Care Personnel."
        Nurs Out, 25 (Sep 1977), 562-567.

3680.   ———. "Nursing Practice Acts." *Am J Nurs*, 74 (Jul 1974),
        1310-1319.

3681.   Kinkela, Gabriella, and Robert Kinkela. "Licensure: What's
        It All About?" *Jr Nurs Admin*, 4 (Mar-Apr 1974), 18-19.

3682.   ———. "Laws for Leaders, Institutional Licensure: Cure-All
        or Chaos?" *J Nurs Admin*, 4 (May-Jun 1974), 16-19.

3683.   Kortright, J.L. "Should Midwives be Registered?" *NY J Gyn
        Obs*, 3 (1893), 197-202; see also *Trans NY State Med Assoc*,
        18 (1893), 416-421.

3684.   Lesnik, Milton J., and Bernice E. Anderson. *Legal Aspects of
        Nursing*. Philadelphia: J.B. Lippincott, 1947.

3685.   Luckes, E.C.E. "State Registration of Nurses." *19th Cent*,
        55 (May 1904), 827-839.

3686.   Mabbott, J.M. "The Regulation of Midwives in New York.
        Am J Obs Dis Wom Child, 60 (1907), 516-527.

3687.   Maister, M. "The Control of Nursing Homes and Midwives; Legal
        Aspects and Education." *J Roy San Inst*, 59 (Jul 1938),
        118-128.

3688. Milike, L., and H. Cohen. *Developments in Health Manpower Licensure and Related Health Personnel Credentialing.* U.S. Dept. of HEW Pub. No. HRA 74-3101. Washington, D.C.: U.S. Government Printing Office, 1973.

3689. Miller, Carol. *Nurses and the Law.* Danville, IL: Interstate Printers and Publishers, 1970.

3690. Mills, Edith W., and Joan Dale. "Florence Nightingale and State Registration." *Int Nurs Rev*, 11 (Feb 1964), 31-36.

3691. "Movement for Licensing Nurses." *Charities & Commons*, 15 (17 Feb 1906), 687.

3692. Murchison, Irene A., and Thomas S. Nichols. *Legal Foundations of Nursing Practice.* London: Collier-Macmillan, 1970.

3693. Murchison, Irene, Thomas S. Nichols, and Rachel Hanson. *Legal Accountability in the Nursing Process.* St. Louis: C.V. Mosby, 1978.

3694. National Center for Health Statistics, U.S. Department of Health, Education and Welfare. *State Licensing of Health Occupations.* PHS Publication No. 1758. Washington, D.C.: U.S. Government Printing Office, 1968.

3695. National Committee on Accrediting. *Part 1: Staff Working Papers: Accreditation of Health Educational Programs.* Washington, D.C.: U.S. Government Printing Office, 1972.

3696. ———. *Study of Accreditation of Selected Health Education Programs. Commission Report.* Washington, D.C.: U.S. Government Printing Office, 1972.

3697. "New Massachusetts Law Restores Autonomy to Board of Nursing." *Am J Nurs*, 76 (May 1976), 831.

3698. "New York State. A Bill for the Registration of Nurses." *Brit J Nurs* (28 Mar 1903), 252.

3699. "New Zealand: The Hospital Nurses Registration Act." *Nurs Rec* (23 Nov 1901), 416-417.

3700. "North Carolina State: An Act to Provide for the Registration of Trained Nurses." *Brit J Nurs* (18 Apr 1903), 314.

3701. "Nurse Practitioners Fight Moves to Restrict Their Practice." *Am J Nurs*, 78 (Aug 1978), 1285-1310.

3702. "Nursing and Midwifery." *So Afr Nurs J*, 16 (Mar 1950), 11-13.

3703. "Nursing Legislation, 1939: What the State Nurses' Associations Accomplished." *Am J Nurs*, 39 (1939), 974-978.

3704.   O'Sullivan, John. *Law for Nurses and Allied Health Profes-
        sionals in Australia.* Sydney: The Law Book Co., Ltd., 1977.

3705.   Palmer, Sophia F. "The Effect of State Registration Upon
        Training Schools." *Am J Nurs*, 5 (Jul 1905), 656.

3706.   *Patterns of Legislation and the Practice of Nurse-Midwifery
        in the United States.* New York: American College of Nurse-
        Midwives, 1974.

3707.   Penka, W. Jean. "History of the Kansas Nurse Practice Act,
        1913-1973." *Kans Nurs*, 48 (Mar 1973), 3-5.

3708.   Peterson, Paul. "Should Institutional Licensure Replace
        Individual Licensure?" *Am J Nurs* (Mar 1974), 446.

3709.   Poole, Henrietta. "The Reasons for the State Registration of
        Trained Nurses." *Nurs Rec* (Aug 1900), 131-133.

3710.   Regenie, S. "Dateline: New York State, 1973." *J Nurs Mid*,
        18 (Summer 1973), 19-23.

3711.   ———. "The New Definition of Nursing in Relation to
        Nurse-Midwifery." *J NY State Nurs Assoc*, 4 (Jul 1973),
        16-19.

3712.   "Registration of Trained Nurses." *Nurs Out*, 73 (14 Mar 1903),
        603-604; see also *Nurs Rec* (Jul 1889), 22-24.

3713.   *Report of the Commission of Inquiry on Health and Social
        Welfare.* Vol. 4. Montreal: Government of Quebec, 1907.

3714.   *Report of the Committee on Nurse Practitioners to the Depart-
        ment of National Health and Welfare, Canada.* Ottawa:
        April, 1972.

3715.   *Report on Licensure and Related Personnel Credentialing.*
        Department of HEW Publication No. HSM 72-11. Washington,
        D.C.: U.S. Government Printing Office, 1971.

3716.   Rockefeller Foundation. *Laws Governing the Practice of Mid-
        wifery (1904-1930).* New York: Rockefeller Foundation, 1931.

3717.   Roemer, Ruth. "Licensing and Regulation of Medical and
        Medical-related Practitioners in Health Service Teams."
        Med Care, 9 (Jan-Feb 1971), 42, 47.

3718.   ———. "The Nurse Practitioner in Family Planning Services:
        Law and Practice." *Fam Plan Pop Rep*, 6(3) (Jun 1977), 28-
        34.

3719.   Roon, Leonore M. "The History of Nursing Legislation in the
        British Commonwealth, 1891-1939." Ph.D. dissertation,
        Radcliffe College, 1952.

3720.   Rothman, Daniel A., and Nancy Lloyd Rothman. *The Professional Nurse and the Law*. Boston: Little, Brown & Co., 1977.

3721.   Rude, Anna E. *The Sheppard-Towner Act in Relation to Public Health*. Washington, D.C.: U.S. Government Printing Office, 1922.

3722.   Sadler, Alfred M., and Blair L. Sadler. "Recent Developments in the Law Relating to Physicians' Assistants." *Vanderbilt Law Rev*, 24 (Nov 1971), 1205.

3723.   Sadler, Blair L. "Licensure for the Physicians Assistant." In *Intermediate-Level Health Practitioners*. Edited by Vernon W. Lippart and Eliz F. Purcell. New York: Josiah Macy Foundation, 1973.

3724.   Sarner, Harvey. *The Nurse and the Law*. Philadelphia: W.B. Saunders, 1968.

3725.   Shannon, M.L. "Nurses in American History. Our First Four Licensure Laws." *Am J Nurs*, 75(8) (Aug 1975), 1327-1329.

3726.   ———. "The Origin and Development of Professional Licensure Examinations in Nursing: From a State-Constructed Examination to the State Board Test Pool Examination." Ed.D. dissertation, Columbia University, 1972.

3727.   Sherman, Toogood F. "The Reason for the State Registration of Trained Nurses." *Nurs Rec* (Aug 1900), 109-112.

3728.   Shryock, Richard H. *Medical Licensing in America 1650-1965*. Baltimore: Johns Hopkins Press, 1967.

3729.   Sigerist, H.E. "The History of Medical Licensure." In *Henry E. Sigerist on the Sociology of Medicine*. Edited by M. Roemer. New York: MD Publications, 1960. Reprint of article in *J Am Med Assoc*, 104 (1935), 1060.

3730.   Society for the State Registration of Trained Nurses. "Deputation to the Prime Minister in Support of State Registration." *Brit J Nurs* (May 1909), 406-411.

3731.   ———. "Meeting to Discuss the College of Nursing Conference on State Registration." *Brit J Nurs* (Apr 1916), 316-317.

3732.   ———. "A Meeting to Discuss the R.B.N.A.'s Redrafted Bill for State Registration." *Brit J Nurs* (Jan 1906), 73-76.

3733.   ———. "Memorandum Prepared by Miss Isla Stewart and Presented to the Public Health Committee of the House of Commons." *Brit J Nurs* (Apr 1904), 310-312.

3734.   ———. "A Reply to the Manifesto Compiled by Sydney Holland." *Brit J Nurs* (Mar 1904), 248-250.

3735.   "The State Board Test Pool Examination." *Am J Nurs*, 52 (May 1952), 613.

3736.   Number deleted.

3737.   "Statutory Status of Six Professions." *Res Bull Nat Educ Assoc*, 16 (Sep 1938), 184-223.

3738.   Steele, Guy. "The Midwife Problem and Its Legal Control." *Maryland Med J*, 48 (Jan 1905), 1-6.

3739.   Stenger, F.E. "Historical Review of the Nurse Practice Act and Susan B. Cook's Contributions to Nursing." *Weather Vane*, 44 (Sep-Oct 1975), 7ff.

3740.   Stewart, I. "State Registration of Nurses." *19th Cent*, 55 (Jun 1904), 987-995.

3741.   Streiff, C.J. *Nursing and the Law*. 2nd ed. Rockville, MD: Aspen System Corp., 1975.

3742.   Studdiford, W.E. "Attempts at Regulation of Midwife Practice." *Am J Obs Dis Wom Child*, 63 (1911), 898-901.

3743.   "The Study of Credentialing in Nursing: A New Approach." *The Report of the Committee*. Vol. 1. Kansas City, MO: American Nurses' Association, 1979.

3744.   Tucker, R., and B. Wetterau. *Credentialing Health Personnel by Licensed Hospitals: The Report of a Study of Institutional Licensure*. Chicago: Rush-Presbyterian-St. Luke's Medical Center, 1975.

3745.   U.S. Department of Health, Education, and Welfare. *Developments in Health Manpower Licensure*. DHEW Publication No. HRA 74-3000. Washington, D.C.: U.S. Government Printing Office, 1973.

3746.   ————. *Report on Licensure and Related Health Personnel Credentialing*. DHEW Publication No. HSM 72-11, 1971.

3747.   Number deleted.

3748.   Van Massenhove, G. "The Status and the Evolution of the Profession." *Nurs* (Brussels), 44 (Jan-Feb 1972), 1-9. (Fr)

3749.   Waller, C.E. "The Social Security Act in Its Relation to Public Health." *Am J Pub Hlth*, 25 (1935), 1186.

3750.   Weisl, Bernard A.G. "The Nurse-Midwife and the New York City Health Code." *West J Surg Obs Gyn*, 71 (Nov-Dec 1963), 266-269.

3751.   West, Roberta Mayhew. "Legislation and Nursing Growth
        Statutory Control Since 1903." *Tr Nurs*, 80 (Jun 1928), 700.

3752.   Willie, Sidney H. *The Nurses' Guide to the Law*. New York:
        McGraw-Hill Book Co., 1970.

3753.   Zimmerman, Anne. "Taft-Hartley Amended: Implications for
        Nursing." *Am J Nurs*, 75 (Feb 1975), 284-287.

12.   NURSING IN INDIVIDUAL COUNTRIES

ALGERIA

3754.   Bull, M.R.   "Health Services in Algeria: The Formation of a New Service for a New Country." *Nurs Mirror*, 128 (10 Jan 1969), 31-33.

ARGENTINA (SEE SOUTH AMERICA)

AUSTRALIA

3755.   Anderson, C.E.   *The Story of Bush Nursing in Victoria*. Melbourne: The Victorian Bush Nurses Association, 1951.

3756.   "Australian Nursing History." *Brit J Nurs*, 55 (Aug 1915), 135-136.

3757.   Avery, L.N.   "Recognition of Professional Status." *Aust Nurs J*, 49 (Aug 1951), 120-122.

3758.   Bauer, F.   "Hospitals and Nursing in Australia." *Kranken-pflege*, 10 (Dec 1966), 525-529.   (Ger)

3759.   Bell, J.   "Nursing Conditions and Problems in Australia." *Nurs Rev*, 1 (1926), 123-127.

3760.   Boorer, D.   "Nursing in Australia." *Nurs Times*, 70 (1974), 844-845.

3761.   Burbridge, G.   "Nursing in Australia." *Am J Nurs*, 48 (1948), 226-228.

3762.   Dock, Lavinia.   "The Progress of Registration in Holland and Australia." *Am J Nurs*, 5 (1905), 318-319.

3763.   Earnshaw, P.A.   "Unwept, Unhonour'd and Unsung." *Queensland Nurs J*, 8 (Sep 1966), 30-37; see also *Med J Aust*, 1 (1966), 427-436.

3764.   Evans, E.P.   "Nursing in Australia." *Int Nurs Rev*, 12 (Jul 1938), 260-264.

3765.   Hagger, J.   "Looking Back Sixty-eight Years (Miss D.M.L. Milhouse)." *Aust Nurs J*, 2 (Mar 1974), 2.

3766.   ————. "Nursing in Melbourne--1910." *Aust Nurs J*, 3(4)
         (Oct 1974), 10.

3767.   Jones, A.L. "Life Times: Ours Not to Reason." *Aust Nurs J*,
         4(11) (Jun 1975), 18-19.

3768.   Kirkcaldie, R.A. *In Gray and Scarlet*. Melbourne: Alexander
         McCubbin, 1922.

3769.   Morris, K.N. "Those Unsinkable Nightingale Nurses." *Aust
         Nurs J*, 1 (Aug 1971), 22-23.

3770.   Morrison, A.A. "The Sociological History of Nursing."
         Aust Nurs J, 63 (May 1965), 106ff.

3771.   "Organized Nursing in South Australia." *Tr Nurs & Hosp Rev*,
         83 (Sep 1929), 357.

3772.   Parsons, R. "Trends in Nursing Education in Colleges of
         Advanced Education." *Lamp*, 30(6) (1975), 6-32.

3773.   Pickhaver, A.M. "The Challenge of Change." *Aust Nurs J*, 3
         (Mar 1975), 12.

3774.   Pidgeon, E.C. "Pioneer Nursing in Australia." *Int Nurs Rev*,
         3 (Oct 1965), 38-42.

3775.   Royal Australian Nursing Federation and the National Florence
         Nightingale Committee of Australia. *Survey Report on the
         Wastage of General Trained Nurses from Nursing in Aus-
         tralia*. Canberra, 1967.

3776.   Savage, Ellen. "Fifty Years Nursing Progress in Australia."
         Nurs J, 49 (Dec 1951), 202-206; 50 (Jan 1952), 2-6.

3777.   South Australian Trainees' Centenary Committee. *Nursing in
         South Australia*. Adelaide: The Committee, 1938.

3778.   Syer, A. "Royal Australian Flying Doctor Service." *Nurs
         Mirror*, 101 (22 Apr 1955), 235.

3779.   Watson, J. Frederick. "Early Nursing Conditions in N.S.W.
         (Australia)." *Aust Nurs J*, 17 (Jan 1919), 21-28.

3780.   White, R. *The Role of the Nurse in Australia*. Canberra:
         National Health and Medical Research Council, 1972.

AUSTRIA

3781.   Moszkowica, L. "Krankenpflege und Krankenpflegeunter-richt
         in Oesterreich." *Wien klin Wchschr*, 38 (1925), 511-513.
         (Ger)

3782.   "Opening Address at the Occasion of the 1st Austrian Nursing
         Congress; from September 7-9, 1974 in Graz." *Osterr
         Krankenpflegez*, 27(11) (Nov 1974), 280-290.   (Ger)

3783. Petschnigg, Lilli. "Nursing in Austria." *Am J Nurs*, 56 (Jan 1956), 61-63.

3784. Pietzcker, Dominika. "Theodor Billroth and the Rudolfiner-haus." *Int Nurs Rev*, 5 (Jul 1930), 356-361. (Ger)

3785. Strobl, Marie Theresa. "Nursing in Germany and Austria, II--Nursing in Austria." *Am J Nurs*, 50 (Nov 1950), 730.

3786. Weiss, Henriette. *Ein Hilferuf fur unserer armen Kranken, Streiflichter aus die Krankenplege in Oesterreich*. Wien: M. Perles, 1903.

BELGIUM AND LUXEMBOURG

3787. Kauffeld, E. "Nursing in the Grand Duchy of Luxembourg." *Int Nurs Rev*, 5 (Jan 1930), 52-54. (Ger)

3788. Murray, Mrs. "Belgian Nursing." *Nurs Times*, 39 (13 Mar 1943), 175.

3789. "The Position of Trained Nursing in Belgium." *Nurs Mirror*, 57 (1 Jul 1933), 264-265.

BOLIVIA (SEE SOUTH AMERICA)

BRAZIL (SEE SOUTH AMERICA)

CANADA

3790. Canadian Nurses' Association. *The First Fifty Years*. Ottawa: Canadian Nurses' Assoc., 1958.

3790.1 ———. *The Leaf and the Lamp*. Ottawa: Canadian Nurses' Assoc., 1968. 105 pp.

3790.2 ———. "Nurses--Their Education and Their Role in Health Programs." *Canad Nurs*, 52 (May 1956), 347-350.

3791. ———. *Nursing and National Health*. Montreal: Canadian Nurses' Assoc.

3792. Carpenter, H. "Canadian Conference on Nursing." *Canad J Pub Hlth*, 49 (1958), 34-37.

3793. ———. "The Canadian Scene." *Int Nurs Rev*, 21(2) (Mar-Apr 1974), 43-48.

3794. ———. "The Role of the Nurse in the Total Health Program." *Int Nurs Rev*, 4 (Oct 1957), 24-30.

3795. Cashman, T. *Heritage of Service: The History of Nursing in Alberta*. Edmonton: The Alberta Association of Registered Nurses, 1966.

3796.   Chittick, Rae. "Forty Years of Growing." *Canad Nurs*, 53
         (Jan 1957), 29-34.

3797.   ————. "Nursing Comes to the Last Frontier." *Canad Nurs*,
         36 (1940), 201-205.

3798.   Clark, M. "Messengers of Mercy to the Women and Children of
         the North." *Canad Nurs*, 69 (Jun 1928), 26.

3799.   Cole, Florence. "The Romance of Nursing and Medicine."
         Canad Nurs, 28 (Apr 1932), 188-190.

3800.   Crosby, Bella. "The History of the Canadian Nurse." *Rapport
         de la Conférence Internationale du Nursing*. Bordeaux,
         1907. pp. 197-199.

3801.   "Early Canadian Nursing." *Jamaican Nurs*, 9 (Sep 1969), 10ff;
         see also *Nurs J India*, 59 (Jun 1968), 183; *So Afr Nurs J*,
         35 (Aug 1968), 7.

3802.   Foran, J.K. *Jeanne Mance or "The Angel of the Colony": The
         Foundress of the Hotel-Dieu Hospital, Montreal*. Montreal:
         Herald Press, 1931.

3803.   Forster, J.M. "The Origin and Development of Nursing in the
         Ontario Hospitals, and the Outlook." *Ontario J Neuro-
         Psychiat* (Toronto) (1923), 31-33.

3804.   Gibson, John Murray, and Mary S. Mathewson. *Three Centuries
         of Canadian Nursing*. Toronto: The Macmillan Co., 1947.

3805.   ————. *The Victorian Order of Nurses for Canada. 50th
         Anniversary*. Montreal: Southam Press, 1947.

3806.   Hilchey, H. "A Living Tradition." *Canad Nurs*, 56 (Oct
         1960), 908-910.

3807.   Hunter, Trenna C. "Just a Mere Fifty Years." *Canad Nurs*,
         54 (1958), 13-15.

3808.   Jones, Ethel. "The First Ten Years." *Canad Nurs*, 54 (1958),
         520-524.

3809.   Jones, Olive Campbell. "A Useful Memorial." *Canad Nurs*, 68
         (Aug 1972), 38-39.

3810.   Jones, P.E. "Symposium on Community Nursing in Canada."
         Nurs Clin No Am, 10 (1975), 691-698.

3811.   Karpoff, Pauline. "Ahran's Ascent." *Canad Nurs*, 51 (1955),
         226.

3812.   Kerr, Sister. "The Heroines of 1639." *Hosp Prog*, 27 (Nov
         1946), 351-358.

3813. Livingston, M. Christine. "The Victorian Order of Nurses for Canada." *Nurs Out*, 6(1) (1958), 42-44.

3814. Loyer, M.A. "Should Nursing Education be Under the Domain of Hospitals?" *Canad Nurs*, 62 (1966), 25-26.

3815. Mathewson, Mary S. "Fifty Years of Nursing at the 'M.G.H.'" *Canad Nurs*, 36 (Apr 1940), 211-215.

3816. McGill University, School for Graduate Nurses, History of Nursing Society, Montreal, Que. *Pioneers of Nursing in Canada*. Ottawa, Ont: Canadian Nurses' Association, 1929.

3817. Merrick, E. "Northern Nurse." *Scholastic*, 43 (10 Jan 1944), 25-26ff.

3818. Mills, T.M. "Nursing Sourdoughs in the Klondike." *Canad Nurs*, 68 (Apr 1972), 51-54.

3819. "More About Canada." *Zambia Nurs J*, 3 (Dec 1968), 13; (Jan 1969).

3820. Morison, J. "Canadian Girls Nursing Uncle Sam." *Canad Nurs*, 59 (Aug 1922), 321-331.

3821. Mussallem, H.K. "Nursing in Canada." *Nurs Times*, 62 (1966), 1626-1629.

3822. ————. "Nursing in Canada from Pioneering History to a Modern Federation." *Int Nurs Rev*, 15 (1968), 29-34.

3823. ————. "Studies on Nursing in Canada." *Int Nurs Rev*, 14 (Jun 1967), 35-42.

3824. "Nursing in Canada." *T Sygepl*, 68 (May 1968), 218-220. (Dan)

3825. "Nursing in Canada: From Pioneering History to a Modern Federation." *Int Nurs Rev*, 15 (1968), 1-29.

3826. "Nursing in Canada in the Early Days." *Nurs Times*, 34 (24 Dec 1938), 1381-1382.

3827. "Nursing in the Early Years in Canada." *ANEC*, 3 (May-Aug 1968), 32-35.

3828. Odell, Elizabeth C. "In Lighter Vein." *Canad Nurs*, 54 (1958), 558-562.

3829. "Pioneer Nursing." *Canad Nurs*, 44 (1948), 92, 126-128.

3830. Richer, Julia. "Les Soeurs de Misericorde." *Garde-Malade Canad-Franc*, 21 (1948), 23-26.

3831. Roswell, G.S. "University Nursing Education--Facts and Trends." *Canad Nurs*, 62 (1966), 31-33.

3832.   Russell, E. Kathleen. "Changes in the Patterns of Nursing."
        Canad Nurs, 54 (Jun 1958), 529-532.

3833.   Sainte-Augustine, Sister, et al. "Nursing among the French
        Canadians in the Province of Quebec, Canada." *Int Counc
        Nurs*, 4 (Jan 1929), 29-33. (Fr)

3834.   Searle, C. "A Review of Nursing in Canada." *So Afr Nurs J*
        (Dec 1962), 25-27; (Jan 1963), 22-24.

3835.   Southcott, M. "Nursing in Newfoundland." *Canad Nurs*, 11
        (Jun 1915), 309-313.

3836.   Steed, M.E. "Trends in Diploma Nursing Education." *Canad
        Nurs*, 64 (1968), 40-41.

3837.   Tougas, Sister Marie-Jeanne. "Definitions of Function."
        Canad Nurs, 46 (Jul 1950), 535-538.

3838.   "Training Days in Canada." *Nurs Times*, 28 (13 Feb 1932),
        159.

3839.   "Voice of the Past." *Canad Nurs*, 55 (Dec 1959), 1133-1138.

3940.   Wilkinson, M. "Four Score and Ten (Nursing in 1909 and 1915)."
        Canad Nurs, 73 (5 Oct 1977), 25-28; (Nov 1977), 14-23;
        (Dec 1977), 16-23.

3841.   Wilson, Jean S., and Sister Allard. "Nursing in Canada."
        Nosokomeion, 10 (Jan 1939), 37-45.

CARIBBEAN COUNTRIES

3842.   Brooks, C. "Historically Speaking: Nurses' Pioneer Group."
        Jamaica Nurs, 9 (Dec 1969), 10-11.

3843.   Cook, B.G. "Island Nurse; County Nurse of San Juan Islands."
        Todays Hlth, 28 (Oct 1950), 22-24.

3844.   Dock, Lavinia, and Eugenia Hilbard. "Historia de la Profes-
        sion de enfermera; a Igunos Hospitales de la isla y las
        Enfermeras de Cuba." *San y benetic Bol Ofic, Haban*, 27
        (1922), 35-44.

3845.   Dorival, Baptist. "The Role of the Nurse in the Past--
        Flash Back--Dominica." *Jamaica Nurs*, 8 (Sep 1968), 11.

3846.   Luty, E. "The Role of the Nurse in the Past--Flash Back--
        With Special Reference to Nursing in Montserrat, St. Croix,
        Dominica and Jamaica." *Jamaica Nurs*, 8 (Sep 1968), 10ff.

3847.   Moorhead, F. "The Role of the Nurse in the Past--Flash Back
        --St. Croix." *Jamaica Nurs*, 8 (Sep 1968), 10.

3848. "Three Hundred Years of Medicine in Jamaica." *Jamaica Nurs*,
      6 (Apr 1966), 18 *passim*.

3949. Tulloch, Edna E. "Historical Perspectives of Nursing in
      Jamaica." *Int Nurs Rev*, 18(1) (1971), 49-58.

CHILE (SEE SOUTH AMERICA)

CHINA

3850. Branch, M. "A Black American Nurse Visits the People's
      Republic of China." *Nurs Forum*, 12 (1973), 402-411.

3851. Chow, M. "Nurses for China's Many." *Ind Woman*, 23 (Dec
      1944), 366-367.

3852. Clawson, D.L. "When the Green and the Yellow Do Not Meet."
      Am J Nurs, 71 (1971), 1971-1973.

3853. "Deepening the Revolution in Medical Education." *Chin Med J*,
      2(2) (1976), 87-92.

3854. Gage, N. "Stages of Nursing in China." *Am J Nurs*, 20 (Nov
      1919), 115-121.

3855. Gray, J. "East Meets West in Canton." *Nurs Mirror*, 142
      (1976), 67-68.

3856. "In China Where Nurses Don't Know 'Impossible.'" *Red Cr
      Courier*, 6 (1 Feb 1927), 16-17; reprinted in *Filipino Nurs*,
      1 (Jul 1927), 42-43.

3857. Lin, E. "Neonatal Nurse Practitioners." *Brit Med J*, 1
      (1975), 115-116.

3858. ———. "Nursing in China." *Am J Nurs*, 38 (Jan 1938), 1-8.

3859. Liu, James K.C., and G.E. Stephenson. *An Outline of the
      History of Nursing*. Shanghai: Nurses' Association of China
      by Kwang Hsueh Publishing House, 1936.

3860. McIntosh, Muriel. "Nursing in China." *Canad Nurs*, 37 (Jan
      1941), 17-20.

3861. Myers, Mary E. *My Hall of Memory*. London: Epworth, 1956.
      90 pp.

3862. Pakkala, K. "Mantsurian Kukkuloilla." *Sairaanjoitaja*, 41
      (1965), 665-667. (Fin)

3863. Pearson, S. "A Peep Behind the Bamboo Curtain: Health Ser-
      vices in China." *Nurs Times*, 69 (1972), 243-244.

3864.   Purwin, L., and R.H. Block. "Nurses for China." *Ind Woman*, 23 (Mar 1944), 66-67.

3865.   "Revolution in Health and Education." *Chin Med J*, 2(2) (1976), 149-154.

3866.   Stanley, M. "China, Then and Now." *Am J Nurs*, 72 (1972), 2213-2218.

3867.   Wang, R. "Nursing in China." *Am J Chin Med*, 2 (Jan 1974), 45.

3868.   Wen, C.P. "Health Care Financing in China." *Med Care*, 14 (3) (1976), 241-254.

COLOMBIA (SEE SOUTH AMERICA)

CUBA (SEE SOUTH AMERICA AND *CARIBBEAN COUNTRIES)*

CZECHOSLOVAKIA

3869.   Mankova, A. "Brief Notes on the History of Nursing in Czechoslovakia." *Int Nurs Rev*, 9 (1934), 213-216.

3870.   Sindlerova, Marta. "The Nurse in Czechoslovakia." *Leag Red Cr Soc Mon Bull*, 15 (Oct 1934), 197-199.

DENMARK

3871.   Broe, E. *Sygeplejens Faglige Udvikling og Historiske Baggrund. 3.* Copenhagen: Busck, 1965. Published originally as *Sygeplejens Historie og Fortsatte Udvikling.*

3872.   Cawford, L. "Health Care in Denmark, Sweden, and Holland." *Nurs Mirror*, 141(14) (1975), 65-67.

3873.   Magnussen, E. "The Great Step. The Victory Struggle for Municipal Authorization." *Sygeplejersken 74 Suppl*, 74 (Oct 1974), 10-15, 47-48. (Dan)

3874.   Norgaard, A. "Common Women and Gentlewomen." *Sygeplejersken*, 68 (Dec 1968), 513-516. (Dan)

3875.   Norrie, Charlotte, "Nursing in Denmark." *Am J Nurs*, 1 (Dec 1900), 183-187.

3876.   Rasmussan, Maria S. "Danish Nursing." *Nurs J India*, 20 (Jan 1929), 18-20.

3877.   *Sjuksköterskan genom tiderna. (Utg. ar Sairaanhoitajien koulutussaatio).* Helsingfors: Soderstrom, 1965.

EAST AND CENTRAL AFRICAN COUNTRIES

3878.   Frewen, E.   "An Account of a Dominican Nurse's Travels to
        Mashonaland in 1892." *Cen Afr J Med*, 5 (1959), 627-628.

3879.   Stanford, D.O.   "Nursing in East and Central Africa--World
        War I." *So Afr Nurs J*, 32 (Oct 1965), 22-24.

EGYPT

3880.   Bell, J.   "Leadership and Responsibility." *Nurs Times*, 69
        (1973), 1542-1543.

3881.   Kuhnke.   "The Doctoress on a Donkey: Women Health Officers in
        Nineteenth Century Egypt." *Clio Medica* (Oxford), 9(3)
        (1974), 193-205.

ETHIOPIA

3882.   Goodman, M.   "Nursing and the WHO." *Am J Nurs*, 49 (1949),
        134-136.

3883.   Magnussen, E.   "Nursing in Ethiopia." *Am J Nurs*, 53 (1953),
        296-297.

3884.   Woolridge, R.   "Nursing in a Famine." *Nurs Times*, 72 (1976),
        166-167.

FINLAND

3885.   Katajamaki, M.   "An Occasion for Our Affairs." English
        abstract. *Sairaanhoitaja*, 49 (12 Jun 1973), 4-10. (Fin)

3886.   Pakkala, K.   "The Interesting Past. The Manchurian Plains."
        Sairaanhoitaja, 41 (2 Oct 1965), 665-667. (Fin)

3887.   ————.   "Pohjolan Jouluruusuja." *Sairaanhoitaja*, 42
        (10 Dec 1966), 838-840. (Fin)

3888.   Valkonen, I.   "Tenth District Association Celebrates 50th
        Anniversary." *Sairaanhoitaja*, 50(4) (25 Feb 1975), 26-28.
        (Fin)

FRANCE

3889.   Badsvaille, M.L.   "Present and Future Position of the Nursing
        Profession in France." *Int Nurs Rev*, 17(2) (1970), 146-147.
        (Fr)

3890.   Barrowclough, F.   "The French Connexion--and Nursing." *Nurs
        Times*, 68 (1972), 735-736.

3891.   Boulton, H.   "Our Nursing Service in France." *19th Cent*, 81
        (Mar 1917), 651-660.

3892.   Burrus, O. "The Nurse in 1976: Who is She?" *Rev Infirm*, 20(4) (1976), 297-304. (Fr)

3893.   Chaptal, L. "Nursing Progress in France." *Am J Nurs*, 29 (1929), 807-810.

3894.   D'Airoles, Mlle. "Nursing in France and Catholic Action." *Cath Nurs* (London), 4 (Feb 1936), 4-6.

3895.   Dock, Lavinia. "The Bordeaux School of Nursing." *Am J Nurs*, 7 (1907), 202-204.

3896.   ————. "The Florence Nightingale School in France." *Am J Nurs*, 18 (1918), 1168.

3897.   ————. "French Nurse Training." *Am J Nurs*, 6 (1906), 316.

3898.   ————. "Nursing in France." *Am J Nurs*, 26 (1926), 35; 32 (1932), 745.

3899.   ————. "Progress in France." *Am J Nurs*, 21 (1921), 393-395.

3900.   ————. "The Revolution in French Hospitals." *Am J Nurs*, 5 (1905), 428-430, 519-522, 693-698, 887-889.

3901.   ————. "Views of Nurse Training and Reforms in French Hospitals." *Am J Nurs*, 4 (1903), 235-239.

3902.   "L'effort d'union des Infirmières du Plan International." *Rev Int Croix Ronge*, 14 (1961), 55-68. (Fr)

3903.   Fautrel, F. "Luxury and Militancy." *Nurs Times*, 69 (1973), 1345-1346.

3904.   *L'infirmière Hospitalière: Guide Théorique et Pratique de l'Ecole Florence Nightingale de Bordeaux.* Paris: Bailliere, 1937. 286 pp. 5th ed., 1947; 6th ed., 1948.

3905.   "International School for Advanced Nursing Education." *Int Nurs Rev*, 14 (Nov-Dec 1967), 11.

3906.   Mordacq, C. "Evolution of the Nursing Profession: From the Professional Idea to that of Nursing Service." *Rev Infirm*, 23 (Mar 1973), 257-261. (Fr)

3907.   "Position of Trained Nursing in France." *Nurs Mirror*, 57 (24 Jun 1933), 242-243.

3908.   Recordon, G. "Le cinquantenaire de l'école des infirmières de l'assistance publique." *Revue de l'Assistance Publique à Paris*, 8 (1957), 423-428.

3909.   Sourdille, A. "L'infirmerie de la maison royale de Saint Cyr." *Hist Med*, 16 (1966), 21-30.

3910.   Stewart, Isla. "La directrice au XXe siècle." *Garde-malade
        Hosp* (Bordeaux) (1906), 3, 19.

3911.   Tenon, J. *Mémoires sur les Hôpitaux de Paris.* Paris:
        Pierres, 1778.

3912.   Xeclainche, X. "La Profession d'infirmière." *Quatre nou-
        velles années d'action Hospitalière Sociale et Médico-
        Sociale, 1956 à 1960.* Paris: Imprimerie Municipale, 1960.

3913.   "Yesterday and Today." *Nurs* (Brussels), 42 (May-Jun 1970),
        35-39.

GERMANY

3914.   "Ambulance Work in the County Districts of Germany." *Sci Am*,
        55 (14 Feb 1903), 226-276.

3915.   Bandau, Adelheid. *Zwölf Jahre als Diakonissin.* Berlin:
        G. Hempel, 1882.

3916.   Buchheim, L. "Wider die Studierenden Frauenzimmer ein
        'Grimmiger Verneiner' Weiblicher Bildung haf das Wort."
        Munch Med Wschr, 103 (1961), 1885-1888.

3917.   Eichhorn, S. "Trends in the Professional Education of
        Doctors, Nurses and Other Paramedical Staff in the German
        Federal Republic." *World Hosp*, 5 (1969), 77.

3918.   Eigenbrod, W. "Eine Kritische Plauderei über interessante
        berufliche Dinge und das Krankenpflegegesetz." *Z Kranken-
        pflege*, 9 (Oct 1965), 438-444.

3919.   Elster, R. "Seventy Years of Initiative for Nursing."
        Z Krankenpflege, 27 (Jan 1973), 4. (Ger)

3920.   Fricke, A. "Agnes Karll." *Int Nurs Rev*, 14 (Jun 1967), 43-
        44.

3921.   Hilbert, Hortense. "Some Historical Aspects of Nursing in
        Germany and in Some German Speaking Countries." *Int
        Aspects Nurs Educ*, New York: Bureau of Publications,
        Teachers College, Columbia University, 1932.

3922.   Hoffmann, W. "Effect of Prosperity upon Nursing." *Deutsch
        Med Wchnsch*, 53 (28 Jan 1927), 201-203. (Ger)

3923.   Horn, P. "Zur krankenpflege in alten perien." *Z Kranken-
        pflege* (Berlin, 1903), 169-173.

3924.   Isliker, R. "Continuity of Nursing." *Z Krankenpflege*, 66
        (Jun 1973), 231-235. (Ger)

3925.   Karll, Agnes. "Die dunkle Periode der Krankenpflege." *Illus
        Monafschr d arztl Polytech*, 32 (1910), 359-365. (Ger)

3926.   Katscher, C. "Current Status of Nursing Education." *Z*
        Krankenpflege, 29(5) (1976), 250-253. (Ger)

3927.   Klose, H. "Testament of a 55 Year Medical Experience: III
        Ethos of the Nursing Profession." *Deutsch Gesundheit*, 13
        (29) (Jul 1958), 1534. (Ger)

3928.   König, Franz. *Die Schwesternpflege der Kranken ein Stück*
        Moderner Culturarbeit der Frau. Berlin: A. Hirschwald,
        1902. 12 pp.

3929.   Kroeger, G. "Nursing in Germany." *Am J Nurs*, 39 (1939),
        483-485.

3930.   Lingner, E. "Krankenpflege im städtischen kinderkrankenhaus."
        Berl Med, 16 (1965), 777-779.

3931.   Piechocki, W. "Gesundheitsfursorge und Krankenpflege in den
        Franckeschen Stiftungen in Halle/Saale." *Acta Hist Leopold*,
        2 (1965), 29-66.

3932.   Rath, G. "Die Göttinger Buchausstellung 'Alte Medizin' mit
        einem Chastischen Kommentar Oslanders zum Frauenstudium."
        Sudhoffs Arch Gesch Med, 46 (1962), 182-184.

3933.   Schilling, F. "Up to Fliedner's Time." *Ztschr f d ges*
        Krankenhaus, 24 (13 Feb 1928), 105.

3934.   Seidler, E. "Die Geschichte der Krankenpflege in Medizin-
        historischer Sicht." *Agnes Karll Schwest*, 17 (1963),
        221-224.

3935.   ————. "Die Krankenpflegeschulen des Franz Anton Mai in
        Mannheim und Heidelberg." *Deutsch Schwest Ztg* (1963),
        Heft 7.

3936.   Setzler, L. "Nursing and Nursing Education in Germany."
        Am J Nurs, 45 (1945), 993-995.

3937.   Soho, K. "Travelogue of a Nurse. 8. Nursing in Germany in
        17-19 Centuries." *Jap J Nurs*, 33 (Nov 1969), 96-97. (Jap)

3938.   Sticker, Anna. "On the Development of Present Day Nursing."
        Deutsch Schwest, 26 (Jul 1973), 282-284.

3939.   ————. *Die Entstehung der neuzeitlichen Krankenpflege*
        Deutsch Quellenstücke aus der ersten Halfte des 19 Jahr-
        hunderts. Stuttgart: Kohlhammer, 1960.

3940.   Stocker, D.A. "Agnes Karll and Congress Days of 1904." *Z*
        Krankenpflege, 27 (Jul 1974), 280-288. (Ger)

3941.   ————. "Independent Professional Nursing Around 1900."
        Z Krankenpflege, 26 (Jul 1973), 282-284. (Ger)

3942. Von Wallnenich, Clementine. *Die Krankenpflege von Mannern durch Frauen. Die Stellung der Oberin im Modernen Kranken-haus.* Munich: J.F. Lehmann, 1902.

GHANA

3943. Kisseih, D. "Developments in Nursing in Ghana." *Int J Nurs Stud*, 5 (1968), 205-219.

3944. "Nursing Service in Ghana." *Ghana Nurs*, 7 (Dec 1971), 13-15.

3945. Pendleton, E.M. "Ghana Looks for the Future." *Bull Am Coll Nurs Mid*, 17 (1972), 78-81.

3946. Swaffield, L. "Blending the Best of Both Worlds--Nursing in Ghana." *Nurs Times*, 70 (1974), 1056.

3947. Twumassi, P.A. "Scientific Medicine--The Ghanian Experience." *Int J Nurs Stud*, 9 (1972), 63-75.

GREAT BRITAIN AND IRELAND

3948. Abel-Smith, B. *A History of the Nursing Profession in Great Britain.* New York: Springer, 1960.

3949. Arthure, H. "Early English Midwifery." *Mid Hlth Visit*, 11(6) (Jun 1975), 187-190.

3950. Auld, M. "Modern Trends in Nursing." *Nurs Mirror*, 142(15) (1976), 49-51, 54-55.

3951. Aveling, J.H. *English Midwives, Their History and Prospects.* Reprint of 1872 edition. London: Eliot, Ltd., 1967.

3952. Bennett, B.A. "The Evolution of the Nursing Profession in Britain: From the First to Second World Wars." *Nurs Mirror*, 110 (20 May 1960), 681-683.

3953. ────. "The Evolution of the Nursing Profession in Britain: 19th and Early 20th Centuries." *Nurs Mirror*, 110 (13 May 1960), 588-590.

3954. ────. "The Evolution of the Nursing Profession in Britain: Post-War Period." *Nurs Mirror*, 110 (27 May 1960), 778-779.

3955. ────. "The Evolution of the Nursing Profession in Britain: Present Trends." *Nurs Mirror*, 110 (3 Jun 1960), 867-868.

3956. Chavasse, J. "Nursing in the Emerald Isle." *Int Nurs Rev*, 15(2) (1968), 183.

3957. Christian, Princess. "The Progress of Nursing in the British Isles." *Prov M J* (Leicester) (1894), xiii, 507; see also *Cong Internat d'hyg et de demog C V 1894.* Budapest, 1896. viii, pt. 6, 433.

3958.   Committee on Nursing, Asa Briggs, Chairman. *Report*. London:
        Her Majesty's Stationery Office, 1972.

3959.   Edwards, Muriel M. "Nurses and the National Health Service."
        Nurs Times (9 Aug 1963), 998-999.

3960.   ————. "Nursing in Britain, 1937-1943." *Am J Nurs*, 44
        (Feb 1944), 125-135.

3961.   Elms, R.R. "Irish Nursing at the Crossroads." *Int J Nurs
        Studies*, 11 (1974), 163-172.

3962.   Emblin, R. "Degree Courses in Nursing." *Nurs Times*, 72
        Part I (7 Oct 1972), 141-143; Part II (14 Oct 1972), 145-
        146.

3963.   Flack, Holly. "Nursing in Ireland from pre-Christian Times
        to the Middle of the Nineteenth Century." *Int Nurs Rev*, 6
        (Sep 1931), 428-441.

3964.   Forbes, Robert. "Professional Responsibility." *Nurs Times*,
        48 (2 Feb 1948), 105-106; (8 Mar 1948), 232-233; (12 Apr
        1948), 371-372; (10 May 1948), 463-464; (14 Jun 1948),
        590-591.

3965.   Forbes, T.R. "The Regulation of English Midwives in the 16th
        and 17th Centuries." *Med Hist*, 8 (1964), 235-244.

3966.   Fox, E.M. "Nursing Progress Over the Years." *Nurs Mirror*,
        46 (Birthday No. 1928), 22, 36-38.

3967.   Fraser, F. "The Nurse in Great Britain." *Canad J Pub Hlth*,
        40 (1949), 292-301.

3968.   *Friendly Letter to Under-Nurses of the Sick--Especially in
        Unions by a Lady*. London: A.W. Bennett, 1861.

3969.   Gordon, J.E. "Domestic Nursing from the Saxons to the
        Stuarts, Part 4." *Mid Hlth Visit*, 6 (Sep 1970), 333-339.

3970.   ————. "Nurses and Nursing in Britain: Care of the Lying-
        in Woman, Part 15." *Mid Hlth Visit*, 8 (Apr 1972), 125-130.

3971.   ————. "Nurses and Nursing in Britain: Care of the Psychia-
        tric Patient." *Mid Hlth Visit*, 7 (Aug 1971), 307-312.

3972.   ————. "Nurses and Nursing in Britain: The Children's
        Nurse, Part 4." *Mid Hlth Visit*, 8 (Feb 1972), 57-61.

3973.   ————. "Nurses and Nursing in Britain: The Mediaeval
        Monastic Tradition, Part 3." *Mid Hlth Visit*, 6 (Aug 1970),
        294-295.

3974.   ————. "Nurses and Nursing in Britain: The 19th Century
        Voluntary Hospitals and Workhouse Infirmaries, Part 16."
        Mid Hlth Visit, 8 (May 1973), 174-179.

3975. ————. "Nurses and Nursing in Britain: The Nurse in the War in the Eighteenth and Nineteenth Centuries, Part 17(1)." *Mid Hlth Visit*, 8 (Jun 1972), 214-217.

3976. ————. "Nurses and Nursing in Britain: The Nurse in the War in the Eighteenth and Nineteenth Centuries, Part 18(2). In the Army." *Mid Hlth Visit* (Jul 1972), 248-257.

3977. ————. "Nurses and Nursing in Britain: Nursing in the Home in the Nineteenth Century, Part 19(1)." *Mid Hlth Visit*, 8 (Aug 1972), 284-287.

3978. ————. "Nurses and Nursing in Britain: The Work of Florence Nightingale, Part 21(1). For the Health of the Army." *Mid Hlth Visit*, 8 (Oct 1972), 351.

3979. ————. "Nurses and Nursing in Britain: The Work of Florence Nightingale, Part 22(2). The Establishment of Nurse Training in Britain." *Mid Hlth Visit*, 8 (Nov 1972), 391-396.

3980. Grey, M. "The Nursing and Midwifery Services of Northern Ireland." *Int J Nurs Studies*, 1 (1964), 145.

3981. Haldane, Elizabeth. *The British Nurse in Peace and War*. London: Murray, 1923.

3982. Healy, E. Nellie. "Nursing in Ireland, 1860-1931." *Int Nurs Rev*, 7 (Jan 1932), 35-53.

3983. Hector, Winifred. *The Work of Mrs. Bedford Fenwick and the Rise of Professional Nursing*. London: Royal College of Nursing, 1973.

3984. Henry, F. "Trends in England and Wales." *Int Nurs Rev*, 9 (Jan-Feb 1962), 31-33.

3985. Henry, M. "The General Nursing Council for England and Wales: Its History and Functions." *Nurs Mirror*, 115 (Mar 1963), 545-547, 549, 561-562.

3986. "The Heritage of British Nursing." *Nurs Mirror*, 89 (30 Jul 1949), 273.

3987. "History of Nursing in Scotland." *Tr Nurs & Hosp Rev*, 83 (7 Sep 1929), 355-357.

3988. Hodkinson, L.J. "A City's Progress in Public Health (Liverpool)." *Nurs Mirror*, 102 (13 Jan 1956), iii.

3989. Hunt, D. "Seventy Years on the QAs Past and Present." *Nurs Mirror*, 134 (7 Apr 1972), 13-16.

3990. Leydon, I. "Development of Nursing Education in Ireland—Training to Meet the Challenges of the Future." *Int J Nurs Studies*, 10 (1973), 95-101.

3991.   Local Government Board, Ireland. "The Abolition of Pauper
         Nursing in Irish Workhouse Infirmaries." *Nurs Rec* (16 Oct
         1897), 309.

3992.   MacDonald, Isabel. *Queens in Nursing History--A Memento of
         Coronation Year.* London: Royal British Nurses Assoc.,
         1953.

3993.   ————. "Royal Nurses in History." *J Roy Inst Pub Hlth*, 17
         (1954), 142-153.

3994.   Maguire, Miss. "Report of an Address." *Queen's Nurs Mag*,
         34 (Jan 1945), 2-5.

3995.   "Manchester District Nursing Service: Centenary of District
         Nursing." *Manchester Nurs Times* (18 Dec 1964), 1667, 1670.

3996.   *"Memories" by a Hospital Nurse, in Twenty-five Chapters.*
         Bristol: John Wright and Sons, 1910.

3997.   Musson, A.E. "Evolution and the Nursing Situation Today."
         Irish Nurs Hosp World, 1 (15 Dec 1931), 22-23; 2 (1 Jan
         1932), 33-35; (15 Jan 1932), 33-35.

3998.   National Council of Trained Nurses of Great Britain and Ire-
         land. "Resolution and Statement Sent to the Secretary of
         State for War Expressing Dissatisfaction with the Organiza-
         tion of the Nursing of Sick and Wounded Soldiers in Military
         Auxiliary Hospitals at Home and Abroad." *Brit J Nurs Supl*,
         (30 Jan 1915), i-vii.

3999.   "Nursing Home (Registration Bill)." *Brit J Nurs*, 73 (Apr
         1925), 69; (Mar 1926), 74-52; (May 1926), 107-108; (Jun
         1926), 129; (Jul 1926), 160-161; (Aug 1926), 184; (Apr 1927),
         75-87; (May 1927), 116; (Aug 1927), 197; see also *Nursing
         Homes (Registration) Bill.* London: HMSO, 1925.

4000.   "Nursing in the Nineties: 1935--Looking Back--1910." *Nurs
         Times*, 31 (4 May 1935), 450-452.

4001.   Nuttal, P. "Nursing in Britain." *Int Nurs Rev*, 12 (Nov-
         Dec 1965), 6.

4002.   ————. "Nursing in England and Wales." *Canad Nurs*, 62
         (1966), 32.

4003.   O'Carrol, M.F. "Restructuring the Health Care System--An
         Irish Solution." *World Hosp*, 7 (1971), 45-49.

4004.   Reidy, M. "The History of Nursing in Ireland." *Int Nurs
         Rev*, 18(4) (1971), 326-333.

4005.   *Report from the Select Committee ... Together with the Pro-
         ceedings of the Committee, Minutes of Evidence, Appendices
         and Index.* Parliament. House of Commons, Select Committee
         on Nursing Homes. London: HMSO, 1926.

4006.   Royal British Nurses' Association. "The Progress of Nursing
        During the King's (George V) Reign, 1910-1935." *Brit J
        Nurs*, 83 (May 1935), 114-115.

4007.   Scanlan, M. "Nursing Education in Ireland." *Int Nurs Rev*,
        16 (Apr 1969), 153.

4008.   Sculco, Cynthia D. "An American Nurse at the London Hospi-
        tal." *Nurs Out*, 24 (Aug 1976), 504-508.

4009.   Spencer, Herbert R. *The History of British Midwifery*.
        London: John Bale Sons & Danielson, 1927.

4010.   Terney, B. "Nursing in Ireland." *Int J Nurs Studies*, 11
        (1974), 111-117.

4011.   Tooley, Sarah A. *A History of Nursing in the British Empire*.
        London: Bousfield, 1906.

4012.   Udell, Florence N. "A Golden Jubilee in the United Kingdom."
        Int Nurs Rev, 13(3) (May-Jun 1966), 17-20.

4013.   Watkin, B. "Nursing in Britain: A Year's Review." *Nurs
        Out*, 12 (1964), 56.

4014.   ————. "Treasure Hunting." *Nurs Mirror*, 142(12) (18 Mar
        1976), 42.

4015.   Wright, M.S. "Nursing: Present Perspectives and Future
        Prospects." *Nurs Mirror*, 139(18) (31 Oct 1974), 53-56.

GREECE

4016.   "American Nurses in Greece." *Hygeia*, 24 (Jan 1946), 47.

4017.   Carr, A. "Nursing in Pre-war Greece." *Am J Nurs*, 42 (1942),
        370-372.

4018.   Ledakis, S. "Nursing Education in Greece." *Int Nurs Rev*, 4
        (Jan 1957), 49-54.

4019.   Messolora, A. "Athena Messolar." *Int Nurs Rev*, 12 (12 Nov
        1965), 70-71.

4020.   ————. "Some Aspects of Nursing in Greece." *Am J Nurs*, 40
        (1940), 635-636.

4021.   Negroponte, Marie. "The Progress of Nursing in Greece."
        League Red Cr Mon Bull, 14 (Sep 1933), 179-180.

4022.   Nicolo, S. "O.R. Nursing in Greece." *AORN J*, 19 (1974),
        114-120.

4023.   Noyes, L. "Establishment of Foreign Training Schools."
        Am J Nurs, 19 (1919), 947-948.

4024.   Papamicrouli, S. "The Greek Red Cross School for Nurses and
        Public Health Nurses." *Int Nurs Rev*, 10 (Oct 1963), 29.

4025.   ————. "Hellenic Red Cross School of Nursing: A Combined
        Program in General and Public Health Nursing." *Int J Nurs
        Studies*, 6 (1969), 27-35.

4026.   ————. "Nursing in Greece." *Int Nurs Rev*, 14 (May-Jun
        1967), 25-28; see also *J Psychiat Nurs*, 7 (1969), 140-142.

HONG KONG

4027.   Choa, G.H. "Speech by the Dr. The Hon. G.H. Choa at the
        Florence Nightingale Day Celebration on Wednesday, 12th May,
        1971 at City Hall." *Hong Kong Nurs J*, 10 (May 1971), 33-34.

4028.   Iu, S. "President's Address at Florence Nightingale Day
        Celebration 12th May 1971, City Hall Theatre." *Hong Kong
        Nurs J*, 10 (May 1971), 27-32; 13 (Nov 1972), 7-9.

4029.   "The Nurse." *Hong Kong Nurs J*, 13 (Nov 1972), 21-27.

4030.   Poon, E.Y. "A Brief History of Nursing in Hong Kong." *Hong
        Kong Nurs J*, 3 (May 1967), 119-123.

4031.   Stratton, D. "History of Nursing in Government Hospitals."
        Hong Kong Nurs J (May 1973), 34-37.

HUNGARY

4032.   Boda, A. "The Heritage of Robert Jones and Agnes Hunt (Report
        of a 6-Month Period of Work at the Orthopedic Clinic of
        Oswetry)." *Magy Traumatol Orthop*, 17(3) (1974), 236-239.
        (Hun)

4033.   "Some Impressions of Nursing in Yugoslavia and Hungary."
        Am J Nurs, 31 (1931), 671-676.

ICELAND

4034.   Bjarnhjedinsson, Christophine. "Nursing in Iceland." *Pac
        Cst J Nurs*, 21 (Mar 1925), 151-152.

4035.   Eiriksdottis, S. "Timant Hjukrunarfelags Islands 40 Ara."
        Tim Hjukrunarfel Isl, 41 (1965), 61-65. (Islandic)

4036.   "Iceland and Its Nursing Service." *Pub Hlth Nurs*, 20 (Sep
        1928), 479-480.

4037.   Thorvaldsson, Sigridur. "Nursing in Iceland" (trans). *ICN*,
        3 (Apr 1928), 114-123. Excerpted in *Am J Nurs*, 29 (Jan
        1929).

INDIA/PAKISTAN

4038.   Ahad, M.A. "Nursing Education in India." *Int Nurs Rev*,
        17(3) (1970), 224-237.

4039.   Aranvaa, T.K. "Nursing in India--1908-1968." *Nurs J India*,
        59 (Nov 1968), 369-371.

4040.   Bachu, A. "Indian Nurse in I.S.A." *Int Nurs Rev*, 20 (Jul-
        Aug 1973), 114-116.

4041.   ———. "The Nurse's Role in Family Planning Service in
        India." *Int Nurs Rev*, 23(1) (1976), 25-28.

4042.   ———. "Problems of Nursing Education in India in an Age of
        Technology." *Int Nurs Rev*, 18 (1971), 85-95.

4043.   Bauman, M.B. "Baccalaureate Nursing in a Selected Number of
        English Speaking Countries." *Int Nurs Rev*, 9(1) (1972),
        12-38.

4044.   Bhatia (nfn). "Our Medical and Nursing Heritage." *Nurs J
        India*, 56 (Jun 1965), 155.

4045.   Burnett, D. "A Nurse Visitor in India." *Pub Hlth Nurs*, 43
        (1951), 408-412.

4046.   Chatterjee, M. "Gandhiji's Interest in Nursing, Medicine and
        Health." *Nurs J India*, 66(10) (Oct 1975), 225, 238.

4047.   Clayton, R.E. "How Men May Live and Not Die in India
        (Florence Nightingale)." *Aust Nurs J*, 2 (Apr 1974), 10-11.

4048.   Devi, L. "Programs for India's Graduate Nurses." *Am J Nurs*,
        56 (1956), 334.

4049.   ———. "Twelve Years of Nursing in India." *Int Nurs Rev*,
        2 (Oct 1955), 49-52.

4050.   Dock, Lavinia. "India." *Am J Nurs*, 4 (1903), 240-244.

4051.   Hartley, D. "Lighted to Lighten." *Nurs J India*, 59 (Nov
        1968), 374-375.

4052.   ———. "Short Survey of Nursing in India." *J Christ M A*,
        16 (Sep 1941), 261-264.

4053.   John, K. "The Advent of Integrated Health Service in India."
        Int J Nurs Studies, 2 (1965), 183-187.

4054.   Kabir, L. "Two Great Ideas, Two Large Hearts--A Birthday
        Tribute." *Nurs J India*, 59 (May 1968), 144.

4055.   Krishnan, S. "Planning Nursing Education for the 70's in
        India." *Int Nurs Rev*, 18(1) (1971), 181-191.

4056.   Libbey, A. "Junior Year in India." *Am J Nurs*, 66 (1966),
        332-334.

4057.   Macry, H. "Nursing in India." *Hosp Prog*, 22 (1941), 283-287.

4058.   Marson, W. "India's Project Number One." *Canad Nurs*, 63
        (1967), 45-49.

4059.   Martin, nfn. "How to Attract the Better Educated Indian
        Girl to Enter the Nursing Profession." *Nurs J India*, 65
        (Jan 1974), 1.

4060.   Nandi, P.K., and Charles P. Loomis. "Professionalization of
        Nursing in India: Deterring and Facilitating Aspects of the
        Culture." *J Asian Afr Stud*, 9 1/2 (1974), 43-59.

4061.   Newman, E.M. "Fifty Years Experience of Nursing." *Nurs J
        India*, 18 (Mar 1927), 69-72.

4062.   "The Nurse and Nursing Seven Decades Ago." *Nurs J India*, 61
        (May 1970), 164.

4063.   Paul, Kurian. "Nursing in India and Its Possible Future
        Development." *Nurs J India*, 36 (Mar 1945), 48-51.

4064.   Pé, A. "Hope for Millions." *Nurs Times*, 61 (1965), 1494-
        1495.

4065.   Prager, Fernan. "In the Footsteps of Florence Nightingale.
        Fernan Prager of the Netherlands is Chief Nurse for Almost
        900,000 Arab Refugees." *Nurs J India*, 46 (May 1955), 186-
        188.

4066.   Radhalaxmi, K.K., and M.N. Rao. "Nursing Under Ancient Jin-
        dian Systems (As Described in Ayurvedic Classics)."
        Indian J Hist Med, 1(1) (1956), 36-40.

4067.   Ramesivara, Rao, G.A.J. "Silver Jubilee of Independence in
        Nursing in Retrospect." *Nurs J India*, 63 (Sep 1972), 298.

4068.   Roy, B. "Follow the Lady with the Lamp." *Nurs J India*, 60
        (Aug 1969), 259.

4069.   Saunby, D. "A Candle-Lighting Service in Kolar, India."
        Am J Nurs, 46 (1946), 873-874.

4070.   Shad, Mohammed A. "Nursing Education in India." *Int Nurs
        Rev*, 17(3) (1970), 224-237.

4071.   Stewart, E. "Nursing in India." *CICIAMS Nouv*, 1 (1975),
        58-60.

4072.   Subba, Reddy, D.V. "Buddha's Discourses on Medicaments,
        Treatment and Nursing." *Indian J Hist Med*, 1(1) (1956),
        41-50.

4073.   Subhadra, V. "An Evaluation of Public Health Services at an
        Urban Health Center." *Int J Nurs Studies*, 7 (1970), 257-
        265.

4074.   Sundaram, S. "Growth of Nursing in India." *Nurs J India*,
        61 (Nov 1970), 353.

4075.   Walton, J. "Where Modern Nursing Began." *Nurs J India*, 62
        (Aug 1971), 247.

4076.   Wilkinson, A. *A Brief History of Nursing in India and
        Pakistan*. New Delhi: Trained Nurses Association of India,
        1958.

IRAN

4077.   Aftab, S. "Nursing and Point Four in Iran." *Nurs World*,
        127 (1959), 8-10.

4078.   Kelly, M.A. "Beliefs of Iranian Nurses and Nursing Students
        about Nurses and Nursing Education." *Int Nurs Rev*, 20
        (Jul-Aug 1973), 108-111.

4079.   Moghadassy, M. "Progress: Postbasic Nursing Education in
        Iran." *Int Nurs Rev*, 19(1) (1972), 3-11.

4080.   Riahi, A. "Nursing Education in Iran." *Int J Nurs Studies*,
        5 (1968), 267-271.

4081.   Ronaghy, H.A. "The Front Line Health Worker: Selection,
        Training and Performance." *Am J Pub Hlth*, 66 (Mar 1976)
        273-277.

4082.   ———. "Migration of Iranian Nurses to United States; A
        Study of One School of Nursing in Iran." *Int Nurs Rev*,
        22(3) (1975), 87-88.

4083.   Salsali, A. "Iran's Nurses." *Am J Nurs*, 61 (1961), 99.

4084.   Setzler, L. "In Iran." *Am J Nurs*, 41 (1941), 520-525.

ISRAEL AND PALESTINE

4085.   Bergman, R. "Israel's Educators in the Diploma Schools of
        Nursing." *Int J Nurs Studies*, 8 (1971), 103-126.

4086.   ———. "Nursing and Organized Groups in Society." *Int Nurs
        Rev*, 12 (Dec 1965), 28-31.

4087.   ———. "Opinion on Nursing." *Int Nurs Rev*, 18(2) (1971),
        195-230; 23(1) (1976), 15-24.

4088.   ———. "Team Nursing in Public Health, Israel." *Int J Nurs
        Studies*, 2 (1965), 261-267.

4089.   Bluestone, M.   "The Hadassah School of Nursing."   *Am J Nurs*,
        28 (1928), 1093-1097.

4090.   Cantor, S.   "Nursing in Israel."   *Am J Nurs*, 51 (1951),
        162-163.

4091.   Golub, S.   "Nursing in Israel."   *Nurs Mirror*, 136 (15 Jun
        1973), 22-25.

4092.   Kaplan, Anna.   "The First Nine Years."   *Hadassah Newsletter*,
        138 (Apr 1938), 127-129.

4093.   Kirschner, Ernestine.   "The Nurse and Her School."   *Hadassah
        Newsletter* (Apr 1939), 157-159.

4094.   Selisberg, A.   "A Modern Training School for Nurses in
        Jerusalem."   *Am J Nurs*, 21 (1921), 721-723.

4095.   Shulamith, L.   "A Nursing School in Palestine."   *Am J Nurs*,
        40 (1940), 880-884.

4096.   Stockler, Rebecca Adams.   *Development of Public Health
        Nursing as Related to the Public Health Needs of the Jewish
        Population of Palestine, 1913 to 1948.*   Ed.D. dissertation,
        Teachers College, Columbia University, 1975.

4097.   Weiss, O.   "Kibbutz Nurses."   *Am J Nurs*, 71 (1971), 1762-1765.

4098.   ———.   "Nurses and Nursing in Israel."   *Nurs Out*, 14 (1966),
        58-60.

ITALY

4099.   Andreoli, A.   "Nursing Education Today."   *Professioni Infer-
        mieristiche*, 28(4) (1976), 121-124.   (Ital)

4100.   Armstrong, F.M.   "The Italian Hospital and Nursing."   *Am J
        Nurs*, 2 (1902), 392-395.

4101.   Baxter, M.   "A Letter from Italy."   *Am J Nurs*, 3 (1903),
        737-738.

4102.   "La Charitas delle Suore del Cottolengo da 50 anni all'
        Ospedale Maria Vittoria di Torino ricordata la ricorrenza
        Unitamenta a guella del 125 Anniversario del Primo Diploma
        Statale per l'abilitazione Professionale di Infermiere."
        G Batt Virol Immun, 58 (1965), 121-128.   (Ital)

4103.   DeTargiani-Giunti, M.   "Notes on the History of Nursing Care
        with a Special Reference to Italy."   *Int Nurs Rev*, 4 (May
        1957), 12-15.

4104.   Enriques, B.   "Les Infirmieres Professionelles en Italie et
        leur Preparation."   *Int Nurs Rev*, 4 (May 1975), 15-18.   (Fr)

4105.   Fitzgerald, A. "Congratulations to Italian Nurses." *Am J Nurs*, 26 (1926), 30.

4106.   Gubert, S. "Nurses in Italy." *Nurs Mirror*, 140(4) (1975), 63-66.

4107.   Huttenback, M. "A Semester in Italy." *Nurs Forum*, 5 (1966), 74-83.

4108.   MacDougall, Eva. "Pioneering in Public Health Nursing in Italy." *Am J Pub Hlth*, 20 (Sep 1930), 1033-1034.

4109.   Saunders, R.G. "Nursing and Social Services in Italy." *Nurs Mirror*, 95(6) (15 Jun 1947), 193-195.

4110.   Sgarra, A. "The Nursing Profession in Italy." *Nurs Mirror*, 105 (1957), 1957-1959.

JAPAN

4111.   Achiwa, Goro. "Linda Richards in Japan." *Am J Nurs*, 68 (Aug 1968), 1716-1719.

4112.   Hayashi, S. "History, Influence of Florence Nightingale on Development of Nursing in Japan." *Rev Int Croix Rouge*, 36 (Apr 1954), 272-278.

4113.   "History of Nursing in Japan. 3. The Japanese Red Cross Nursing School. 3. Chinese-Japanese War and the Red Cross Nurses (1894-1896)." *Jap J Nurs*, 36 (Jan 1972), 74-80. (Jap)

4114.   "History of Nursing in Japan. 4. The Japanese Red Cross Nursing School. 4. Boxer Insurrection and the Japanese Red Cross Nurses." *Jap J Nurs*, 36 (May 1972), 368-375. (Jap)

4115.   Inouye, N. "Nursing in Japan." *Rev Inform Bull League Red Cr Soc*, 12 (Jan 1949-1951; Feb 1951), 9-12.

4116.   Ishihara, A. "Journey of the Japanese History of Nursing: Hokaido, Sapora City." *Jap J Nurs*, 30 (Aug 1966), 1. (Jap)

4117.   ———. "Journey of the Japanese History of Nursing: Osaka Castle." *Jap J Nurs*, 30 (Nov 1966), 1. (Jap)

4118.   ———. "A Journey of the Japanese History of Nursing: 10. Taikaku Temple--Kyoto City." *Jap J Nurs*, 30 (Oct 1966), 1. (Jap)

4119.   ———. "Journey of the Japanese History of Nursing: Todai Temple." *Jap J Nurs*, 30 (Jun 1966), 1. (Jap)

4120.   ———. "A Journey of the Japanese History of Nursing: Tokyo Tsukiji." *Jap J Nurs*, 30 (Sep 1966), 1. (Jap)

4121.   ————. "A Journey Through the Japanese History of Nursing.
         Yasaka Shinto Shrine." *Jap J Nurs*, 30 (Jul 1966), 1. (Jap)

4122.   "Japanese Literature on History of Nursing." *Jap J Nurs Educ*,
         10 (Jul 1969), 26-29. (Jap)

4123.   Kanai, K., et al. "Concepts of Health and Illness Described
         by Nightingale." *Compr Nurs Q*, 10(4) (Nov 1975), 63-79.

4124.   Kinoshita. Y. "Japanese Nursing History." *Jap J Nurs*, 11
         (Nov 1965), 124-131; (Dec 1965), 114-120; 12 (Jan 1966),
         122-129; (Feb 1966), 124-130; (Mar 1966), 123-129; (Apr
         1966), 142-148; (May 1966), 131-138; (Jun 1966), 135-147.
         (Jap)

4125.   McGee, A.N. "American Nurses in Japan." *Cent Mag*, 60 (Apr
         1905), 905.

4126.   Nakazato, R. "History of Establishing Nursing Education in
         Modern Japan." *Kango*, 26 (Apr 1974), 103-108; (Mar 1974),
         86-90; (Feb 1974), 59-64.

4127.   ————. "History of Nursing Education at the Dawn of Modern
         Japan." *Kango*, 26 (Jan 1974), 88-93.

4128.   "An Outline of the History of Nursing in Japan." *Aust Nurs J*,
         6 (1977), 23-26.

4129.   "People During the Formative Years of Modern Nursing in
         Japan." *Jap J Nurs*, 32 (May 1968), 77-81; (Jun 1968),
         89-93.

4130.   Richards, Linda. "Nursing Progress in Japan." *Am J Nurs*, 2
         (Apr 1902), 491-494.

4131.   Standlee, Mary W. *The Great Pulse: Japanese Midwifery and
         Obstetrics Through the Ages*. Rutland, VT: Charles E.
         Tuttle, 1959.

4132.   Takahashi, M. "Book Review by Discussion. On the Revised
         Edition of 'Bedside Nursing' by Chika Ozeki." *Jap J Nurs
         Res*, 8(1) (Winter 1975), 62-76. (Jap)

4133.   Takahashi, T. "Beginning of Professional Nursing in Japan."
         Jap J Nurs Res, 5 (Spring 1972), 265-292. (Jap)

4134.   Tomoika, J. *Kangofu Gendaishi (Modern History of Nursing)*.
         Tokyo: Jgaku Shoin (Kango Kyoyo Shinsho), 1966. (Jap)

4135.   Yamane, N. "In Search of Unknown Nursing Literature: (2) A
         Nursing Textbook of the Edo Period. *Byoke Suchi*." *Jap J
         Nurs Educ*, 16(7) (Jul 1975), 425-431; 16(8) (Aug 1975),
         495-499. (Jap)

4136.   ———. "Unknown Nursing Literature: (4) Nursing Literature
          Used in the Early Stage of Nursing Education in the Early
          1900s." *Jap J Nurs Educ*, 16(9) (Sep 1975), 580-585. (Jap)

KOREA

4137.   Bauer, F. "Entwickelungsgeschichte der Schwesternschaft von
          Korea." *Z Krankenpflege*, 10 (Mar 1966), 116-118.

4138.   ———. "The Story of the Development of Nursing in Korea."
          Deutsch Schwestern, 18 (10 Oct 1965), 376-379. (Ger)

4139.   "Fifty Years of Nursing Profession Reflected in the Mass
          Media." *Korean Nurs*, 12 (25 Apr 1973), 58-61. (Kor)

4140.   Hong, S.Y. "Cherishing the Memory of F. Nightingale: Greet-
          ing 150th Birthday Commemoration." *Korean Nurs*, 9 (25 Dec
          1970), 8-10. (Kor)

4141.   "The Nursing Profession Yesterday and Today." *Korean Nurs*,
          12 (Apr 1973), 55-57. (Kor)

LEBANON

4142.   Cardwell, V. "Public Health Nursing in Lebanon." *Pub Hlth
          Nurs*, 35 (1943), 430-434.

4143.   Edwards, M. "Health Services in Lebanon." *Nurs Times*, 60
          (1964), 848.

4144.   Mango, M. "The British Nurse Midwife with WHO." *Nurs Mirror*,
          99 (26 Jun 1954), iv-v.

4145.   Mitchell, A. "Unique Mental Hospital in the Middle East."
          Nurs Mirror, 99 (23 Apr 1954), vii-ix.

4146.   Rifka, G.E. "Nursing Manpower in Lebanon." *Int Nurs Rev*,
          17(3) (1970), 195-205.

4147.   Shahla, Sarah G. "Nursing in Syria." *Am J Nurs*, 30 (Dec
          1930), 1515-1518.

4148.   Stevens, E. "Nursing in Syria." *Nurs Times*, 23 (1927),
          1063.

4149.   Thomas, G.M. "Nursing in Lebanon." *Int Nurs Rev*, 22 (Sep-
          Oct 1975), 138-143.

MEXICO (SEE SOUTH AMERICA)

MOROCCO

4150.   Moutow, L. "A Glimpse at the Nursing Profession in Morocco."
         Int Nurs Rev, 22(1) (1975), 23-24.

4151.   Rogers, C. "Morocco: An Exotic Land." *AORN J*, 21 (1975),
         324-330.

NETHERLANDS

4152.   Cawford, L. "Health Care in Denmark, Sweden and Holland."
         Nurs Mirror, 141(4) (1975), 65-67.

4153.   Dane, Corrie. *Geschiedenis van de ziekenverpleging*. Lochen:
         De Tijdstroom, 1967. (Dut)

.4154.   DeHaan, M.C. "The Student of the Intermediate Professional
         Nursing Education in Training and Practice, Nursing Educa-
         tion in Future Perspective." *Tijdschrift vior Ziekenver-
         pleging*, 29(9) (1976), 408-417. (Dut)

4155.   Hooykaas, S. "Nursing in the Netherlands." *Am J Nurs*, 46
         (1946), 760-762.

4156.   Kruysee, M. "The Training of Nurses in the Wilhelmina
         Hospital, Amsterdam, Holland." *Am J Nurs*, 2 (1901), 136-
         137.

4158.   Meij-De leur, A.P.M. van der. *Van olie en wijn Geschiedenis
         van verplugkunde en Sociale Zorg*. Amsterdam: Agon Elsvier,
         1971. (Dut)

4159.   Meijer-Neels, E. "Part-time Nursing in Holland." *Nurs
         Mirror*, 106 (17 Jan 1976), 1149-1150.

4160.   Melk, H.H. "A Friendly Comparison." *Am J Nurs*, 30 (1930),
         1103-1109.

4161.   ———. "A Glimpse into Nursing and Nursing Education in
         Holland." *Int Nurs Rev*, 7 (8 Mar 1932), 185-188.

4162.   Ministry of Public Health and Environmental Hygiene. *Mental
         Health in the Netherlands*. The Hague: The Ministry, 1972.

NEW ZEALAND

4163.   Boyd, E. "Postbasic Nursing Education in New Zealand."
         Int Nurs Rev, 17(1) (1970), 43-52.

4164.   Bridges, E.R. "Nursing in New Zealand." *Am J Nurs*, 39
         (1939), 1205-1212.

4165.   *Great Days in New Zealand Nursing*. London: George G. Harrap
         & Co., 1961.

4166. Holdgate, E. "President's Address 1969." *New Zeal Nurs J*,
       62 (Jun 1969), 5-11.

4167. Lambie, M.I. "A Wealth of Information: Facts Relating to Our
       Nursing History which Every Nurse Should Know." *New Zeal
       Nurs J*, 53 (Jul 1960), 8-17.

4168. Maclean, Hester. *Nursing in New Zealand, History and
       Reminiscences.* Wellington: Tolan Print Co., 1932.

4169. Mordacq, C. "Constraints and Opportunities in a Nursing
       Career." *Int Nurs Rev*, 20 (Jul-Aug 1973), 112-113.

4170. New Zealand Department of Health. *Historical Development of
       Nursing in New Zealand 1840-1946.* Wellington: Department
       of Health, 1947.

4171. "Nursing in New Zealand." *Am J Nurs*, 47 (1947), 216-217.

4172. Rattray, J. *Great Days in New Zealand Nursing.* London:
       George G. Harrap & Co., 1961.

4173. *Report of the Nursing Council of New Zealand.* Wellington:
       Nursing Council of New Zealand, 1976.

4174. Shadbolt, Y.T. "Nursing Education in New Zealand." *New Zeal
       Nurs J*, 68(1) (1975), 19-22.

4175. Thomson, M. "Change in Nursing Education." *New Zeal Nurs J*,
       68(12) (1975), 22-23.

NIGERIA

4176. Beckingham, A.C. "History, Trends and Planning for Research
       in Nursing." *Niger Nurs*, 6(2) (Apr-Jun 1974), 39-40.

4177. Birch, J.A. "Nigeria in Peace and War." *Int J Nurs Studies*,
       8 (1971), 145-152.

4178. Chokrieh, A.C. "Change in Nursing in Nigeria." *Int Nurs Rev*,
       22(3) (1975), 71-79.

4179. Clemence, B.A. "Baccalaureate Nursing Education in Nigeria."
       Int Nurs Rev, 18(1) (1971), 40-48.

4180. Davis, A.J. "Health Problems and Nursing Practice in Sub-
       Saharan Africa." *Int J Nurs Studies*, 12 (1975), 61-64.

4181. Davitz, L.J. "Becoming a Nurse in Nigeria." *Am J Nurs*, 82
       (1972), 2026-2028.

4182. Dosunmu, N.E. "Nursing as a Career in Nigeria." *Int Nurs
       Rev*, 20(1) (1973), 30.

4183.   Duke, E.O. "History of Nursing in Nigeria." *Aust Nurs J*,
         65 (Feb 1967), 34-36.

4184.   Hamilton, J. "Nursing in Northern Nigeria." *Nurs Times*, 62
         (1966), 259-260.

4185.   "History of Nursing in Nigeria." *Aust Nurs J*, 65 (Feb 1967),
         34.

NORWAY

4186.   Gordon, Karen Allyn Rhea Stray. *Health Services in Transi-
         tion: Health Personnel in Primary Care: A Look at Nursing
         in Norway*. Ph.D. dissertation, Yale University, 1976.

4187.   Tomasgaard, J. "Vi moter Bergljot Larsson." *Sykepleien*, 51
         (1 Oct 1965), 488-490. (Nor)

4188.   Wyller, Ingrid. *Sykepleiens Historie i Norge*. Oslo: Land of
         Kirke, 1951, 1964. (Nor)

4189.   ————. *Sykepleiens Verdenchistorie*. Oslo: Land of Kirke,
         1969. (Nor)

PHILIPPINES

4190.   Lara, Hillario. "Development of Hygiene and Preventive Medi-
         cine (Public Health) in the Philippines." *Filipino Nurs*,
         12 (Oct 1937), 9-12.

4191.   "Nurse Administrator, Philippine Bureau of Health, Traces
         Progress Since 1919 in this Province." *Filipino Nurs*, 13
         (Apr 1938), 8-11.

4192.   Tupas, Anastacia. *History of Nursing in the Philippines and
         Manila*. Manila: University Press, 1952.

POLAND

4193.   Klodziński, S. "Jadwiga Dabrowska-Belońska (Dabrowsak-
         Belońska J)." *Prezegl Lek*, 31 (1974), 232-237. (Pol)

4194.   Krzywicka-Kowalik, K. "The Shape of the Fatherland During my
         Years of Labor." *Pieleg Polozna*, 7 (1976), 24-25. (Pol)

4195.   Lewandowski, S. "Organizacje Zawodowe Pieleniarek w Okresie
         Miedzywojennym." *Pieleg Polozna*, 8 (1966), 14-15. (Pol)

4196.   Migalska, A. "September Days." *Pieleg Polozna*, 9 (Sep
         1972), 23-24. (Pol)

4197.   Serafin, K. "Stories from Lódź." *Pieleg Polozna*, 3 (1976),
         24-25. (Pol)

4198.   Suwaia, Z. "Our Thirty Years." *Pieleg Polozna*, 4 (1976),
        1-3. (Pol)

4199.   Tarnowska, Maria. "The History of Nursing in Poland."
        Filipino Nurs, 11 (Jan 1936), 39-40, 52.

PORTUGAL

4200.   Correia, Fernando da Silva. *Origens' e formacão das Misri-
        córdias Portuguesas*. Lisbon: Torres, 1944.

RHODESIA

4201.   Ross, W.F. "The Advanced Clinical Nurse and the Health
        Team." *Cen Afr J Med*, 21 (1975), 243-245.

4202.   Snelgrone, F.W. "A School to be Proud of." *Int Nurs Rev*,
        21 (1974), 9-12.

4203.   Whitaker, B. "Mpilo Central Hospital." *Int J Nurs Studies*, 3
        (1966), 53-55.

RUMANIA

4204.   Anscombe, Ella. "Nursing in Roumania." *Brit J Nurs*, 72
        (Jul 1924), 160-161.

4205.   Fitzroy, Yvonne. *With the Scottish Nurses in Roumania*.
        London: Murray, 1918.

4206.   Reiner, A. "Scurt Istoric al Presei Personalului Medius
        Sanitar Intre Anii 1900 si 1939." *Munca Sanit*, 14 (Sep
        1966), 568-570. (Rum)

SENEGAL

4207.   Dieng, I. "Evolution of the Nursing Profession in Senegal."
        Int Nurs Rev, 21(6) (Nov-Dec 1974), 172-173.

SOUTH AFRICA

4208.   Bauman, M.B. "Baccalaureate Nursing in a Selected Number of
        English Speaking Countries." *Int Nurs Rev*, 19(1) (1972),
        12-38.

4209.   Beal, B. "Bantu Nursing." *Am J Nurs*, 70 (1970), 547-550.

4120.   Bridges, D. "A Journey to Africa." *Int Nurs Rev*, 2 (Apr
        1955), 7-13.

4211.   Bull, M.R. "Training South Africa's Nurses." *Nurs Mirror*,
        133 (24 Dec 1971), 18-20.

4212.   Epstein, S.P. "Links in Memory's Golden Chain." *So Afr
        Nurs J*, 32 (Nov 1965), 23-30.

4213.   Grobellaan, A. "South African Experiments with the Basic
        Collegiate Program." *Am J Nurs*, 58 (1958), 1401-1402.

4214.   Harrison, P.H. "Coloured Nursing Progress in South Africa."
        So Afr Nurs J, 36 (Nov 1969), 27.

4215.   Kark, Sydney L. "The Nurse in Health Centre Practice, Her
        Functions and Training." *So Afr Nurs J*, 16 (30 Jun 1950),
        9-11.

4216.   Kretzmar, Noel. "An Introduction to the History of Medicine
        on the Diamond Fields of Kimberly, South Africa." *Med
        Hist*, 18(2) (1974), 155-162.

4217.   Laxarus, B. "The History of Nursing--Its Importance in
        Training." *So Afr Nurs J*, 17 (5 Oct 1929), 2.

4218.   Lechemere, K.M. "Nursing in South Africa Thirty Years Ago."
        Cath Nurs, 9 (8 Jun 1941), 6.

4219.   Marais, J. "Nursing in Mau Mau Time." *So Afr Nurs J*, 40
        (Nov 1973), 25-26.

4220.   Minde, M. "One Hundred Years of Mental Nursing." *So Afr
        Nurs J*, 20 (Mar 1954), 37.

4221.   Pask, M.M.F. "Reminiscences of a Pioneer South African
        Nurse. I. Early Days." *So Afr Nurs J*, 36 (Sep 1969), 7.

4222.   ————. "Reminiscences of a Pioneer South African Nurse.
        II. The New Somerset Hospital." *So Afr Nurs J*, 36 (Sep
        1969), 9.

4223.   ————. "Reminiscences of a Pioneer South African Nurse.
        III. Marie." *So Afr Nurs J*, 36 (Oct 1969), 35.

4224.   ————. "Reminiscences of a Pioneer South African Nurse.
        IV." *So Afr Nurs J*, 36 (Nov 1969), 29-31; 37 (Jan 1970),
        17-19; (Feb 1970), 29-30; (Mar 1970), 30-31.

4225.   Pope, Georgina Fane. "Nursing in South Africa During the
        Boer War." *Brit J Nurs* (20 Sep 1902), 232-234.

4226.   Roberts, H. "Nursing in Johannesburg." *Nurs Mirror*, 129
        (19 Sep 1969), 39-41.

4227.   Searle, Charlotte. "Developments in Nursing Education at
        South African Universities." *Int J Nurs Studies*, 6 (1969),
        107-113.

4228.   ————. "Episodes in Our Nursing History; 1--Contribution
        from Natal to the Nightingale Fund, 1956." *So Afr Nurs J*
        (Oct 1963), 11.

4229.   ———. "Fifty Years of Nursing Service in South Africa
        1914-1964." *So Afr Nurs J* (Nov 1964), 32-55.

4230.   ———. *The History of the Development of Nursing in South
        Africa.* Cape Town: C. Struik (Pty) Ltd., 1965.

4231.   ———. "The History of the Development of Nursing in South
        Africa, 1652-1960." *So Afr Nurs J*, 33 (Jan 1966), 9.

4232.   ———. "Nursing Education in South Africa." *Int Nurs Rev*,
        41 (1957), 49-62.

4233.   ———. "A Review of Nursing Education in South Africa."
        Int Nurs Bull, 9 (Winter 1953), 5-10.

SOUTH AMERICA

4234.   Aguiar Horta, W.D. "Historic Evaluation of Nursing Students
        of the Nursing School of the University of the São Paulo."
        Rev Enferm Nov Deimens, 1(4) (Sep-Oct 1975), 198-202. (Por)

4235.   Alcointara, Herrera J. "Historical Notes Relating to Nursing
        in Mexico." *Span Med Rev Mex*, 40 (Dec 1960), 547-555.
        (Spa)

4236.   Aznarez, E.P. "History--Nurses and Servants of Women's
        Hospital During the Tyranny." *Prensa Med Argent*, 28
        (8 Jan 1961), 133-136. (Spa)

4237.   Bareira, I. "Changes in the Image of the Nurse in Brazil."
        Int Nurs Rev, 23 (Mar-Apr 1976), 43-47.

4238.   Beck, Frances S. "Background to Nursing in Bolivia." *Int
        Nurs Rev*, 13 (Apr 1966), 21-25.

4239.   ———. "Impressions of a Visit to Latin America." *Int Nurs
        Rev*, 6 (Apr 1959), 53-59.

4240.   Bejarano, J., and Jaramillo, A.A. "History and Development
        of Nursing in Colombia." *Rev Fac de Med Bogotá*, 17 (Jul
        1948), 1075-1079. (Spa)

4241.   Chagas, A. "Modern Nursing in Latin America." *Am J Nurs*,
        53 (1953), 34-36.

4242.   De Alcantara, G. "Nursing in Brazil." *Am J Nurs*, 53 (1953),
        576-579.

4243.   "Development of Nursing Service in Brazil." *Am J Nurs*, 22
        (1922), 560.

4244.   Galiano, S. "Brief History of Nursing in Nicaragua." *Int
        J Nurs Studies*, 12(4) (1975), 223-229.

4245.   Goncalves da Silva, M. "Historico de Faculdade de Enfermagem
        Madre Maria Teodora." *Rev Brasil Enferm*, 18 (Dec 1965),
        550-552. (Por)

4246.   Guanes, H. "Nursing Education in Brazil." *Int Nurs Rev*, 5
        (1958), 32-33.

4247.   Hentsch, Y. "Nursing in Latin America." *Am J Nurs*, 43
        (1943), 440-442.

4248.   Jackson, J. "Nursing in Brazil." *Am J Nurs*, 2 (1901), 56-57.

4249.   Number deleted.

4250.   Molina, Teresa Maria. *Historia de la Enfermeria*. Buenos
        Aires: Intermedica, 1973.

4251.   Moreno, G.T. "Mexican Nurses' Association: Change for
        Development." *Int Nurs Rev*, 19(4) (1972), 370-376.

4252.   Mussallem, H.K. "A Glimpse of Nursing in Cuba." *Canad Nurs*,
        69 (1973), 23-30.

4253.   "The Nurse from the Sixteenth to the Twentieth Century in
        Mexico." *Enfermeras*, 18 (1971), 7-10. (Spa)

4254.   O'Hara, H. "Public Health Nursing in Latin America." *Pub
        Hlth Nurs*, 42 (1950), 73-78.

4255.   Paixão, Walisk. *Págenas de História de Enfermagem*. 2nd ed.
        revised. Rio de Janeiro: B. Buccini, 1960. (Por)

4256.   Parsons, E. "Modern Nursing in Brazil." *Am J Nurs*, 27
        (1927), 443-449.

4257.   Pérez, Riblé R. "Address Presented at the Convention of the
        Panamerican Federation of Male and Female Nurses in Vina
        del Mar, Chile; Dec 7-12, 1975." *Bol Col Prof Enferm PR*,
        2(5) (Mar 1976), 16-19. (Spa)

4258.   Ponte, M.L. "A Rapid Glance at Brazilian Postgraduate Edu-
        cation." *Int J Nurs Studies*, 4 (1967), 37-46.

4259.   Pontes, C. de. "History of Nursing, Alfredo Pinto School of
        Nursing, The Pioneer of Nursing Schools in Brazil." *Rev
        Brasil Enferm*, 24 (Apr-Jun 1971), 199-214. (Por)

4260.   Portilla, Rueda. "Evolution of Nursing Care and Health Ser-
        vice in Colombia." *ANEC*, 5(13) (Oct 1974), 25-28.

4261.   Porto-Alegre, Idalia de Aranjo. "The Evolution of the Nurs-
        ing School in Brazil." *League Red Cr Soc Month Bull*, 16
        (Jul 1935), 128-129; reprinted *Brit J Nurs*, 83 (Sep 1935),
        242; *Filipino Nurs*, 12 (Jan 1937), 32-33.

4262. "Progress in Nursing Education in Latin America." *Int Nurs Rev*, 14 (Jan-Feb 1967), 64.

4263. Prestrepo, R. "Nursing in Colombia." *Canad Nurs*, 65 (1969), 37.

4264. Pullen, B. "Nursing in Brazil." *Am J Nurs*, 35 (1935), 345-350.

4265. Rets, M.A. "Reminiscences of Brazilian Nursing." *Rev Brasil Enferm*, 30 (1977), 73-75. (Por)

4266. Romero, H. "Development of Medicine and Public Health in Chile. I." English Abstract. *Rev Med Chile*, 100 (Jul 1972), 853-876.

SPAIN

4267. Martinez Navarro, J.F. "Social Factors in the Origin of Nursing in Spain." *Rev Sanid Hig Publica* (Madrid), 49(4) (Apr 1974), 343-356. (Spa)

SWEDEN

4268. Adler, S.P. "Swedish Student Nurses: A Descriptive Study." *Nurs Res*, 18 (1969), 363-365.

4269. Andrell, M. "Nursing in Sweden." *Am J Nurs*, 40 (1940), 1136-1141.

4270. Axelsson, S., and U. Nicolausson. "Community Health Nursing --Farthest Outpost of Health and Medical Services." *Curr Swed*, 144 (1977), 1-7.

4271. Berglind, H. "Occupation Activity of a Swedish RN." *Int J Nurs Studies*, 2 (1965), 251-260.

4272. Cawford, L. "Health Care in Denmark, Sweden and Holland." *Nurs Mirror*, 141(4) (1975), 65-67.

4273. Detlow-Berg, A.L. "Medical History in Helsingfors." *T Sverige Sjukskot*, 43(1) (Jan 1976), 4-5. (Swe)

4274. Dillner, Elisabet. *Eight Decades.* Stockholm: Svensk Sjukskoterske Forenings Forlag, 1949.

4275. ————. "Nursing." *Medicinal Vosendet i Sweirge 1813-1962.* English Abstract. Stockholm: A.B. Nordiska Bokhandelns Forlag, 1963. pp. 618-644. (Swe)

4276. Dunbar, V. "Nursing in Northern Europe." *Am J Nurs*, 37 (1932), 123-130.

4277.   Lobban, Marjorie. "Nursing Museum in a Swedish Hospital."
        Nurs Mirror (5 Oct 1956), vii-ix.

4278.   "The Nursing Profession--A Large Piece of Cultural History."
        T Sverige Sjukskot, 36 (24 Sep 1969), 1014-1015.

4279.   "The Nursing Profession--A Piece of Cultural History."
        T Sverige Sjukskot, 37 (Jan 1970), 111-113.

4280.   Olsen, Marie. "Nursing in Sweden." *Am J Nurs*, 32 (Oct
        1932), 1059-1062.

4281.   Rodhe, Estrid. "Nursing of the Sick." *Canad Nurs*, 5 (Aug
        1909), 506-510.

SWITZERLAND

4282.   Dummermuth-Helfer, M. "75th Anniversary of Lindenhof, Bern."
        Z Krankenpflege, 67(8-9) (Aug-Sep 1974), 340-341. (Ger)

4283.   Freudweiler, E. "The Nursing of the Sick in Switzerland."
        Tr Nurs, 79 (Sep 1927), 270-272.

4284.   Naef, Nelly. "The Development of Nursing in Switzerland up
        to the Middle of the 19th Century" (trans). *ICN*, 2 (Jan
        1927), 19-35.

4285.   Studer-Von Goumoens, Elisabeth. "Development of Nursing
        Switzerland Since 1850" (trans). *ICN*, 3 (Jul 1928), 230-
        241.

TAIWAN

4286.   Chang, G.T. "Maternity Care in Free China." *Bull Am Coll
        Nurs Mid*, 18 (1968), 139-142.

4287.   Li, S.F. "Public Health Nursing in Taiwan, Republic of
        China." *Am J Pub Hlth*, 56 (1966), 492-498.

4288.   Mei-Li, L.L. "The Education and Role of Nurses in Taiwan."
        Int Nurs Rev, 20 (Nov-Dec 1973), 176-177.

THAILAND

4289.   Fitzgerald, Alice. "Nursing in Siam." *Am J Nurs*, 29 (Jul
        1929), 817-821.

TURKEY

4290.   Sehsurazoglu, B.N. "A Survey of Nursing in Anatolian, Turks
        and Nursing History (Istanbul)." *Tip Fakultesi Mecmurasi*,
        23 (1960), 240-250. (Turk)

4291.   Türer, Asuman. "Turkey--Cradle of Modern Nursing." *Int Nurs Rev*, 16(1) (1969), 64-68.

4292.   Wheeler, C.T. "Trained Nurse in Turkey." *Outlook*, 84 (1 Sep 1906), 32-35.

4293.   VanZandt, J. "A Training School of Nurses in the Turkish Empire." *Am J Nurs*, 9 (1909), 274-276.

UNITED STATES

4294.   "American Nursing--Fifty Years Ago." *Tr Nurs & Hosp Rev* (1940), 105, 298-301.

4295.   Bard, H. "Commencement Address--September 10, 1967." *Alum Mag* (Baltimore), 66 (Dec 1967), 100-102.

4296.   "The Birth of the American Trained Nurse." *Nurs Mirror*, 119 (3096) (Oct 1964), xii-xiii.

4297.   Brown, Esther Lucille. *Nursing as a Profession*. New York: Russell Sage Foundation, 1936.

4298.   Bullough, Bonnie, and Vern Bullough. "The Origins of Modern American Nursing: The Civil War Era." *Nurs Forum*, 2 (1963), 13-27.

4299.   Carnegie Commission on Higher Education. *Higher Education and the Nation's Health: Policies for Dental and Medical Education*. New York: McGraw-Hill Book Co., 1970.

4300.   Chayer, Mary Ella. "American Nursing--History and Interpretation." *Nurs Out*, 2 (Jun 1954), 295-296.

4301.   "The Cold Affusion--The Way It Was." *Nurs Clin No Am*, 3 (Jun 1968), 373ff.

4302.   Day, P.E. "A Symposium on Nursing in America: Nursing History in the States." *Nurs Mirror*, 143(2) (8 Jul 1976), 47-48.

4303.   Dodge, Bertha Sanford. *The Story of Nursing*. Boston: Little, Brown & Co., 1954, 1965.

4304.   Donegan, Janet B. *Midwifery in America, 1760-1860: A Study in Medicine and Morality*. Ph.D. dissertation, Syracuse University, 1972.

4305.   Duffy, John. *The Healers: A History of American Medicine*. New York: McGraw-Hill Book Co., 1976; Urbana: University of Illinois, 1978. 385 pp.

4306.   Emmons, Arthur B., and James L. Huntington. "The Midwife: Her Future in United States." *Am J Obs Dis Wom Child*, 65 (Mar 1912), 393-404.

4307.   Fishbein, Morris. *A History of the American Medical Associa-*
        tion, 1847-1947. Philadelphia: W.B. Saunders, 1947.

4308.   Fitzpatrick, M. Louise. "Nurses in American History,
        Nursing and the Great Depression." *Am J Nurs*, 75
        (Dec 1975), 2188-2190.

4309.   Flexner, Abraham. *Medical Education in the United States and*
        Canada: A Report to the Carnegie Foundation for the
        Advancement of Teaching. Bulletin No. 4. Boston: P.B.
        Updike, 1910.

4310.   Jensen, Joan M. "Politics and the American Midwife Contro-
        versy." *Frontiers*, 1 (Spring 1976), 19-33.

4311.   Jones, F.M. "History of Nursing in America." *Nurs J India*,
        20 (Apr 1929), 93-100.

4312.   Kalish, Philip A., and Beatrice Kalish. *The Advance of*
        American Nursing. Boston: Little, Brown & Co., 1978.

4313.   Litoff, Judy Barett. *American Midwives: 1860 to Present.*
        Westport, CT: Greenwood Press, 1978.

4314.   McGee, Anita N. "The Growth of the Nursing Profession in the
        United States." *Tr Nurs*, 24 (1900), 441-445.

4315.   Macy Foundation. *The Midwife in the United States.* New
        York: Josiah Macy, Jr. Foundation, 1968.

4316.   Mary Collett, Mother. "The Trend of the Nursing Profession."
        Bull Am Hosp Assoc, 5 (Jan 1931).

4317.   "Medical Education in the United States." *J Am Med Assoc*, 79
        (1922), 629-633.

4318.   Merrick, Elliott. *Northern Nurse.* New York: Charles
        Scribner's Sons, 1942.

4319.   Norwood, W.F. *Medical Education in the U.S. Before the Civil*
        War. Philadelphia: University of Pennsylvania Press, 1944.

4320.   Packard, F.R. *History of Medicine in the United States.* 2nd
        ed. 2 vols. New York: P.B. Hoeber, 1931.

4321.   Richards, Linda. "Progress in Twenty Years (1875-1895)."
        Tr Nurs, 100 (Apr 1938), 360-361.

4322.   ————. "Thirty Years of Progress." *Am J Nurs*, 4 (Jan
        1904).

4323.   Roberts, Mary M. *American Nursing: History and Interpreta-*
        tion. New York: Macmillan Co., 1954.

4324.   Rogers, Caroline. "The Birth of Our Profession in America."
        AORN J, 11 (Jun 1970), 73-76.

4325.   Shoemaker, Sister M. Theophane. *History of Nurse-Midwifery in the United States.* Washington, D.C.: Catholic University Press, 1947.

4326.   Shyrock, Richard H. *Medicine in America: Historical Essays.* Baltimore: Johns Hopkins Press, 1966.

4327.   Sigerist, Henry E. *American Medicine.* New York: W.W. Norton, 1934.

4328.   Stewart, Isabel Maitland. "A Half-Century of Nursing Education." *Am J Nurs,* 50 (Oct 1950), 617-620.

4329.   ————. "Isabel M. Stewart Recalls the Early Years (1900-1920)." *Am J Nurs,* 60 (Oct 1960), 1426-1430.

4330.   Thomas, Margaret W. *The Practice of Nurse-Midwifery in the United States.* U.S. Dept. H.E.W., Children's Bureau Pub. No. 436. Washington, D.C.: U.S. Government Printing Office, 1965.

4331.   Walsh, James J. *History of Medicine in New York.* New York: National American Society, 1919; New York: P.J. Kennedy and Sons, 1929.

4332.   Weispfenning, I. "Development and Current Aspects of the Nursing Profession in the USA." *Z Krankenpflege,* 29(6) (1 Jun 1976), 325-328. (Ger)

UNION OF SOVIET SOCIALIST REPUBLICS

4333.   Abdellah, Faye. "Nursing and Health Care in the U.S.S.R." *Am J Nurs,* 73 (Dec 1973), 2096-2099.

4334.   Agaev, E.R. "The Journal 'Fel'dsher i Akusherka'--Forty Years Old." *Feldsher Akush,* 41(1) (1976), 5-11. (Rus)

4335.   ————. Borodulin VI. "30-Letie Zhurnal--'Fel'dsher i akusherka'?" *Feldsher Akush,* 31(1) (1966), 4-11. (Rus)

4336.   Akkerman, B.I. "The Life and Work of Feldsher G.V. Sidochenko." *Feldsher Akush,* 38(3) (1973), 43-45. (Rus)

4337.   Albin, E. "Nursing in the U.S.S.R." *Am J Nurs,* 46 (1946), 525-528.

4338.   Armstrong, J. "Health Services in the USSR." *Nurs Times,* 61 (1965), 1592.

4339.   Bogoiavlenskii, N.A. "Feldshers in the History of Russian Culture." *Feldsher Akush,* 31(1) (1966), 54-59. (Rus)

4340.   Brizhak, B.E. "Revolutionary L.A. Volkenshtein in Sakhalin." *Sohetsk Zdravoorhr,* 8 (1975), 81. (Rus)

4341.   Chikin, Sia. "Revolutionary Activities of Feldshers Who Used
        to Work with V.I. Lenin." *Feldsher Akush*, 35(2) (1970),
        3-5. (Rus)

4342.   Crowe, Margaret. "Nursing History in Russia." *Nurs Mirror*,
        78 (19 Feb 1944), 309.

4343.   Curtis, John Shelton. "Russian Nightingale." *Am J Nurs*, 68
        (May 1968), 1029-1031.

4344.   ————. "Russian Sisters of Mercy in the Crimea, 1954-1955."
        Slavic Rev, 25 (Mar 1966), 84-100.

4345.   Dionesor, S.M. "The History of Midwifery Training at the
        Beginning of the Nineteenth Century in Russia." *Sovetsk
        Zdravoohr*, 20(6), 67-72. (Rus)

4346.   Dyachenko, D.P. "Geroicheskie traditsii fel'dsherar Kam-
        chatki." *Feldsher Akush*, 30(11) (1965), 26-30. (Rus)

4347.   Ensberger, M. "Nursing in Russia." *Nurs Out*, 11 (1963), 883.

4348.   Hoffman, I. "Progress in Russia." *Am J Nurs*, 14 (1913),
        197-198.

4349.   Holliday, J. "Glimpses of Nursing in Russia." *Nurs Out*, 6
        (1958), 496-497.

4350.   Ikonnikova, J. "Nurses in the Soviet Union." *Int Nurs Rev*,
        10 (Jul-Aug 1963), 17.

4351.   Kachalova, P. "Nurses at the 50th Anniversary of the USSR."
        Med Sestra, 31 (Dec 1972), 34-35. (Rus)

4352.   Kaderova, V. "Reminiscence of Old Nurses." *Zdrav Prac*, 21
        Suppl (Jun 1971), 33-42. (Cze)

4353.   Kolybina, Olga. "Nursing in the USSR." *Int J Nurs Studies*,
        4 (Aug 1967), 257-261.

4354.   Kuz'min, M.K. "A Feldsher of Chapaev's Division." *Feldsher
        Akush*, 32(11) (1967), 18-20. (Rus)

4355.   Leitz, D. "Nursing in the Soviet Union." *Nurs Mirror*, 117
        (31 Jan 1964), 64-66.

4356.   Morris, K.H. "Profile of a Russian Nurse." *Am J Nurs*, 66
        (1966), 549-551.

4357.   Morris, R.M. "Letter: Jane Helena Daly." *Cen Afr J Med*,
        21(4) (Apr 1975), 88. (Rus)

4358.   Muller, J.E. "The Soviet Health System—-Aspects of Relevance
        for Medicine in the United States." *New England J Med*, 286
        (30 Mar 1972), 693-702.

4359. Mussallem, K.H. "A Glimpse of Nursing in the USSR." *Canad Nurs*, 63 (1967), 27–33.

4360. Nesterendo, A.T. "Company Feldshers and Soviet Power." *Feldsher Akush*, 32 (Nov 1967), 11–13. (Rus)

4361. Powell, A. "Nurse Training in USSR." *Nurs Times*, 60 (1964), 481.

4362. Quinn, S.E. "Nursing in the Soviet Union." *Int Nurs Rev*, 15(1) (1968), 75–86.

4363. Rozova, K.A. "First Pages of the History of Soviet Feldshers." *Feldsher Akush* (Apr 1970), 47–51. (Rus)

4364. Sagalov, G.M. "O Nashem Zhurnale." *Feldsher Akush*, 1 (1960), 21–22. (Rus)

4365. Shmarov, A.A. "Meditsinskie Sestry Kronshtadtskoga Gospitalia." *Med Sestra*, 25 (Feb 1966), 50–51. (Rus)

4366. Sidel, W. "Feldshers and Feldsherism: The Role and Training in the Feldsher in the U.S.S.R." *New Directions for Nurses*. Edited by Bonnie and Vern Bullough. New York: Springer, 1971. pp. 40–50.

4367. Slomimskaia, I.A. "Their Distinguished Names are Never to be Forgotten." *Feldsher Akush*, 1 (1967), 25–28. (Rus)

4368. Svetliakor, A.G. "Iz istori podgotovki fel'dsherkoskusherskikh kadrov v Rossii." *Feldsher Akush*, 31(3) (1966), 44–47. (Rus)

4369. Velikoretski, A.N. "Clinical Subjects in the Journal 'Fel'dsher i Akusherka' During 10 Years (1966–1975)." *Feldsher Akush*, 41(1) (1976), 52–60. (Rus)

4370. ————. "Klinicheskaia tematika zhurnala 'Fel'dsher i akusherka' za 30 let." *Feldsher Akush*, 31(1) (1966), 12–16. (Rus)

4371. Voropai, A.V. "Slava vam, voennye fel'dshera." *Feldsher Akush*, 30(11) (1965), 22–26. (Rus)

4372. Zhuk, A.P. "Soviet Feldsher and the Problem of 'Feldsherism.'" *Feldsher Akush*, 12 (1966), 35–38. (Rus)

VIETNAM

4373. Lam Thi Hal. "Vietnam to U.S." *Am J Nurs*, 55 (Dec 1955), 1469.

YUGOSLAVIA

4374.   Benson, E. "Nursing in Servia ... Early Days." *Am J Nurs*,
        74 (1974), 472-474.

4375.   ————. "Vignette of Nursing in Yugoslavia." *Nurs Out*, 17
        (1969), 36-38.

4376.   Ingram, R. "Nursing in Yugoslavia." *Am J Nurs*, 30 (1930),
        139-145.

4377.   Milena, P. "The Development of Nursing in the Northern Part
        of Jugoslavija (SR--Solvenija)." *Int J Nurs Studies*, 9
        (Aug 1972), 151-158.

4378.   "Some Impressions of Nursing in Yugoslavia and Hungary."
        Am J Nurs, 31 (1931), 671-676.

4379.   Urbancic, D. "Nursing in Yugoslavia." *Am J Nurs*, 56 (1956),
        585-587.

ZAMBIA

4380.   Baxter, A.J. "A Long Journey to Kasama ... On Foot."
        Zambia Nurs J, 2 (Jun 1966), 14-18.

13. INDIVIDUAL STATES (UNITED STATES)

CALIFORNIA

4381. "Again the Woman Question." *Nurs J Pac Cst*, 5 (Jan 1909), 3.

4382. Brocon, Charlotte B. "Obstetric Practice Among the Chinese
       in San Francisco." *Pac Med Surg J*, 26 (Jul 1883), 15-21.

4383. *California State Nurses' Association and the Economic Security
       of Its Members*. Sacramento: California State Nurses'
       Association, 1943.

4384. "Editorial Comment (Eight Hour Day)." *Pac Cst J Nurs*, 9
       (Jun 1913), 243.

4385. Estep, Katherine A. "The Pioneer Nurse." *Nurs J Pac Cst*, 1
       (Dec 1904), 54-57.

4386. "Impressions of Pacific Coast Training Schools." *Nurs J Pac
       Cst*, 2 (Mar 1906), 19-20.

COLORADO

4387. Popiel, E.S. "Colorado Schools of Nursing. Try to Remember
       Our Heritage." *Colo Nurs*, 68 (May 1968), 9-13.

4388. ————. "Try to Remember Our Heritage." *Colo Nurs*, 66
       (Jun-Jul 1966), 21-23.

DELAWARE

4389. Sargent, C.A. "Midwifery in Delaware." *Del State Med J*, 5
       (Aug 1933), 176-177.

FLORIDA

4390. Hanson, Henry, and Lucile S. Blackly. "Present Status of
       Midwifery in Florida." *So Med J*, 25 (Dec 1932), 1252-1258.

4391. Paylor, Mary Margaret. "A History of Nursing Education in
       Florida from 1893-1970." Ed.D. dissertation, Florida State
       University, 1975.

GEORGIA

4392.   Georgia State Nurses Association. *Highlights of Georgia
        State Nurses Association in Action 1907-1957.* Atlanta:
        Georgia Nurses' Association, 1958.

HAWAII

4393.   Lewis, Frances R. Hegglund. *History of Nursing in Hawaii.*
        Node, WY: Germann-Kilmer Co., 1969.

INDIANA

4394.   Allen, Dotaline E. *History of Nursing in Indiana.* Indiana-
        polis: Wolfe, 1950.

4395.   Meyers, Mary A. "Early History of Nursing in Indiana."
        Mont Bull Ind Board Hlth, 48 (1945), 28, 45-47.

KANSAS

4396.   *Lamps on the Prairie, A History of Nursing in Kansas. Com-
        piled by the Writers Program of the Work Projects Adminis-
        tration in the State of Kansas, Sponsored by the Kansas
        State Nurses' Association.* Emporia Gazette Press, 1942.
        292 pp.

4397.   Mulvany, Esther Ring. *Lamps Still Aglow: A History of Kansas
        Nursing.* North Newton, KS: Mulvany, 1956; Hillsboro, KS:
        Mennonite Publishing House, 1976.

KENTUCKY

4398.   Breckinridge, Mary. "Hard-Riding Nurses of Kentucky." *Lit
        Digest*, 96 (Mar 1928), 29-30.

4399.   ————. †*Wide Neighborhoods: A Study of Frontier Nursing
        Service.* New York: Harper, 1952.

LOUISIANA

4400.   King, Edward L. "Fifty Years of Obstetrics in New Orleans."
        Obs Gyn, 19(6) (Jun 1962), 826-830.

4401.   Wall, Emma L. "Nursing Conditions in Louisiana." *Am J Nurs*,
        15 (May 1915), 654-655.

MASSACHUSETTS

4402.   Howard, Anne T., and Dorrian Apple. *Nursing Needs and Re-
        sources in Massachusetts.* Boston: Massachusetts League
        for Nursing, 1960.

4403. Huntington, James L. "The Midwife in Massachusetts: Her
       Anomalous Position." *Bost Med Surg J*, 168 (Mar 1913),
       418-421.

MINNESOTA

4404. Hartley, E.C., and Ruth E. Boynton. "A Survey of the Midwife
       Situation in Minnesota." *Minn Med*, 7 (Jun 1924), 439-446.

4405. Winberg, O.K. "County Nurse in Minnesota." *Am City* (T and
       C ed.), 21 (Sep 1919), 228.

MISSISSIPPI

4406. Ferguson, James H. "Mississippi Midwives." *J Hist Med*, 5
       (1950), 85-95.

4407. Price, B.M. "Nurses at Corinth in 1862." *Mississippi RN*, 32
       (Jul 1970), 9-10.

MISSOURI

4408. Christ, Edwin. *Missouri's Nurses: The Development of the
       Profession, Its Associations, and Its Institutions.*
       Jefferson City, MO: Missouri Nurses' Association, 1958.

4409. Trenholme, Louise Irby. *History of Nursing in Missouri.*
       Columbia: Missouri State Nurses's Association, 1926. 140
       pp.

NEBRASKA

4410. Nebraska Professional Nursing Organizations. *A Report of the
       Survey to Measure Nursing Needs and Resources in Nebraska,
       1950-1951.* Lincoln: Nebraska Professional Nursing Organi-
       zations, 1952.

NEW JERSEY

4411. Fondiller, S. "30 Years of Nursing History at Atlantic City
       Conventions, 1946-1976." *So Am Nurs*, 8(2) (31 Jan 1976),
       6-7.

4412. Levy, Julius. "The Maternal and Infant Mortality in Mid-
       wifery Practice in Newark, New Jersey." *Am J Obs*, 77
       (1918), 41-51.

NEW YORK

4413. Crowell, Elizabeth. "The Midwives of New York." *Charities*,
       17 (5 Jan 1907), 671-677.

4414.   Pryor, J.H. "The Status of the Midwife in Buffalo." *New York Med J*, 11 (Aug 1884), 129–132.

NORTH CAROLINA

4415.   Warren, E.W. "History of Nursing in North Carolina. Your Share." *Tar Heel Nurs*, 33 (Mar 1971), 48–49.

4416.   Wyche, Mary Lewis. *The History of North Carolina*. Chapel Hill: University of North Carolina Press, 1938.

NORTH DAKOTA

4417.   Bower, Sister Carita. "The Women in White March Across the Prairies." *Prairie Rose*, 22 (Jan-Feb-Mar 1953), 4; (Apr-May-Jun 1953), 2.

OHIO

4418.   Austin, Anne L. "Development of Nursing in Ohio." *Ohio Archaeol Hist Q*, 50 (1941), 351–365.

4419.   Bower, Irene M. *Public Health Nursing in Cleveland (Ohio)*. Cleveland: Western Reserve University, 1930. 120 pp.

4420.   Logan, Laura. "Nursing in Cincinnati, 1820-1920." *Univ Cincin Med Bull* (1920), 68–86.

4421.   Rodabaugh, James H., and Mary Jane Rodabaugh. *Nursing in Ohio: A History*. Columbus: Ohio State Nurses' Association, 1951.

OKLAHOMA

4422.   Crockett, Bernice Norman. *The Origin and Development of Public Health Nursing in Oklahoma, 1830-1930*. Ph.D. dissertation, University of Oklahoma, 1953.

PENNSYLVANIA

4423.   Henry, Frederick P. *Standard History of the Medical Profession in Philadelphia*. Chicago: Goodspeed Brothers, 1897.

4424.   Morton, T.G. *The History of the Pennsylvania Hospital, 1751-1895*. Philadelphia: Times Printing House, 1897.

4425.   Royer, B.F. "Midwives in Pennsylvania." *Penn Med J*, 16 (Jan 1913), 289–294.

4426.   West, Roberta Mayhew. *History of Nursing in Pennsylvania*. Harrisburg: Pennsylvania State Nurses' Association, 1926, 1939.

TENNESSEE

4427.   "Aunt Sarah: Tennessee's Champion Midwife." *Newsweek*, 48
        (Aug 1956), 54.

TEXAS

4428.   Crowder, E.W. "On Nursing in Texas. Anyone Here for His-
        tory." *Texas Nurse*, 48(8) (Sep 1974), 4.

UTAH

4429.   McKean, C. "The Tale of a Nurse." *Utah Nurs*, 23 (Fall
        1972), 3-4.

VERMONT

4430.   Bogie, Edythe. "The History of Nursing in Vermont." *Am J
        Nurs*, 42 (Apr 1942), 421-424.

4431.   Kelley, Madeline V. "Mountain Nurse." *Survey*, 68 (15 Oct
        1932), 512-513.

4432.   Vermont State Nurses' Association. *We Who Serve: A Story of
        Nursing in Vermont*. Montpelier: The Association, 1941.

VIRGINIA

4433.   Faris, Jessie Wetzel. "Two Hundred Years of Nursing in
        Richmond (VA)." *Am J Nurs*, 37 (Aug 1937), 847-849.

4434.   Plecker, W.A. "The Midwife Problem in Virginia." *Virginia
        Med Semi Monthly*, 19 (Dec 1914), 456-458. See also Nos.
        2679-2682.

WEST VIRGINIA

4435.   Bond, D.H. *A Half Century of Nursing in West Virginia, 1907-
        1957*. Charleston: West Virginia State Nurses' Association,
        1957.

4436.   Reid, Mary E. *A History of Nursing in West Virginia, 1907-
        1941*. Edited by Margaret J. Steele. Charleston: West
        Virginia State Nurses' Association, 1941.

WISCONSIN

4437.   Cooper, Signe S. *Wisconsin Nursing Pioneers*. Madison:
        University Extension, University of Wisconsin, Department
        of Nursing, 1968.

4438.   Van Kooy, Nelly. "Development of Public Health Nursing in
        Wisconsin." *Pub Hlth Nurs*, 14 (Feb 1922), 87-89.

14. RELIGIOUS NURSING AND SISTERHOODS

4439. Appleton, Nigel J.W. "Bethany Homestead, Northampton: A
        Case Study in Christian Social Concern." *J United Ref
        Chur His Soc*, 1(2) (1974), 61-66.

4440. Ayres, Anne. *Evangelical Sisterhoods. In Two Letters to a
        Friend*. Edited by W.A. Muhlenberg. New York: T. Whittaker,
        1867. Reprinted *The Letters on Protestant Sisterhoods*.
        New York: R. Craighead, 1956.

4441. Barton, George. *Angels of the Battlefield: A History of the
        Labors of the Catholic Sisterhoods in the Late Civil War*.
        Philadelphia: Catholic Art Publishing Co., 1897.

4442. Borczon, Robert S. "In Depth Organization Chart of the Fran-
        ciscan Sisters of the Poor (US)." *Hosp Prog*, 46 (Nov 1965),
        86-91.

4443. Brooks, M.M. "Contributions of Methodist Hospitals to Nursing
        During the Last 40 Years." *Tr Nurs*, 80 (Jun 1928), 709-711.

4444. Bunford, A.M. *Ninety (90) Years a Mission, 1857-1947*. The
        Ranyard Mission (India), 1947.

4445. Callahan, Barbara. "The Doctors Mayo and the Sisters."
        Hosp Prog, 46 (Jul 1965), 65-74.

4446. Campbell, G.A. *The Knights Templars, Their Rise and Fall*.
        London: Duckworth, 1937.

4447. *The Catholic Encyclopedia*. New York: Robert Appleton, 1908-
        1914. Lists various orders; updated in the *New Catholic
        Encyclopedia*. See No. 4483.

4448. Celano, Thomas de. *Vite Prima and Vita Secundo*. 2 vols.
        Florence: College of S. Bonaventura, 1926-1927. Life of
        St. Francis.

4449. "Centennial Commemoration of the Sisters of Misericorde of
        Montreal." *Hosp Prog*, 28 (1947), 391-392.

4450. *Conferences de S. Paul aux Filles de la Charité*. Paris,
        1881.

4451. Daly, C.B. "Nursing--A Christian Profession." *IR Nurs News*
        (Winter 1972), 19-22.

4452.   Daughters of Charity of St. Vincent de Paul, Los Angeles.
        *One Hundred (100) Years of Service--The Daughters of Charity
        of St. Vincent de Paul 1856-1956*. Los Angeles: Daughters
        of Charity, 1956.

4453.   Delatte, Paul. *The Rule of Saint Benedict*. Translated by
        Dom Justin McCann. Latrobe, PA: The Archabbey Press, 1950.

4454.   Doyle, Ann. *Nursing by Religious Orders in the U.S. (1809-
        1928)*. Reprinted from *Am J Nurs*, 9 (Jul 1929), 775-786;
        (Aug 1929), 959-969; (Sep 1929), 1085-1095; (Oct 1929),
        1197-1207; (Nov 1929), 1331-1343; (Dec 1929), 1466-1484.

4455.   Dwyer, J.D. "Nuns in the Canal Zone." *Hosp Prog*, 45 (Nov
        1964), 44-48.

4456.   Elizabeth Clare, Sister. "The Sisters of Providence in the
        Northwest: An Historical Survey." *Alaska Med*, 4 (1962),
        60-61.

4457.   Emanuel, Cyprian W. *The Charities of St. Vincent de Paul*.
        Ph.D. dissertation, Catholic University of America, 1923.

4458.   Fedden, Marguerite. *Sisters' Quarters, Salonika*. London:
        Grant Richards, 1921.

4459.   Fitzgerald, Sister Mary Isabel. *The Philosophy of St. Thomas
        of Aquinas in Relation to the Spiritual Aspects of Nursing*.
        M.S. thesis, Catholic University of America, 1938.

4460.   Fowler, Franklin T. "The History of Southern Baptist Medical
        Missions." *Baptist Hist & Heritage*, 10(4) (1975), 194-203.

4461.   Fritschel, H.L. "History, Contribution of Lutheran Deacon-
        esses to Nursing During Last 40 Years." *Tr Nurs*, 80
        (Jun 1928), 714.

4462.   "Future of Nursing." *Christian Nurs*, 230 (Jun 1970), 16ff.

4463.   Gallison, Marie. *The Ministry of Women: 100 Years of Women's
        Work at Kaiserwerth 1836-1936*. London: Lutterworth Press,
        1936.

4464.   Gately, Sister M.J. *The Sisters of Mercy*. New York: The
        Macmillan Co., 1931.

4465.   Gillgannon, Mary McAuley. *The Sisters of Mercy as Crimean
        War Nurses*. Ph.D. dissertation, University of Notre Dame,
        1962.

4466.   Goldes, Christian. *History of the Deaconess Movement in the
        Christian Church*. Cincinnati: Jennings & Pye, 1903.

4467.   Gooch, Robert. "Protestant Sisters of Charity." *Blackwood's
        Edinburgh Mag* (Nov 1825), 732-735; see also *The London Med
        Gaz*, 1 (1827), 55-58.

4468.   Goodall, Francis P. "The Society of Catholic Medical Mission-
        aries of Philadelphia: Twenty-Five Years of Pioneering."
        Rec Am Cath His Soc Phila, 61 (1950), 237-247.

4469.   Gowan, Sister M. Olivia, and Sister M. Maurice Sheehy.
        "Contribution of Religious Communities to Nursing Educa-
        tion." *Tr Nurs & Hosp Rev*, 100 (1938), 404-409, 652-655,
        700.

4470.   *History of Nursing and Society.* Compiled by a Sister of
        Charity of Emmitsburg, Maryland. Bridgeport, CT: 1929.

4471.   Holloway, S.W. "The All Saints Sisterhood at University
        College Hospital, 1862-1899." *Med Hist* (Apr 1959), 146-
        156.

4472.   Howson, J.S. *Deaconesses or the Official Help of Women in
        Parochial Work and in Charitable Institutions.* An essay
        reprinted with large additions from *Q Rev* (Sep 1860).
        London: Longmans Green and Roberts, 1862.

4473.   Jameson, A.B. *Sisters of Charity, Catholic and Protestant,
        Abroad and at Home.* London: Longmans, 1855; Boston: Ticknor
        and Fields, 1858.

4474.   Keeler, Floyd. *Catholic Medical Missions.* New York: Mac-
        millan Co., 1925.

4475.   Keller, H. "75th Anniversary of the Deaconate and Nursing
        Station, Zurich." *Z Krankenpflege*, 67(10) (Oct 1974), 385.
        (Ger)

4476.   Khan, P. "Origin of Nursing and Christian Ideals." *Nurs J
        India*, 63 (Feb 1972), 48.

4477.   King, E.J. "The Grand Priory of the Order of the Hospital
        of St. John of Jerusalem." *England: A Short History.*
        London: Fleetway Press, 1924.

4478.   *Leaves from the Annals of the Sisters of Mercy.* 1: 3 vols.
        New York: Catholic Public Society, 1881-1893. Vol. 1:
        Ireland; Vol. 2: England, The Crimea, Scotland, Australia
        and New Zealand; Vol. 3: America.

4479.   Mazzeo, M. "Medical Aid Inspired by Christianity: Beginning
        of Participation of Laymen in Medical Aid Activities."
        Ann San Pubb Roma, 17(6) (Nov-Dec 1956), 1143-1178. (Ital)

4480.   Monteith, Mary Coby. "Seventh-Day Adventist Schools of
        Nursing." *Am J Nurs*, 51 (Feb 1951), 113-115.

4481.   Murphy, Denis G. *They Did Not Pass By. The Story of the
        Early Pioneers of Nursing.* London: Longmans Green & Co.,
        1956.

4482.   Nelson, S. "The Influence of Christianity on the Care of the
        Sick Up to the End of the Middle Ages." *So Afr Nurs J*, 40
        (Aug 1973), 18-19.

4483.   *New Catholic Encyclopedia*. Washington, D.C.: Catholic Uni-
        versity, 1967. An update on nursing orders. See also
        No. 4447.

4484.   Noall, Claire. "Mormon Midwives." *Utah Hist Q*, 10 (1942),
        84-144.

4485.   "Nurses' Settlement in Richmond." *Charities & Commons*, 16
        (7 Apr 1906), 47.

4486.   Pauline, Sister, Sister Christiana, and Alphonse Schwitalla.
        "The Sisters of the Poor of St. Francis, 1845-1945." *Hosp
        Prog*, 27 (1946), 51-58.

4487.   Potter, H.G. *Sisterhoods and Deaconesses at Home and Abroad*.
        New York: E.P. Dutton, 1873.

4488.   *Practical Thoughts on Sisterhoods*. New York: T. Whittaker,
        1864.

4489.   Robinson, J.M. *Deaconesses in Europe and Their Lessons for
        America*. New York: Hunt and Eaton, 1889.

4490.   *St. Clare and Her Order: A Story of Seven Centuries*. Edited
        by the author of *"The Enclosed Nun."* London: Mill and Boon,
        1912.

4491.   Schermerhorn, Elizabeth Wheeler. *On the Trail of the Eight-
        Pointed Cross. A Study of the Heritage of the Knights
        Hospitallers in Feudal Europe*. New York: G.P. Putnam's
        Sons, 1940.

4492.   Schwitalla, A.M., and M.R. Kneifi. "Catholic Schools of
        Nursing in U.S. and Canada at Beginning of 1934." Prepared
        under Auspices of Council on Nursing Education, Catholic
        Hospital Association of U.S. and Canada. *Hosp Prog*, 15
        (Apr 1934), 147-210; 16 (Jan 1935), 1-51; 17 (Feb 1936), 1;
        see also *QCIM*, 918.

4493.   Sherman, R.B. "The Sign of the Cross in Nursing Insignia."
        Alum Mag (Baltimore), 71 (Jul 1972), 5.

4494.   Sherwood, G.H. "Sister of Charity, Pioneer." *Catholic World*,
        133 (Aug 1931), 585-593.

4495.   "Sisters in the History of Nursing." *America*, 92 (6 Nov
        1954), 144.

4496.   Skardon, Alvin W. *Church Leader in the Cities: William
        August Muhlenberg*. Philadelphia: University of Pennsylvania
        Press, 1971.

4497.   Smith, Lena Mae. "Deaconess." *Mennonite Encyclopedia*.
         4 vols. Scottsdale, PA: Mennonite Publishing House, 1955-
         1959. Vol. 2, pp. 22-25.

4498.   Stanley, Mary. *Hospitals and Sisterhoods*. London: Murray,
         1854.

4499.   *Two Letters on Protestant Sisterhoods*. 3rd ed. New York:
         R. Craighead, 1856.

4500.   Thoburn, J.M. *The Deaconesses and Their Vocation*. New York:
         Hunt and Eaton, 1893.

4501.   Walsh, James J. *These Splendid Sisters*. New York: J.H.
         Sears, 1927.

4502.   Walton, Harold, and Kathryn Jensen Nelson. *Historical
         Sketches of the Medical Work of Seventh Day Adventists*.
         Washington, D.C.: Review and Herald Publishing Co., 1948.

4503.   Wheeler, Henry. *Deaconesses: Ancient and Modern*. New York:
         Hunt and Eaton, 1889.

4504.   "With the Migrants in California, Missionary Nurses."
         Mission Rev, 62 (Jul 1939), 371-372.

15. RED CROSS, WHO, AND
INTERNATIONAL NURSING

4505.   Ackerson, Jeanie L. "Progress Means Change." *Nurs World*,
133 (Mar 1959), 10-13.

4506.   Alperin, Shirley Hope. "Nursing Assignment: The United
Nations." *Nurs World*, 132 (Sep 1958), 12.

4507.   Bakewell, Charles M. *The Story of the American Red Cross in
Italy*. New York: Macmillan Co., 1920.

4508.   Barton, C. *The Red Cross in Peace and War*. Meriden, CT:
J. Publishing Co., 1912.

4509.   Barton, Clara H. *The Story of the Red Cross*. New York:
Appleton-Century-Crofts, 1904.

4510.   Best, S.H. *The Story of the British Red Cross*. London:
Cassell, 1938.

4511.   Bicknell, E.P. *Pioneering with the Red Cross*. New York:
Macmillan Co., 1935.

4512.   Billington, M.F. *The Red Cross in War: Woman's Part in the
Relief of Suffering*. London: Hodder & Stoughton, 1914.

4513.   Boardman, Mabel T. "Rural Nursing Service of the Red Cross."
Am J Nurs, 13 (Sep 1913), 937-939.

4514.   ————. *Under the Red Cross Flag at Home and Abroad*.
Philadelphia: J.B. Lippincott, 1915. 2nd ed., 1917.

4515.   British Red Cross Society. *The Proudest Badge: The Story of
the Red Cross*. 5th ed. London: British Red Cross Society,
1966.

4516.   British Red Cross Society and the Order of St. John of
Jerusalem. *Red Cross and St. John: The Official Record of
the Humanitarian Services of the War Organization of the
British Red Cross Society and Order of St. John of Jerusa-
lem, 1939-1947*. Compiled by P.G. Cambray and G.G.B. Briggs.
London: British Red Cross Society, 1949.

4517.   Clement, Fannie F. "American Red Cross and Nursing."
Survey, 29 (18 Jan 1913), 517-518.

4518.   ———. "Prospective Red Cross Rural Nursing in the Rocky
         Mountains." *Am J Nurs*, 13 (Jul 1913), 768-771.

4519.   Cole, A.M.F. "French Red Cross Nurses." *Cath World*, 87
         (Jul 1908), 522-530.

4520.   Creelman, Lyle, Agnes Chagas, and Virginia Arnold. *The First
         Ten Years of WHO*. Geneva: WHO, 1958.

4521.   ———. "WHO and Professional Nursing." *Am J Nurs*, 54
         (Apr 1954), 448-449.

4522.   Dardenne, Mme. "The Red Cross in the Congo." *Rev Info Bull
         Leag Red Cr Soc*, 12 (Jul 1931), 235-239.

4523.   Davidson, Henry P. *The American Red Cross in the Great War,
         1917-1919*. New York: Russell Sage Foundation, 1943.

4524.   DeMarsh, K.G. "Red Cross Outpost Nursing in New Brunswick."
         Canad Nurs, 69 (Jun 1973), 24-27.

4525.   Dock, Lavinia, Sarah Pickett, and Clara Noyes. *History of
         American Red Cross Nursing*. New York: The Macmillan Co.,
         1922.

4526.   Dulles, Foster Rhea. *The American Red Cross: A History*. New
         York: Harper and Brothers, 1950.

4527.   Dunant, Henri. *A Memory of Solferino*. Washington, D.C.:
         American National Red Cross, 1939. Original edition, *Un
         Souvenir de Solferino* was published in 1859. Many editions
         and translations were made.

4528.   Number deleted.

4529.   Elliman, Virginia B. "American Red Cross Nursing Services--
         50th Anniversary." *Nurs Out*, 7(3) (Mar 1959), 148-151.

4530.   Fox, Elizabeth G. "Red Cross Public Health Nursing After the
         War." *History of American Red Cross Nursing*. New York:
         Macmillan Co., 1922. pp. 1293-1351.

4531.   Gumpert, Martin. *Dunant: The Story of the Red Cross*. New
         York: Oxford University Press, 1938.

4532.   Hentsch, Yvonne. "Influence of the Red Cross on Professional
         Nursing." *Information Bulletin for Red Cross Nurses*.
         Geneva, May-Aug 1947.

4533.   International Red Cross. *The Ceaseless Challenge: Souvenir
         of the Red Cross Centenary 1863-1963*. Interspan Press
         Service, Ltd., 1963.

4534.   Kernodle, Portia B. *The Red Cross Nurse in Action, 1882-1948*.
         New York: Harper and Brothers, 1949.

4535.   Korson, George. *At His Side: The Story of the American Red Cross Overseas in World War II*. New York: Coward-McCann, 1945.

4536.   League of Red Cross Societies. *Collected Papers Relating to the League 1863-1963*. Geneva: The League, 1963.

4537.   ⸻. *Important Dates in the History of the League of Red Cross Societies*. Geneva: The League, 1963.

4538.   ⸻. *Red Cross Nursing Around the World*. Geneva: The League, 1963.

4539.   ⸻. *Red Cross Nursing: Report Presented to the XIV International Red Cross Conference, The Hague*. Paris: The League, 1928.

4540.   Lippman, Helen Byrne. "The Future of the Red Cross Volunteer Nurses Aide Corps." *Am J Nurs*, 45 (Oct 1945), 811-812.

4541.   Noyes, C.D. "Red Cross Nurse in the West Indies." *Bull Pan Am Union*, 53 (Nov 1921), 440-448.

4542.   Oliver, Beryl. *The British Red Cross in Action*. London: Faber and Faber, 1966.

4543.   Paul, E.H. "Nursing Program of the Indian Red Cross Society." *Int J Nurs Studies*, 4 (1967), 56-62.

4544.   Pearson, Elizabeth. "British Red Cross Nursing Service--At Home and Abroad." *Nurs Times* (29 Apr 1955), 456-463.

4545.   Pickett, S.E. *The American National Red Cross--Its Origin, Purposes, and Service*. New York: Century, 1923.

4546.   "Red Cross Nurses: A Viable Force in California Since 1907." *Calif Nurs*, 72(2) (Jun 1976), 12-13.

4547.   Rundle, Henry. *With the Red Cross in the Franco-German War A.D. 1870-1871: Some Reminiscences*. London: Laurie, 1911.

4548.   Schmidt-Meinecke, S. "One Hundred (100) Years of Red Cross Nursing Society in Hamburg." *Deutsch Schwester*, 22 (Dec 1969), 657-658.   (Ger)

4549.   Skimming, Sylvai. *Sand in My Shoes: The Tale of a Red Cross Welfare Officer with the British Hospitals Overseas in the Second World War*. Edinburgh: Oliver and Boyd, 1945.

4550.   Weigand, E. "Nurses of the German Red Cross." *Am J Nurs*, 49 (1949), 218-219.

16. ECONOMICS OF NURSING
(WORKING CONDITIONS, NUMBER OF NURSES, COLLECTIVE BARGAINING, HEALTH CARE DELIVERY, HEALTH MANPOWER)

4551. American Medical Association. *Voluntary Prepayment Medical Benefit Plans*. Chicago: American Medical Association, 1953.

4552. Ball, Frank W. "My Industrial Hospitalization." *Nurs World*, 129 (Jun 1955), 22-24.

4553. Corning, Peter A. *Social Security Programs Throughout the World*. Washington, D.C.: U.S. Government Printing Office, 1967.

4554. Dickenson, M. "Industrial Relations in the Queensland Nursing Service. The Anatomy of an Attitude." *Aust Nurs J*, 5(1) (Jul 1975), 23-27.

4555. Dickerson, O.D. *Health Insurance*. Homewood, IL: Richard D. Irwin, Inc., 1959.

4556. Downey, Gregg W. "Healthcare Planning Gets Muscles." *Mod Hlth Care*, 3 (Mar 1975), 32-37.

4557. Dublin, Louis I. *Health Work Pays*. New York: Metropolitan Life Insurance Co., 1925. 11 pp.

4558. Dublin, Louis I., and Alfred J. Lotka. *Twenty-Five Years of Health Progress*. New York: Metropolitan Life Insurance Co., 1937.

4559. Dykstra, A.J. "The First 5 Years. Development of an Economic Security Program." *Int Nurs Rev*, 12 (Apr 1965), 46-55.

4560. *The Economic Status of Registered Professional Nurses, 1946-1947*. Bulletin 931, Department of Labor, Bureau of Labor Statistics. Washington, D.C.: U.S. Government Printing Office, 1947.

4561. "Editorial Comment." *Pac Cst J Nurs*, 9 (Jun 1913), 243.

4562. "The Eight-Hour Day for Nurses." *Tr Nurs & Hosp Rev*, 53 (1914), 37.

4563.   "Employment Conditions for Registered Nurses" (editorial).
         Am J Nurs, 46 (Jul 1946), 437–438.

4564.   Ewing, O.R. *The Nation's Health: A Report to the President*.
         Washington, D.C.: U.S. Government Printing Office, 1948.

4565.   Falk, I.S., C.R. Korem, and M.D. Ring. *Costs of Medical
         Care*. Chicago: The University of Chicago Press, 1933.

4566.   ———. *Security Against Sickness: A Study of Health Insur-
         ance*. New York: Doubleday, 1936.

4567.   Fein, Rashi. *The Doctor Shortage: An Economic Analysis.
         (Studies in Social Economics)*. Washington, D.C.: The
         Brookings Institution, 1967.

4568.   Fishbein, Morris. "The Committee on the Costs of Medical
         Care." *J Am Med Assoc*, 99 (1932), 1950.

4569.   Field, Mark G. *Soviet Socialized Medicine: An Introduction*.
         New York: Free Press, 1967.

4570.   Fox, Elizabeth G. "The Economics of Nursing." *Am J Nurs*, 29
         (Sep 1929), 1037–1044.

4571.   Geister, Janet M. "Nurses Out of Work." *Survey*, 65 (15 Dec
         1930), 320–321.

4572.   Health Policy Advisory Committee. *The American Health
         Empire: Power, Profits and Politics*. New York: Random
         House, 1970.

4573.   Holly, H. "Wanted: A Day's Work for a Day's Pay." *Nev Nurs
         Assoc Newslett* (Winter 1967), 1 *passim*.

4574.   Jacox, Ada. "Collective Action and Control of Practice by
         Professionals." *Nurs Forum*, 10(3) (1971), 239–257.

4575.   Jammé, Anne C. "The California Eight-Hour Law for Women."
         Am J Nurs, 19 (1919), 525–530.

4576.   Kleingartner, Archie. "Nurses, Collective Bargaining and
         Labor Legislation." *Labor Law J*, 18 (Apr 1967), 236–245.

4577.   Kramer, Marlene. *Reality Shock: Why Nurses Leave Nursing*.
         St. Louis: C.V. Mosby Co., 1974.

4578.   "L.V.N. Group Asks More Pay, Rescinds No Strike Policy."
         Hosp, 43 (16 Nov 1969), 107.

4579.   McCormick, Virginia. "Are There Too Many Nurses?" *Survey*,
         64 (15 Jul 1930), 349–350.

4580.   Marshall, E.D., and E.B. Moses. *RNs 1966: An Inventory of
         Registered Nurses*. New York: American Nurses' Association,
         1969.

4581.   *Medical Care for the American People: The Final Report of the
        Committee on the Costs of Medical Care.* Chicago: Univer-
        sity of Chicago Press, 1932.

4582.   Miller, Anna J. "Salaries in 1935." *Pub Hlth Nurs* (Jun
        1935), 344-346.

4583.   Miller, Jon D., and Stephen M. Shortell. "Hospital Unioni-
        zation: A Study of Trends." *Hosp*, 43 (16 Aug 1969), 67-72.

4584.   Mittman, Ben, and Beatrice Bumgarner. "What Happened in San
        Francisco." *Am J Nurs*, 67 (Jan 1967), 80-84.

4585.   "The National Survey." *Am J Nurs*, 41 (Aug 1941), 929-930.

4586.   *The NRA and Nursing.* New York: American Nurses' Association,
        1933.

4587.   "Nurses and Labor Laws." *Tr Nurs & Hosp Rev*, 52 (1914), 37.

4588.   "Nurse Membership in Unions" (editorial). *Am J Nurs*, 37
        (Jul 1937), 766-767.

4589.   Nuttal, Peggy D. "The British National Health Service."
        Nurs Out, 25 (Feb 1977), 98-102.

4590.   "The Open Forum, The WPA and Nursing." *Am J Nurs*, 38 (Jun
        1938), 733-735.

4591.   Parkhurst, Genevieve. "Wanted--100,000 Girls for Sub-Nurses."
        Pict Rev (Oct 1921), 15, 82.

4592.   ————. "White Cap Famine." *Pict Rev* (Sep 1921), 2, 72-75.

4593.   "Personnel Shortage Closes Thousands of Hospital Beds."
        Southern Hosp, 15 (1947), 44.

4594.   Peters, Dorothy. "The Kewanee Story." *Am J Nurs*, 61 (Oct
        1961), 74-79.

4595.   Petry, L., M. Arnstein, and R. Gillan. "Surveys Measure
        Nursing Resources." *Am J Nurs*, 49 (Dec 1949), 770-772.

4596.   Phillips, Donald F. "Health Planning: New Hope for a Fresh
        Start." *Hosp J Am Hosp Assoc*, 49 (16 Mar 1975), 35-38.

4597.   Reid, Leslie D. "The Trouble with Nursing: No Nurses."
        Mod Hosp, 88 (Jan 1957), 58-60.

4597.1 Reverby, Susan, and David Rosner. *Health Care in America:
        Essays in Social History.* Philadelphia: Temple Univer-
        sity Press, 1979.

4598.   Rogers, Pamela J. "Pay-as-you-eat. A Transition in the
        System of Material Rewards in the Nursing Profession of the
        United Kingdom." *Nurs Times*, 65 (20 Nov 1969), 193ff.

4599.   Rose, Marie L. "What About Our Own Catastrophe." *Am J Nurs*,
        32 (Jan 1932), 62-63.

4600.   Roth, Aleda V., and Alice R. Walden. *The Nation's Nurses: A
        1972 Inventory of Registered Nurses*. Kansas City, MO:
        American Nurses' Association, 1974.

4601.   Schutt, Barbara G. "The Right to Strike." *Am J Nurs*, 68
        (Jul 1968), 1455.

4602.   Schwitalla, Alphonse M. "The Present Economic Objectives of
        the Nursing Profession." *Am J Nurs*, 33 (Dec 1933), 1135-
        1142.

4603.   Scott, William C. "Shall Professional Nurses' Associations
        Become Collective Bargaining Agents for Their Members?"
        Am J Nurs, 44 (Mar 1944), 231-232.

4604.   Scott, William C., and Donald W. Smith. "Taft-Hartley Act
        and the Nurse." *Am J Nurs*, 56 (Dec 1956), 1556.

4605.   Sinai, Nathan, Odin W. Anderson, and Melvin L. Dollar.
        Health Insurance in the United States. New York: The
        Commonwealth Fund, 1946.

4606.   *The Size and Shape of the Medical Care Dollar*. U.S. Depart-
        ment of Health, Education and Welfare, Social Security
        Administration. Washington, D.C.: U.S. Government Print-
        ing Office, 1970.

4607.   Sleeper, Ruth. "Stretching the Nurse." *Hosp*, 28 (Mar 1954),
        80-81, 184-186.

4608.   Smith, Donald W. "The Wagner-Murrary-Dingell Bill, Senate
        Bill 1050, H.R. 3293." *Am J Nurs*, 45 (Nov 1945), 933-936.

4609.   "Social Security Official Estimates National Nurse Shortage
        at 40,000." *Mod Hosp*, 72 (1949), 146.

4610.   Somers, Herman Miles, and Anne Ransay Somers. *Doctors,
        Patients and Health Insurance*. Washington, D.C.: The
        Brookings Institution, 1961.

4611.   Taft, W.H. "Wanted 30,000 Nurses." *Ladies Home J*, 35 (May
        1918), 22.

4612.   Titus, Shirley. "Economic Facts of Life for Nurses." *Am J
        Nurs*, 52 (Sep 1952), 1109-1112.

4613.   U.S. Bureau of Labor Statistics. *The Economic Status of
        Registered Professional Nursing*. Washington, D.C.: U.S.
        Government Printing Office, 1947.

4614.   U.S. Department of Health, Education, and Welfare: Division
        of Nursing. *Health Manpower Source Book; 2. Nursing*

          Personnel. Public Health Publication No. 263, Section 2
          revised. Washington, D.C.: U.S. Government Printing
          Office, 1969.

4615.   U.S. Public Health Service. *Toward Quality in Nursing:*
          Needs and Goals. Report of the Surgeon General's Consul-
          tant Group on Nursing. Washington, D.C.: U.S. Government
          Printing Office, 1963.

4616.   Vonderheid, A.E. "The Grand Nursing Revolution of 1966 from
          My Historical Perspective." *Calif Nurs*, 72(2) (Jun 1976),
          35.

4617.   Williamson, A.A. "California and the Eight-Hour Law."
          Tr Nurs & Hosp Rev, 53 (1914), 257.

4618.   Wolfe, Samuel, ed. *Organization of Health Workers and Labor*
          Conflict. Farmingdale, NY: Baywood, 1978. 155 pp.

4619.   Woodward, Ella S. "Federal Aspects of Unemployment Among
          Professional Women." *Am J Nurs*, 34 (Jun 1934), 534-538.

4620.   ————. "The WPA and Nursing." *Am J Nurs*, 37 (Sep 1937),
          994-997.

4621.   Yett, D.E. *An Economic Analysis of the Nurse Shortage.*
          Lexington, MA: D.C. Heath, 1975.

4622.   Zimmerman, Anne. "The ANA Economic Security Program in
          Retrospect." *Nurs Forum*, 10(3) (1971), 312-321.

4623.   ————. "Taft-Hartley Amended; Implications for Nursing:
          The Industrial Model." *Am J Nurs*, 75 (Feb 1975), 284-288.

17. SOCIOLOGY

MEN IN NURSING

4624.   Aldag, Jean C. "Male Nurse Interest and Personality Charac-
        teristics." Ph.D. dissertation, Washington University,
        1970.

4625.   Boorer, David J. "Men Nurses in Britain." *Nurs Out*, 16
        (Nov 1968), 24-26.

4626.   Bush, Patricia J. "The Male Nurse: A Challenge to Tradi-
        tional Role Identities." *Nurs Forum*, 15 (1976), 390-405.

4627.   Craig, L.N. "Opportunities for Men Nurses." *Am J Nurs*, 40
        (Jun 1940), 666-670.

4628.   Crummer, Kenneth T. "Men Nurses—A Survey of the Present
        Day Situation of Graduate Men Nurses." *Am J Nurs*, 28
        (May 1928), 467-469.

4629.   "Have Times Changed? The *Nursing Mirror* June 15, 1907. Male
        Nurses and Nursing." *Nurs Mirror*, 141(10) (4 Sep 1975), 75.

4630.   "Men as Nurses." *America*, 94 (22 Oct 1955), 89.

4631.   Nash, Herbert J. "Men Nurses in New York State." *Tr Nurs &
        Hosp Rev* (Aug 1936), 123.

4632.   O'Hanlon, George. "Men Nurses in General Hospitals." *Am J
        Nurs*, 34 (Jan 1934), 16-19.

4633.   Russell, William L. "Men Nurses in Psychiatric Hospitals."
        Am J Nurs, 34 (Jan 1934), 19-24.

4634.   Schoenmaker, Adrian. "Nursing's Dilemma: Male Versus Female
        Admissions Choice." *Nursing Forum*, 4 (1976), 406-412.

4635.   Schoenmaker, Adrian, and David M. Radosevich. "Men Nursing
        Students: How They Perceive Their Situation." *Nurs Out*,
        24(5) (May 1976), 298-301.

4636.   Stout, P.S. "A Plea for Male Nurses." *New York Med J*, 103
        (1916), 1225.

4637.   Tuttle, G.T. "The Male Nurse." *Am J Insanity*, 63 (1906),
        192.

4638. Whitte, Frances W. "Opportunities in Graduate Education for
       Men Nurses." *Am J Nurs*, 34 (Feb 1934), 133-135.

                        MINORITIES IN NURSING

4639. Blackburn, Laura. "Meeting Local Hospital Needs." *Tr Nurs*,
       98 (Feb 1937), 176-178.

4640. Branch, Marie Foster, and Phyllis Perry Paxton. *Providing
       Safe Care for Ethnic Peoples of Color*. New York: Appleton-
       Century-Crofts, 1976.

4641. Bullough, Bonnie, and Vern Bullough. *Poverty, Ethnic Iden-
       tity and Health Care*. New York: Appleton-Century-Crofts,
       1972.

4642. Bureau of Health Resources Development. *Minorities and
       Women in Health Fields: Applicants, Students, and Workers*.
       DHEW Publication No. HRS 75-22, Washington, D.C.: U.S.
       Government Printing Office, 1974.

4643. Carnegie, Mary Elizabeth. "Are Negro Schools of Nursing
       Needed Today?" *Nurs Out*, 12 (Feb 1964), 52-56.

4644. ————. "The Impact of Integration on the Nursing Profes-
       sion: An Historical Sketch." *Negro Hist Bull*, 28(7)
       (1965), 154-155, 168.

4645. Cogan, L. *Negroes for Medicine: Report of a Macy Conference*.
       Baltimore: Johns Hopkins Press, 1968.

4646. Downing, L.C. "Early Negro Hospitals, With Special Refer-
       ence to Nurses' Training Schools." *J Nat Med Assoc*, 33
       (1941), 13-18.

4647. Elmore, Joyce Ann. "Black Nurses: Their Service and Their
       Struggle." *Am J Nurs*, 76 (Mar 1976), 435-437.

4648. Franklin, Rabbi Leo. "Orthodox Jewish Customs in Their
       Relation to the Nursing Profession." *Am J Nurs*, (Oct 1913),
       11-18.

4649. Gage, Nina D., and Alma C. Haupt. "Some Observations on
       Negro Nursing in the South." *Pub Hlth Nurs*, 24 (Dec 1932),
       674-680.

4650. Gunter, Laurie M. "The Effects of Segregation on Nursing
       Students." *Nurs Out*, 9 (Feb 1961), 74-76.

4651. Haupt, Alma C. "A Pioneer in Negro Nursing." *Am J Nurs*, 35
       (Sep 1935), 857-859.

4652. McMurdy, Robert. "Negro Women as Trained Nurses, Experiment of a Chicago Hospital." *Survey*, 31 (8 Nov 1913), 159-160.

4653. Miller, Helen Sullivan. *The History of Chi Eta Phi Sorority Inc., 1932-1967*. Washington, D.C.: Association for the Study of Negro Life and History, 1968.

4654. Morais, H.M. *History of the Negro in Medicine*. New York: Publishers Co., 1968.

4655. National Association of Colored Graduate Nurses, The. *Four Decades of Service*. New York: The National Association of Colored Graduate Nurses, Inc., 1945.

4656. "Paradox (Only 308 Negro Nurses in the Army and Not One in the Navy)." *Survey*, 81 (Feb 1945), 50-51.

4657. Staupers, Mabel K. *No Time for Prejudice: A Story of the Integration of Negroes in Nursing in the United States*. New York: Macmillan Co., 1961.

4658. ————. "Story of the National Association of Colored Graduate Nurses." *Am J Nurs*, 51, 222-223.

4659. Taylor, Susie King. *Reminiscences of My Life in Camp*. New York: Arno Press, 1968.

4660. ————. "Teenage Civil War Nurse: Susie King Taylor." *Ebony*, 25 (Feb 1970), 96ff.

4661. Thoms, A.B., and C.E. Bullock. "Development of Facilities for Colored Nurse Education." *Tr Nurs & Hosp Rev*, 80 (1928), 722.

4662. Thoms, Adah M. *Pathfinders--A History of the Progress of Colored Graduate Nurses*. New York: Kay Printing House, 1929.

NURSING AND WOMEN

4663. "Again the Woman Question." *Nurs J Pac Cst*, 5 (Jan 1909), 3.

4664. Ashley, Jo Ann. *Hospitals, Paternalism, and the Role of the Nurse*. New York: Teacher's College Press, 1976.

4665. ————. "Nurses in American History: Nursing and Early Feminism." *Am J Nurs*, 75(9) (Sep 1975), 1465-1467.

4666. Austin, George Lowell. *Perils of American Women, or a Doctor's Talk with Maiden, Wife and Mother*. Boston: Lee and Shepard, 1883.

4667.   Austin, Margaret. "History of Women in Medicine: A Symposium.
         Early Period." *Bull Med Libr Assoc*, 44 (1956), 12-15.

4668.   Balfour, Margaret I. *The Work of Medical Women in India*.
         London: n.p., 1929.

4669.   Bass, E. "These Were the First. (Women Doctors)." *J Am Med
         Wom Assoc*, 9 (1954), 34-95.

4670.   Bauer, F. "The Woman's Historical Role in Russian Medicine.
         I." *Z Krankenpflege*, 11 (Feb 1967), 68-78; "II." 11 (Mar
         1967), 112-119; "III." 11 (Jun 1967), 255-263.   (Ger)

4671.-
4672.   Numbers deleted.

4673.   Blackwell, Elizabeth. *Pioneer Work in Opening the Medical
         Profession to Women: Autobiographical Sketches*. London and
         New York: Longmans, Green and Co., 1895.

4674.   Blake, John B. "Women and Medicine in Antebellum America."
         Bull Hist Med, 39 (1965), 99-123.

4675.   Boothe, Viba B., ed. *Women in the Modern World*. Philadel-
         phia: American Academy of Political and Social Science,
         1929.

4676.   Brand, K.L., et al. "Perils and Parallels of Women and
         Nursing." *Nurs Forum*, 14(2) (1975), 160-174.

4677.   Breckinridge, Sophonisba. *Women in the Twentieth Century*.
         New York: McGraw-Hill Book Co., 1933.

4678.   Bullough, Bonnie. "Barriers to the Nurse Practitioner Move-
         ment: Problems of Women in a Woman's Field." *Int J Hlth
         Serv*, 5(2) (1975), 225-233.

4679.   Bullough, Bonnie, and Vern Bullough. "Sex Segregation in
         Health Care." *Nurs Out*, 23 (Jan 1975), 40-45.

4680.   Bullough, Vern L., with a final chapter by Bonnie Bullough.
         The Subordinate Sex: A History of Attitudes Towards Women.
         Urbana, IL: University of Illinois Press, 1973; Baltimore:
         Penguin Books, 1974.

4681.   Bullough, Vern, and Martha Voght. "Women, Menstruation, and
         Nineteenth Century Medicine." *Bull Hist Med*, 47 (Jan-Feb
         1973), 66-82.

4682.   Burstyn, Joan N. "Education and Sex: The Medical Case Against
         Higher Education for Women in England, 1870-1900." *Pro-
         ceedings of the American Philosophical Society*, 117(2)
         (Apr 1973), 79-89.

4683.   Chavasse, Pye Henry. *Woman as a Wife and Mother*. Philadel-
         phia: W.B. Evans, 1870.

4684. Christy, Teresa. "Equal Rights for Women: Voices from the Past." *Am J Nurs*, 71 (1971), 288-293.

4685. ————. "The Fateful Decade 1890-1900." *Am J Nurs*, 75 (Jul 1975), 1163-1166.

4686. Cleland, Virginia. "Sex Discrimination: Nursing's Most Pervasive Problem." *Am J Nurs*, 71 (Aug 1971), 1542-1547.

4687. ————. "To End Sex Discrimination." *Nurs Clin No Am*, 9 (Sep 1974), 563-571.

4688. Cockram, E.J. "Tribute to Sabine (Women in Medicine in 16-17 Centuries)." *J Med Wom Fed*, 43 (1961), 86-96.

4689. Davidson, R. "Women and Nursing." *Nurs Sci*, 3 (1965), 327-337.

4690. Dexter, Elizabeth A. *Career Women of America: 1776-1840*. Francetown, NH: M. Jones, 1950.

4691. ————. *Colonial Women of Affairs: Women in Business and Professions in America Before 1776*. Boston: Houghton Mifflin, 1931.

4692. Dock, Lavinia L. "The Relation of the Nursing Profession to the Woman Movement." *Nurs J Pac Cst*, 5 (1909), 197-201.

4693. ————. "Some Urgent Social Claims." *Am J Nurs*, 7 (Jul 1907), 895-901.

4694. Dube, W.F. "Women Enrollment and Its Minority Component in U.S. Medical Schools: Datagram." *J Med Educ*, 51 (Aug 1976), 691-693.

4695. Ehrenreich, Barbara, and Deidre English. *Complaints and Disorders: The Sexual Politics of Sickness*. New York: The Feminist Press, 1973.

4696. Flexner, Eleanor. *Century of Struggle: The Woman's Rights Movement in the United States*. Cambridge, MA: Harvard University Press, 1959.

4697. Gordon, Linda. *Woman's Body, Woman's Right: A Social History of Birth Control in America*. New York: Grossman Publishers, 1976.

4698. Grissum, Marlene, and Carol Spengler. *Womanpower and Health Care*. Boston: Little, Brown & Co., 1976.

4699. Harland, Marion. *Eve's Daughters: Or Common Sense for Maid, Wife and Mothers*. New York: John R. Anderson and Henry S. Allen, 1882.

4700. Hole, Christina. *The English Housewife in the Seventeenth Century*. London: Chatto and Windus, 1953.

4701.   Hurd-Mead, Kate Campbell. *A History of Women in Medicine*.
         Haddam, CT: Haddam Press, 1938.

4702.   ———. *Medical Women of America*. New York: Froben Press,
         1933.

4703.   "Journal's Attitude on the Suffrage Question." *Am J Nurs*, 8
         (Sep 1908), 956-957.

4704.   Karmaukhova, E.I. "The Beginning of Medical Education for
         Women in Russia." *Sovetsk Zdravoohr*, 19(5) (1960), 37-41.
         (Rus)

4705.   Kaufman, Martin. "The Admission of Women to 19th Century
         American Medical Societies." *Bull Hist Med*, 50 (1976),
         251-260.

4706.   Kleinert, Margaret Noyes. "Medical Women in New England.
         History of the New England Women's Medical Society."
         J Am Med Wom Assoc, 11 (1956), 63-64, 67.

4707.   Lejeune, F. "History, Women Through the Ages as Healer and
         Physician's Aide." *Wien Klin Wchnschr*, 55 (1 May 1942),
         341-344. (Ger)

4708.   Lima, L.L. "Nursing's Contribution Toward Participation of
         Women in the 19th Century." *Rev Brasil Enferm*, 21 (Aug
         1968), 152-162. (Por)

4709.   Little, M. "Some Pioneer Medical Women of the University of
         Sydney." *Med J Aust*, 2 (1958), 341-350.

4710.   "Mobilizing Women as Nurses." *Lit Digest*, 57 (27 Apr 1918),
         33.

4711.   Molina, W.F. "History--Role of Women in Welfare and Social
         Service Work." *Rev Med Peruanoa*, 13 (Jul 1941), 420-432.
         (Spa)

4712.   Mosher, Clelia Duel. *Health and the Woman Movement*. 2nd rev.
         ed. New York: Woman Press, 1918.

4713.   North, Franklin H. "A New Profession for Women." *Cent Mag*
         (Jul 1882), 38-47.

4714.   Parker, W.W. "Woman's Place in the Christian World: Superior
         Morally, Inferior Mentally to Man; Not Qualified for Medi-
         cine or Law; The Contrariety and Harmony of the Sexes."
         Trans Med Soc Virginia, 23 (1892), 86.

4715.   Patrineli, H. "Address by the President of the Hellenic
         National Graduate Nurses' Association." *Hellen Adelphe*, 23
         (Jun 1968), 6. (Grk)

4716.   Paull, E.H.   "The Golden Jubilee of the Lady Hardinge Medical
        College and Hospital, New Delhi."   *Nurs J India*, 57 (1966),
        204-205.

4717.   Quist, G.   "Ladies Only--Until 1948 (Royal Free Hospital
        School of Medicine)."   *Med News* (10 Jan 1964), 7, 29.

4718.   "Reminiscences of the First Woman Student of Madras Medical
        College."   *Indian J Hist Med*, 2(1) (1957), 63-66.

4719.   Roberts, Joan T., and Thetis M. Group.   "The Woman's Movement
        and Nursing."   *Nurs Forum*, 12(3) (1973), 303-322.

4720.   Rosenberg, Charles E.   "Sexuality, Class and Role in Nine-
        teenth-Century America."   *Am Q*, 25 (May 1973), 131-154.

4721.   Sanger, Margaret.   *Motherhood in Bondage*.   New York:
        Brentano's, 1928.

4722.   ————.   *My Fight for Birth Control*.   London: Faber & Faber,
        1932.

4723.   Smith-Rosenberg, Carroll.   "The Hysterical Woman: Sex Roles
        and Role Conflict in Nineteenth-Century America."   *Soc Res*,
        39 (Winter 1972), 652-678.

4724.   Smith-Rosenberg, Carroll, and Charles Rosenberg.   "The Female
        Animal: Medical and Biological Views of Woman and Her Role
        in Nineteenth-Century America."   *J Am Hist*, 60 (Sep 1973),
        332-356.

4725.   Smuts, Robert W.   *Women and Work in America*.   New York:
        University Press, 1959.

4726.   Strachey, Ray.   *The Cause, A Short History of the Women's
        Movement in Great Britain*.   London: G. Bell & Sons, 1928.

4727.   Thomas, G. Morton.   "Removal of the Ovaries as a Cure for
        Insanity."   *Am J Insanity*, 49 (1892-1893), 397-401.

4728.   Walsh, Mary Roth.   *Doctors Wanted: No Women Need Apply*.   New
        Haven, CT: Yale University Press, 1977.

4729.   ————.   "Feminism: A Support System for Women Physicians."
        J Am Med Wom Assoc (Jun 1976).

4730.   Wilson, Victoria.   "An Analysis of Femininity in Nursing."
        American Behavioral Scientist, 15(2) (Nov 1971), 213-220.

4731.   *Woman's Work in the Field of Medicine*.   New York: The
        College of Midwifery, 1883.

4732.   Woody, T.   *A History of Women's Education in the United
        States*.   2 vols.   Lancaster, PA: Science Press, 1929.

NURSE-PHYSICIAN RELATIONSHIPS

4733.   Beard, Richard Olding. "Fair Play for the Trained Nurse."
         Pict Rev (Feb 1922), 28, 95-96.

4734.   Bishop, W.J. "Dr. Thomas Fuller's Ideal Nurse." *Nurs
         Mirror*, 99 (18 Jun 1954), 759.

4735.   Burosh, Phyllis. "Physician's Attitudes Toward Nurse-Mid-
         wives." *Nurs Out*, 23(7) (Jul 1975), 452-456.

4736.   Burstyn, Joan N. "Education and Sex: The Medical Case Against
         Higher Education for Women in England 1870-1900." *Proceed-
         ings Amer Philosophical Soc*, 117(2) (Apr 1973), 79-89.

4737.   Davison, W.C. "History--Nursing as Foundation of Medicine."
         North Carolina Med J, 4 (Apr 1943), 141-143.

4738.   Flores, Florence. "The Nurse: Handmaiden or Partner?"
         Boston Med Q, 8(2) (1957), 52-55.

4739.   Frisch, J. "Robert Gersung's Views on Qualifications of
         Nurses." *Wien Med Wehnschr*, 79 (27 Apr 1929), 583-586.
         (Ger)

4740.   Geyman, John P. "Is There a Difference Between Nursing Prac-
         tice and Medical Practice." *J Fam Prac*, 5 (Dec 1977), 935-
         936.

4741.   Goering, Paula P. "Nurse-Doctor Relationships in a Psychia-
         tric Setting." *Doc. Year: 1974*. Vol. No. 52, Abstract
         No. 01025. Toronto: Queen Street Mental Health Centre.

4742.   Mayo, Charles H. "Do You Covet Distinction." *Am J Nurs*, 22
         (Jan 1922), 251-252. Reprinted in *New Directions for
         Nurses*, edited by Bonnie and Vern Bullough. New York:
         Springer, 1971. pp. 87-94.

4743.   ———. "Wanted--100,000 Girls for Sub-Nurses: An Answer to
         the Nursing Problem." *Pict Rev* (Oct 1921), 15.

4744.   Noyes, Clara D. "Sub-Nurses? Why Not Sub-Doctors?" *Pict Rev*
         (Dec 1921), 28, 79-80.

4745.   Nuckolls, Katherine B. "Who Decides What the Nurse Can Do?"
         Nurs Out, 22 (Oct 1974), 626-631.

4746.   "Requirements of a Nurse, 1730 AD." *Canad Nurs*, 41 (Jan
         1945), 58.

4747.   St. Thomas' Hospital London. "The Doctors Versus the Nurses
         --Correspondence from the Archives." *Nurs Times* (15 Jun
         1962), 783-784.

4748. "The Sister Profession" (editorial). *Canad Med Assoc J*, 85 (1961), 90-91.

4749. Stein, Leonard. "The Doctor-Nurse Game." *Archives of Gen Psychia*, 16(6) (1967), 699-703. Reprinted in *Am J Nurs*, 68 (Jan 1968), 101-105; *New Directions for Nurses*, edited by Bonnie and Vern Bullough. New York: Springer, 1971. pp. 129-137.

4750. Thompson, William Gilman. "The Overtrained Nurse." *New York Med J*, 83 (1906), 845.

4751. Thomstad, Beatrice, Nicholas Cunningham, and Barbara H. Kaplan. "Changing the Rules of the Doctor-Nurse Game." *Nurs Out*, 23 (Jul 1975), 422-427.

4752. "The Trained Nurse and Her Position" (editorial). *J Am Med Assoc*, 37 (12 Oct 1901), 982.

4753. Tucker, William. "The Nurses' Role Through the Physician's Eyes. A Historical Review." *Virginia Med Monthly*, 101 (Jun 1974), 449-451.

4754. Wood, T. "The Practice of Medicine by Nurses: An Opinion." *Canad Med Assoc J*, 114 (1976), 947.

4755. Worcester, Alfred. "Is Nursing Really a Profession?" *Am J Nurs*, 2 (Aug 1902), 908-912.

4756. Wright, Dr. "A Doctor Looks at Nursing." *Canad Nurs*, 53 (Feb 1957), 104-109.

NURSING ORGANIZATIONS

4757. American Nurses Association. *Perspective on the Code for Nurses*. Kansas City, KS: American Nurses Association, 1978.

4758. Amundson, Norman E. "Will the Supervisor Issue Destroy the Nurses Association as a Professional Organization?" *J Nurs Admin* (Jul-Aug 1973), 6, 61.

4759. "The ANA and the Wagner-Murray-Dingell Bill, S1606." *Am J Nurs*, 46 (Jun 1946), 375-376.

4760. *ANA in Washington: A Brief History of the Federal Legislative Concerns of ANA During the Period of 1951-1971*. New York: American Nurses' Association, 1972.

4761. "ANA is Denied Place on JCAH Council for Long-Term Care." *Am J Nurs*, 77 (Jan 1977), 7-8.

Sociology

4762. Arnold, V. "ICN 75th Anniversary: The Past: Way to the Future." *Int Nurs Rev*, 21(3-4) (May-Aug 1970), 68-76.

4763. ————. "ICN 75th Anniversary: Years of Growth in International Service to Nursing." *Int Nurs Rev*, 21(3-4) (May-Aug 1974), 96-102, 104-106.

4764. Association of Queen's Nurses. "Nurses--Their Education and Role in Health Programs." *Queen's Nurs Mag*, 45 (Aug 1956), 119-122.

4765. "The Biennial." *Am J Nurs*, 34 (Jun 1934), 603-627; 38 (Jun 1938), 673-699; 46 (Nov 1946), 728-746. Reports of the meetings of the American Nurses' Association appear every even numbered year under various titles. These are listed here because of title. See the *Journal*.

4766. Bill, S.A. "A Glimpse into AAIN's Past." *Occup Hlth Nurs NY*, 23(12) (Dec 1975), 20-22.

4767. Blair, Mary Stewart. "Social Trends and Nursing Organization." *Am J Nurs*, 34 (Feb 1934), 141-148.

4768. Boysen, J.E. "From the Crimea to the Planets." *Am Assoc Industr Nurs J*, 15 (Jun 1967), 15-17.

4769. "Brazilian Nurses' Association." *Aust Nurs J*, 2 (Sep 1972), 9.

4770. Breay, Margaret, and Ethel Gordon Fenwick. *The History of the International Council of Nurses, 1899-1925*. Geneva: The International Council of Nurses, 1931.

4771. Bridges, Daisy C. "Events in the History of the International Council of Nurses." *Am J Nurs*, 49 (Sep 1949), 594-595.

4772. ————. *A History of the International Council of Nurses, 1899-1964*. Philadelphia: J.B. Lippincott, 1967.

4773. ————. *Outstanding Events in the History of the I.C.N.* Stockholm: International Council of Nurses, 1949.

4774. Bullough, Bonnie, and Vern Bullough. "The Problem of Goal Changes." *Nurs Forum*, 4 (1965), 79-92.

4775. Christy, T.E. "The First 50 Years of the American Nurses' Association." *Kango*, 24 (Feb 1972), 50-58. (Jap)

4776. Committee on the Structure of National Nursing Organizations. *New Horizons in Nursing*. New York: The Macmillan Co., 1950.

4777. Corcoran, Janet. "NSNA's First Six Years." *Am J Nurs*, 59 (1959), 695-698.

4778. Dock, L. "ICN: Report on Affiliation of National Councils, 1904." *Int Nurs Rev*, 21(3-4) (May-Aug 1974), 88.

4779. Fenwick, E.B. "President's Address: First ICN Congress 1901." *Int Nurs Rev*, 21(3-4) (May-Aug 1974), 91-93.

4780. Fitzpatrick, M.L. *The National Organization for Public Health Nursing 1912-1952: Development of a Practice Field.* New York: National League for Nursing, 1975; Ph.D. dissertation, Columbia University, 1972.

4781. Flanagan, Lydia. *One Strong Voice: The Story of the American Nurses' Association.* Kansas City, KS: The American Nurses' Association, 1976.

4782. Fleming, W.J. "Nursing; An Account of the Dresden Nursing Association, Albert Verein." *Glasgow M J*, vii(4) (1875), 220-227.

4783. Gardner, Mary S. "The National Organization for Public Health Nursing." *Visit Nurs Q*, 4 (1912), 13.

4784. Geister, Janet M. "Miss Geister Accepts A.N.A. Position" (editorial). *Am J Nurs*, 26 (Dec 1926), 954.

4785. "Give or Get $5 (History of American Nurses' Foundation, Inc.)." *Am J Nurs*, 60 (1960), 495.

4786. Goodnow, Minnie. "Beginning and Growth of Nursing Organizations." *Tr Nurs*, 80, 128-686, 788.

4787. *Handbook on the Structure of National Nursing Organizations.* New York: Committee on the Structure of National Nursing Organizations, 1949.

4788. "Historic Retrospective: Danish Nursing Council Founded in a Room in Kopenhagen." *Sygeplejersken*, 74 (Oct 1974), Supl., 4-8. (Dan)

4789. "History of Organized Nursing in New Zealand." *Tr Nurs & Hosp Rev*, 83 (Sep 1929), 359.

4790. "The ICN and Nursing Education." *Am J Nurs*, 50 (Jul 1950), 385-386.

4791. "ICN Presidents: Leaders Who Have Forged the Future." *Int Nurs Rev*, 21(3-4) (May-Aug 1974), 77-79.

4792. "ICN Statement of Nursing Education, Nursing Practice and Service and Social and Economic Welfare of Nurses." *Am J Nurs*, 69 (Oct 1969), 2177-2179.

4793. "The ICN's Eleventh Quadrennial Congress, May 23-June 1, 1957." *Nurs Out*, 5 (May 1957), 468-471.

4794.   "ILO/WHO Group Draws Up Instrument of Personnel Practices
        Recommended for Adoption for Nurses Worldwide." *Am J Nurs*,
        74 (Feb 1974), 189.

4795.   International Congress of Charities, Correction and Philan-
        throphy, Chicago, Illinois, 1893, 3rd Section. *Nursing of
        the Sick*, Isabel A. Hampton et al. Reprint. New York:
        McGraw-Hill Book Co., 1949.

4796.   Lugo, O.R. "Historic Sketch of the Benefits Obtained by the
        Association of Male and Female Nurses of Puerto Rico Since
        Its Beginning Until the Present Time." *P Rico Enferm*, 49
        (Mar 1974), 12-32. (Spa)

4797.   Martin, Leota. "National Organization for Public Health
        Nursing." *Pac Cst J Nurs*, 10 (Apr 1914), 149-153.

4798.   McIver, Pearl. "Some Findings of the N.O.P.H.N. Survey of
        Public Health Nursing of Significance to State Health
        Administrators." *Pub Hlth Rep*, 49 (1934), 1081.

4799.   Merrill, Bertha Estelle. *The Trek from Yesterday--A History
        of Organized Nursing in Minneapolis, 1883-1936*. Minnea-
        polis: Nurses' Association, 1944.

4800.   Moreno, G.T. "Mexican Nurses' Association: Charge for
        Development." *Int Nurs Rev*, 19 (1972), 370-376.

4801.   Muller, M. "Founding Texas Nurses' Association Member Talks
        of Early Days." *Bull Texas Nurs Assoc*, 43 (Jun 1970),
        12-13.

4802.   Munson, Helen W., and Katharine Stevens. *The Story of the
        National League of Nursing Education*. Philadelphia: W.B.
        Saunders, 1934.

4803.   Mussallem, Helen K. "Canadian Nurse Studies NLN Accreditation
        Program (News)." *Nurs Out*, 5 (Nov 1957), 669-670.

4804.   Nahm, Helen. "The Accreditation Program in Nursing." In
        The Nursing Program in the General College. Edited by
        Sister M. Olivia Gowan. Washington, D.C.: The Catholic
        University of America, 1954.

4805.   "National Committee for Improvement of Nursing Services."
        Am J Nurs, 54 (1954), 322-323.

4806.   National League for Nursing. *Nurses for a Growing Nation*.
        New York: The League, 1957.

4807.   "National Student Nurse Association." *Am J Nurs*, 53 (1953),
        978-983.

4808.   "Notes from Headquarters, American Nurses Association."
        Am J Nurs, 33 (Oct 1933), 1101.

4809. "Nursing Organizations in the Past." *Nurs Times*, 56 (Feb 1960), 241-242.

4810. Nyquist, Ann S. "Minnesota Organization for Public Health Nursing." *Minn Reg Nurs*, 13 (1940), 22-23.

4811. "On Accreditation." *Am J Nurs*, 60 (Oct 1960), 1475-1478. Prepared by the National League for Nursing staff and Marion Sheahan.

4812. "One Hundred (100) Years of Organized Nursing." *Sykepleien*, 55 (15 Nov 1968), 655-656. (Dan)

4813. "An Outline of the History of the Queensland Bush Nursing Association." *Queensland Nurs J*, 8 (Nov 1966), 13-14.

4814. Oxley, N.F. "Guild of St. Barnabas for Nursing; Its Growth in 42 Years." *Tr Nurs*, 80 (Jun 1928), 716.

4815. Parmentier, J. "The National Federation of Belgian Nurses." *Pub Hlth Nurs*, 24 (Nov 1932), 633-634.

4816. Penka, J. "National Academy of Nursing Launched." *Kans Nurs*, 48 (Mar 1973), 3-5.

4817. Petry, Lucile. "Minnesota League of Nursing Education--1930-1950." *Minn Reg Nurs*, 13 (1940), 25-26.

4818. Piemonte, Robert Victor. *A History of the National League of Nursing Education 1912-1932: Great Awakening in Nursing Education.* Ed.D. dissertation, Columbia University, 1976.

4819. "The Professional Organization and Its Influence on Nursing." *Queensland Nurs J*, 10 (Oct 1968), 5-19.

4820. Queensland Bush Nursing Association. "An Outline of the History of the Queensland Bush Nursing Association." *Queensland Nurs J*, 8 (1966), 13-14.

4821. Rankiellour, Caroline M. "The Minnesota Nurses' Association 1930 to 1940." *Minn Reg Nurs*, 13 (1940), 10-14.

4822. Raymond Rich Associates. "Report on the Structure of Organized Nursing." *Am J Nurs*, 46 (Oct 1946), 648-661.

4823. "Seventy-Fifth (75th) Anniversary of the Danish Nursing Council, 1899-1974." *Sygeplejersken*, 74 (27 Oct 1974), Supp. 1-48. (Dan)

4824. Sgarra, A. "Organization of the Nursing Profession in Italy." *Int Nurs Rev*, 2 (Apr 1955), 48-54.

4825. Shiraishi, K. "History and Current Status of the International Council of Nurses." *Jap J Nurs*, 37 (Apr 1973), 418-423. (Jap)

4826.   Simpson, C.E. "Soul's Sincere Desire Attained; Record of the
        Nurses' Association of China." *Mission Rev*, 49 (Oct 1926),
        808-810.

4827.   Smith, Gloria R. "From Invisibility to Blackness: The Story
        of the Black Nurses' Association." *Nurs Out*, 23(4) (Apr
        1975), 225-229.

4828.   Society for the State Registration of Trained Nurses. "Pro-
        ceedings of a Public Meeting Held at Morley Hall on May 30th
        Organized by the Society." *Nurs Rec* (Jun 1902), 453-458.

4829.   Stallknecht, K. "Seventy-Fifth (75th) Anniversary of the
        Danish Nursing Council." *Sykepleien*, 61(23) (5 Dec 1974),
        1180-1181, 1206. (Dan)

4830.   Sticker, A. "1903--January 11, 1973. Founding of the Profes-
        sional Organization of German Nurses: In Memory of Agnes
        Karl." *Z Krankenpflege*, 27 (Jan 1973), 5-11. (Ger)

4831.   Swort, Arlowayne. *The A.N.A.: The Formative Years, 1875-
        1922*. Ed.D. dissertation, Columbia University, 1974.

4832.   "A Tentative Plan for One National Nursing Organization."
        Am J Nurs, 48 (May 1948), 321-328.

4833.   Thompson, Julia. *The ANA in Washington*. Kansas City, MO:
        The American Nurses' Association, 1972.

4834.   Thomson, Elnora E. "Address to House of Delegates, ANA."
        *Proceedings 28th Convention of American Nurses' Associa-
        tion*. New York: The Association, 1930. pp. 5-8.

4835.   Tompkins, F. "NSNA's First 20 Years." *Imprint*, 19 (Oct
        1972), 10-11.

4836.   Walsh, Margaret E. "NLN: Twenty-five Years of Nursing
        Leadership." *Nurs Out*, 25 (Apr 1977), 248-249.

4837.   White, A. "I.C.N.: Past, Present, and Future." *IR Nurs J*,
        4 (Aug-Sep 1971), 7-9.

4838.   Widmer, Carolyn. "Sigma Theta Tau: Golden Anniversary."
        Nurs Out, 20 (Dec 1972), 786-788.

4839.   Zimmerman, Anne. "ANA--Its Record on Social Issues."
        Am J Nurs, 76 (1976), 588-590.

                    NURSING ROLE, ETHICS, ISSUES, DIRECTIONS

4840.   Abdellah, Faye, Irene Beland, Lamdea Martin, and Ruth Matheney.
        Patient-Centered Approaches to Nursing. New York: Macmillan
        Co., 1960.

Nursing Role, Ethics, Issues, Directions   *349*

4841.   Annello, Michael. "Responsibility for Change and Innovation
        in Professional Nursing." *Int Nurs Rev*, 16(3) (1969), 208-
        221.

4842.   Baly, Monica E. *Nursing and Social Change*. London: Heine-
        mann, 1973.

4843.   Benne, Kenneth D., and Warren Bennis. "Role Conflict in
        Nursing: What is Real Nursing?" *Am J Nurs*, 59 (Mar 1959),
        196-198, 380-383.

4844.   Bowar-Ferres, Susan. "Loeb Center and Its Philosophy of
        Nursing." *Am J Nurs*, 75 (May 1975), 810-815.

4845.   Brown, Esther Lucile. *Nursing for the Future: A Report Pre-
        pared for the National Nursing Council*. New York: Russell
        Sage Foundation, 1948.

4846.   ————. *Nursing Reconsidered--A Study of Change: Part I--
        The Professional Role in Institutional Nursing*. Philadel-
        phia: J.B. Lippincott Co., 1970.

4847.   ————. *Nursing Reconsidered--A Study of Change: Part II--
        The Professional Role in Community Nursing*. Philadelphia:
        J.B. Lippincott, 1971.

4848.   Bullough, Bonnie, and Vern Bullough, eds. *Expanding Horizons
        for Nurses*. New York: Springer, 1977.

4849.   ————. *Issues in Nursing*. New York: Springer, 1966.

4850.   ————. *New Directions for Nurses*. New York: Springer,
        1971.

4851.   Chaska, Norma L., ed. *The Nursing Profession: Views Through
        the Mist*. New York: McGraw-Hill Book Co., 1978.

4852.   Christensen, V.A. "International Trends: Nursing in a
        Changing World." *VA J Psychiatr Nurs*, 12(6) (Nov-Dec
        1974), 39-43.

4853.   "Code of Ethics as Applied to Nursing." *Int Nurs Rev*, 21
        (3-4) (May-Aug 1974), 103-104.

4854.   Committee on the Function of Nursing. *A Program for the
        Nursing Profession*. New York: Macmillan Co., 1948.

4855.   Connolly, Arlene Frances. *The Application of Role Theory
        Concepts to a Historical Examination of the Head Nurse,
        1873-1969*. Ed.D. dissertation, Boston University, 1971.

4856.   Crowder, E. "Manners, Morals, and Nurses: An Historical
        Overview of Nursing Ethics." *Tex Rep Biol Med*, 32(1)
        (Spring 1974), 173-180.

4857.   Cutler, Mary Jane. "Nursing Leadership and Management: An
         Historical Perspective." *Nurs Adm Q*, 1(1) (Fall 1976),
         7-19.

4858.   Damatirca, F., et al. "Image and Work of Nurses Through the
         Ages (History, Literature, Arts, Ethics)." *Munca Sanit*,
         21 (Dec 1973), 741-744. (Rum)

4859.   Dietz, Lena Dixon. *Professional Problems for Nurses*. 2nd ed.
         Philadelphia: F.A. Davis, 1937.

4860.   Donaghue, S. "Humanist Traditions in Nursing Development."
         Aust Nurs J, 4(11) (Jun 1975), 26-30.

4861.   Donovan, Mary C. "Professional Ideals and the Creed of Ser-
         vice to Humanity." *Nurs World*, 124 (Aug 1950), 368-369.

4862.   Folta, Jeannette R., and Edith S. Deck. *Sociological Frame-
         work for Patient Care*. 2nd ed. New York: John Wiley,
         1979. 510 pp.

4863.   Freeman, Howard E., Sol Levine, and Leo G. Reeder. *Handbook
         of Medical Sociology*. Englewood Cliffs, NJ: Prentice-Hall,
         1963; 1972.

4864.   Goodrich, Annie W. *The Social and Ethical Significance of
         Nursing*. New York: Macmillan Co., 1932.

4865.   Goostray, S. "Challenge and Change." *Bull Massachusetts
         Nurs Assoc*, 36 (Summer 1967), 3-6.

4866.   Group, T.M., et al. "Exorcising the Ghosts of the Crimea."
         Canad Nurs, 70(10) (Oct 1974), 31-35.

4867.   "Half Angel, Half Draft Horse: Nurse is Now Half Angel, Half
         Assistant Doctor." *Mod Hosp*, 100 (Sep 1963), 107-109.

4868.   Hardy, Margaret E., and Mary E. Conway, ed. *Role Theory:
         Perspectives for Health Professionals*. New York: Appleton-
         Century-Crofts, 1978.

4869.   Headberry, J.E. "Florence Nightingale and Modern Nursing."
         J West Aust Nurs, 32 (Jan 1966), 7-16; see also *UNA Nurs J*,
         64 (Mar-Apr 1966), 80-87.

4870.   Henderson, Virginia. "Excellence in Nursing." *Am J Nurs*,
         69 (Oct 1969), 2133-2137.

4871.   Hughes, Everett C., Helen MacGill Hughes, and Irwin Deutscher.
         Twenty Thousand Nurses Tell Their Story. Philadelphia:
         J.B. Lippincott Co., 1958.

4872.   Johns, Ethel, and Blanche Pfefferkorn. *An Activity Analysis
         of Nursing*. New York: Committee on the Grading of Nursing
         Schools, 1934.

4873. Johnson, Dorothy E. "Development of Theory: A Requisite for
       Nursing as a Primary Health Profession." *Nurs Res*, 23(5)
       (Sep-Oct 1974), 372-374.

4874. ————. "The Nature of a Science of Nursing." *Nurs Out*, 7
       (1959), 291-294.

4875. ————. "A Philosophy of Nursing." *Nurs Out*, 7 (1959),
       198-200.

4876. Kawakami, T., et al. "Nursing Theory. 6. Notes on Nursing
       by Florence Nightingale." *Jap J Nurs*, 36 (Jun 1972), 760-
       763. (Jap)

4877. ————. "Nursing Theory. 7. Notes on Nursing by Florence
       Nightingale. 2." *Jap J Nurs*, 36 (Jul 1972), 885-889. (Jap)

4878. Kelly, Lucie Young. *Dimensions of Professional Nursing*. 3rd
       ed. New York: Macmillan Co., 1975.

4879. King, Arthur G. "The Changing Role of the Nurse." *Hosp
       Topics*, 46 (Jun 1964), 89, 92.

4880. Kinlein, M. Lucile. "The Self-Care Concept." *Am J Nurs*, 77
       (Apr 1977), 598-601.

4881. Kodama, K. "Thoughts on Translation of Florence Nightingale's
       'Notes on Hospitals.'" *Compr Nurs Q*, 5 (Spring 1970),
       18-20. (Jap)

4882. Kreuter, Frances R. "What is Good Nursing Care?" *Nurs Out*,
       5 (1957), 302-304.

4883. "Lady Nurses." *Godey's Lady's Book and Magazine*, 82 (1871),
       188-189. Reprint. Austin, *Source Book*. pp. 431-432, See
       No. 50.

4884. Lanara, V.A. "Philosophy of Nursing and Current Nursing
       Problems." *Int Nurs Rev*, 23(2) (Mar-Apr 1976), 48-54.

4885. ————. "Philosophy of Nursing Care and Contemporary Nursing
       Problems." *Hellen Adelphe*, 51 (Mar-May 1975), 27-34. (Gr)

4886. Larsson, B. "The Nurse in Civic Life." *Int Nurs Rev*, 21
       (3-4) (May-Aug 1974), 94-95.

4887. Laver, E.M. "1939-And New to the Role." *Nurs Mirror*, 140
       (22) (Jun 1975), 76-77.

4888. Leininger, Madeleine. "Two Strange Health Tribes: The Ghis-
       trun and Enicidem in the United States." *Human Organ*, 35
       (3) (Feb 1976), 253-261.

4889. MacIver, Pearl. "Nursing Moves Forward." *Am J Nurs*, 52
       (Jul 1952), 821-823.

4890. Marram, Gwen D., M.W. Schlegel, and E.O. Bevis. *Primary
       Nursing: A Model for Individualized Care.* St. Louis:
       C.V. Mosby, 1974.

4891. "Matrimony Is Not the Goal of the Trained Nurse." *Lit Digest*,
       55 (1917), 84.

4892. Mauksch, Hans O. "Nursing Dilemma in the Organization of
       Patient Care." *Nurs Out*, 5 (Jan 1957), 31-33.

4893. Mauksch, Ingeborg G. "How Did It Come to Pass." *Nurs Forum*,
       10(3) (1971), 258-272.

4894. Merton, Robert K. "The Search for Professional Status."
       Am J Nurs, 60 (May 1960), 662-664.

4895. Meyer, S. "Knowledge and Co-responsibility at a Higher
       Level." *Sykepleien*, 62(1-2) (20 Jan 1975), 23-24. (Dan)

4896. Miller, N. "The Nurse in Contemporary Society." *New Zeal
       Nurs J*, 69 (May 1976), 23-27.

4897. Nahm, Helen. "Tribute to the Past--Prelude to the Future."
       Int Nurs Rev, 13 (Jul-Aug 1966), 14-23.

4898. Nelson, Josephine. *New Horizons in Nursing.* New York:
       Macmillan Co., 1950.

4899. Nightingale, Florence. "Notes on Nursing: What It Is and
       What It Is Not. 1." *Compr Nurs Q*, 9 (Spring 1974), 92-98.
       (Jap)

4900. ———. "Notes on Nursing: What It Is and What It Is Not.
       2." *Compr Nurs Q*, 9(2) (Summer 1974), 85-99. (Jap)

4901. ———. *Notes on Nursing; What It Is and What It Is Not.*
       New York: D. Appleton & Co., 1860. 114 pp. Reprints.
       New York: Appleton-Century-Crofts, 1960. Other editions.

4902. O'Dwyer, E.M. "Concepts of Professionalism." *World IR Nurs*,
       4 (Dec 1975), 9.

4903. Ramphal, Marjorie. "Peer Review." *Am J Nurs*, 74 (Jan 1974),
       63-67.

4904. Reissman, Leonard. *Change and Dilemma in the Nursing Profes-
       sion.* New York: G.P. Putnam's Sons, 1957.

4905. Reiter, Francis. *The Improvement of Nursing Practice.* New
       York: ANA Publication, 1961.

4906. Rogers, Martha. *Reveille in Nursing.* Philadelphia: F.A.
       Davis, 1964.

4907. Saunders, Lyle. "The Changing Role of Nurses." *Am J Nurs*, 54 (Sep 1954), 1094-1098.

4908. Schulman, Sam. "Basic Functional Roles in Nursing: Mother Surrogate and Healer." *Patients, Physicians and Illness.* Edited by E. Gartly Jaco. Glencoe, IL: The Free Press, 1958.

4909. Spalding, H.S. *Talks to Nurses: The Ethics of Nursing.* New York: Benziger, 1920.

4910. Stewart, Isabel M. "Which Way Are We Going in Nursing?" *Survey*, 46 (18 Jun 1921), 409-410.

4911. Strauss, Anselm. "The Structure and Ideology of American Nursing." *The Nursing Profession: Five Sociological Essays.* Edited by F. Davis. New York: John Wiley, 1966.

4912. Titus, H. "The Public Image of Nurses--Today and Yesterday." *Nurs News* (Hartford), 42 (Jan 1968), 14-15.

4913. Todd, Arthur J. "Nursing as a Learned Profession--A Sociologist's View." *Pub Hlth Nurs*, 11 (Jan 1919), 13-18.

4914. Tucker, Katherine. "The Nurse: A New Social Force." *Survey*, 55 (1 Nov 1925), 151-152.

4915. Williams, K. "Ideologies of Nursing: Their Meanings and Implications." *Nurs Times*, 70 Suppl. (8 Aug 1974).

18. PRACTICAL NURSING:
STRATIFICATION OF THE NURSING ROLE

4916.   Ashton, K. "To Every Nurse's Aid." *Nurs Times*, 72(8)
        (26 Feb 1976), 288-289.

4917.   Bertrand, Alvin Lee. *A Study of Practical Nurse Education
        and Practical Nursing in Louisiana 1950-1955*. Baton Rouge:
        State Department of Education, 1956.

4918.   Bullough, Bonnie, and Vern Bullough. "The Causes and Conse-
        quences of the Differentiation of the Nursing Role." In
        Varieties of Work Experience. Edited by Phyllis L. Stewart
        and Muriel G. Cantor. Cambridge, MA: Schenkman, 1974.
        pp. 292-300.

4919.   Carpenter, Frances B. "A Memo From Yesterday." *J Pract Nurs*,
        17 (Aug 1967), 22.

4920.   Deming, Dorothy. *The Practical Nurse*. New York: The Common-
        wealth Fund, 1947.

4921.   ———. "Practical Nursing and the Changing Professional
        Attitude." *Am J Nurs*, 46 (Jun 1946), 366-370.

4922.   ———. "Practical Nursing—A Success Story." *Nurs World*
        (May 1951), 183-204.

4923.   ———. "Practical Nursing Then and Now." *Am J Nurs*, 50
        (Oct 1950), 621-623.

4924.   Federal Security Agency. *Practical Nursing*. Washington, D.C.:
        U.S. Government Printing Office, 1947.

4925.   Johnston, Dorothy F. *History and Trends of Practical Nurs-
        ing*. St. Louis: C.V. Mosby, 1966.

4926.   Kerr, Elizabeth E., and others. *Practical Nursing in Iowa:
        A Profile. A Study of the Developments, Trends and Current
        Status of Practical Nursing in Iowa*. Iowa City: Division
        of Medical Affairs, Iowa University, 1968. 133 pp.

4927.   Leone, Lucile Petry. "Increasing and Using Nursing Auxilia-
        ries." *Hosp*, 17 (1943), 37.

4928.   ———. "Nursing Service in Hospitals." *Chicago-Cook County
        Health Survey*. New York: Columbia University Press, 1949.

4929.   ———. "Training of Practical Nurses for Hospital Staffs
         Urged." *Hosp Manag*, 62 (1946), 74.

4930.   ———. "Trends and Problems in Practical Nurse Education."
         Am J Nurs, 56 (Jan 1956), 51-53.

4931.   Putnam, H.C. "Attendants and Nursemaids: Less Expensive and
         Less Expert Service Needed; Classes by Philanthropic Organ-
         izations; Medical Institutions for the Sick--the Proper
         Ones to Give Such Instruction; This Grade of Helpers Would
         Raise the Standing of Graduate Nurses." *J Am Med Assoc*, 38
         (1902), 1364.

4932.   Reiner, A. "Brief Outline of the Press of the Ancillary
         Health Personnel From 1900 to 1939." *Munca Sanit*, 14
         (Sep 1966), 568-570. (Rum)

4933.   Reynolds, Raymond J. "Practical Nurse Education in Massa-
         chusetts." Master's Thesis, Yale University, 1952.

4934.   Ruth, Viola H. "History of the Practical Nurse in Arizona."
         Nurs World, 127 (Aug 1953), 31-32.

4935.   Stevenson, Neva. "Curriculum Development in Practical Nurse
         Education." *Am J Nurs*, 64 (Dec 1964), 81-86.

4936.   Stone, Francis. "Is There Need for Another Class of Sick
         Attendants Besides Nurses?" *Am J Nurs*, 17 (Jun 1917),
         991-993.

4937.   Tomlinson, Robert M., et al. *Practical Nursing in Illinois--
         A Profile*. Illinois State Board of Vocational Education
         and Rehabilitation. Urbana, IL: Dept. of Vocational and
         Technical Education, University of Illinois, 1968.

4938.   Torrop, Hilda M. "Are Practical Nurses the Answer?" *Hosp*,
         26 (Jul 1952), 56-57.

4939.   ———. "How Much Nursing Service Should an Orderly Give?"
         Am J Nurs, 37 (Jan 1937), 15-17.

4940.   ———. "A True Fairy Tale." *J Pract Nurs*, 23 (Jun 1973),
         18-21.

4941.   "Trained Attendants and Practical Nurses." *Am J Nurs*, 44
         (Jan 1944), 7-8.

4942.   "Training Program Announced for 10,000 Nurses' Aides."
         Hosp Mgmt, 52 (1941), 44.

4943.   Tucker, Georgia Lee. "The Licensed Practical Nurse in Today's
         Setting or the Licensed Practical Solution." *J Prac Nurs*,
         22 (Aug 1972), 24-26.

4944. U.S. Office of Education. *Practical Nursing.* Vocational
        Education Division, Misc. #8. Washington, D.C.: U.S.
        Government Printing Office, 1947, 1950.

4945. Van Matre, Alma F. "Highlights in the Development of Prac-
        tical Nursing." *Prac Nurs Dig*, 2 (Jul 1955), 12-14.

19. HOSPITALS AND NURSING HOMES

4946. Angell, E.B. "The Modern Hospital: Its Value to the Patient and to Physician." *Am J Nurs*, 1 (Jul 1901), 703-712.

4947. Baltz, K.E. "Historical Notes on Twelve General Hospitals (U.S.); History of Nursing Service." *Q Bull Northwestern Univ Med Sch*, 21 (1947), 269-273.

4948. "Bart's (London, England St. Bartholomew Hospital)." *Nurs Mirror*, 136 (18 May 1973), 11-15; (25 May 1973), 15-16.

4949. Bernheim, Bertram. *The Story of Johns Hopkins*. Surrey, England: Windmill Press, 1949.

4950. Bowditch, N.I. *A History of the Massachusetts General Hospital, 1810-1851. With a Continuation, 1851-1872 by George E. Ellis*. Boston: Bowditch Fund, 1872.

4951. Brand, V., et al. "Dr. Steele's Report to the Governors 1871." *Guys Hosp Rep*, 120 (1971), 181-183.

4952. Briele, L., M. Moring, and C. Quentin. *Collection de documents pour servir à l'histoire des hopitaux de Paris*. 4 vols. Paris: Imprimerie Nationale, 1881-1887.

4953. Carson, Maude B. "Improving Standards in Nursing Homes." *Pub Hlth Nurs*, 39 (Jun 1947), 312-314.

4954. Cassie, Ethel. "The Registration and Inspection of Nursing Homes." *Pub Hlth* (London), 47 (Jun 1934), 294-297.

4955. "Chalmers Hospital, Edinburgh--1864-1964." *Nurs Times*, 60 (18 Sep 1964), 1215.

4956. Clay, Rotha Mary. *The Medieval Hospitals of England*. London: Methuen and Co., 1909.

4957. Cobbe, Frances Power. "Workhouse Sketches." *Macmillan's Mag*, 3 (Nov 1860-Apr 1861), 448-461.

4958. Commission on Hospital Care. *Hospital Care in the United States*. New York: The Commonwealth Fund, 1947.

4959. Corwin, E.H.L. *The American Hospital*. New York: The Commonwealth Fund, 1946.

4960.   Coxhead, E. "Miss Nightingale's Country Hospital." *Nurs Times*, 64 (10 May 1973), 615-617.

4961.   Davis, M.M., and A.R. Warner. *Dispensaries: Their Management and Development*. New York: Macmillan Co., 1918.

4962.   Davis, Michael M. *Clinics, Hospitals and Health Centers*. New York: Harper & Brothers, 1927.

4963.   DeWitt, Katherine. "Hospital Sketches." *Am J Nurs*, 6 (Apr 1906), 455-459.

4964.   Faxon, Nathaniel W. *The Hospital in Contemporary Life*. Cambridge, MA: Harvard University Press, 1949.

4965.   Frances, Bobbie Collen, Blanche Madero, Krikor Soghikean, and Sidney R. Garfield. "Kaiser-Permanente Experiment in Ambulatory Care." *Am J Nurs*, 71 (Jul 1971), 1371-1374.

4966.   Freidson, Eliot. *The Hospital in Modern Society*. New York: The Free Press of Glencoe, 1963.

4967.   Gask, G.E., and J. Todd. "The Origins of Hospitals." *Science, Medicine and History*. Edited by E.A. Underwood. 2 vols. Oxford: Oxford University Press, 1953.

4968.   "The History of St. Martin's Hospital." *Queensland Nurs J*, 8 (1966), 16-18.

4969.   Homersham, E. Margery. "The Registration and Inspection of Nursing Homes." *J Roy San Inst*, 24 (Apr 1903), 649-652.

4970.   *Hospital Services in the U.S.S.R.* Washington, D.C.: U.S. Department of Health, Education and Welfare, 1966.

4971.   "Hospitals--Yesterday and Today." *Nurs Out*, 8 (May 1960), 260-261.

4972.   Howland, R. "Salisbury's First Nursing Home." *Cen Afr J Med*, 10 (1964), 419-421.

4973.   Imbert, Jean. *Les Hopitaux en Droit Canonique*. Paris: J. Vrin, 1947.

4974.   Kenesly, Annesley. "In a Cholera Hospital at Hamburg." *Nurs Rec* (22 Sep 1892), 185-186.

4975.   Kinnaman, Joseph H. "The Nursing Home--A Medical Facility." *Am J Pub Hlth*, 39 (Sep 1949), 1099-1105.

4976.   LaMotte, Ellen N. "The Hotel-Dieu of Paris: An Historical Sketch." *Med Libr & Hist J* (1906), 225.

4977.   Lancet Sanitary Commission for Investigating the State of the Infirmaries of Workhouses. "The Findings of the Lancet Commission for Investigating the Care of the Sick in the

Workhouse Infirmaries, Presented Among Other Matters, Observations of the Conditions in Nursing and Suggested Appropriate Remedies." *Lancet* (1 Jul 1865), 14-22.

4978. Larrabee, E. *The Benevolent and Necessary Institution: The New York Hospital, 1771-1971.* Garden City, NY: Doubleday, 1971.

4979. LeSage, Albert. "Cinquantenaire de la fondation de l'Association des Gardes-malades, Hôpital Notre-Dame, 1898-1948." *Garde-Malade Canad-Franc*, 21 (1948), 353-361. (Fr)

4980. Lewis, Edith P. "The New York City Hospital Story." *Am J Nurs*, 66 (Jul 1966), 1526-1533.

4981. Loretta Bernard, Sister. "A Century of Progress." *Hosp Prog*, 16 (Apr 1935), 158-163.

4982. *Manual of Essentials of Good Hospital Nursing Service.* New York: American Hospital Association and National League of Nursing Education, 1926, 1936.

4983. Maria Corona, Sister. "The Catholic Hospital as an Educational Agency for the Profession of Nursing." *Hosp Prog*, 22 (Sep 1941), 288-291.

4984. Maroney, Kathrine Appel. "How a Small Hospital Can Nurse Its Patients Without a School." *Am J Nurs*, 32 (Jun 1932), 640-642.

4985. Marsh, Edith L. "The Care of the Chronically Ill." *Am J Nurs*, 41 (Feb 1941), 161-166.

4986. Mary Felician, Sister. "The Catholic Hospital in the History of Nursing Education." *Hosp Prog*, 11 (Oct 1930), 447-449.

4987. Maxson, Edwin R. *Hospitals: British, French, and American.* Philadelphia: Privately printed, 1868.

4988. Maxwell, A.C. "The Field Hospital at Chickamauga Park." *Tr Nurs & Hosp Rev*, 23 (1899), 3.

4989. Miller, Sydney R. "Private Nursing Homes." *STH Med J*, 16 (Aug 1923), 633-636.

4990. Morris, E.W. *The History of the London Hospital.* London: Edward Arnold, 1910.

4991. Myers, Grace Whiting. *A History of the Massachusetts General Hospital, June 1872 to December 1900.* Boston: Griffith-Stilling Press, 1929.

4992. New York Infirmary. *The New York Infirmary: A Century of Devoted Service.* New York: New York Infirmary, 1954.

4993. Nightingale, Florence. "Notes on Hospitals." *Compr Nurs Q*,
       6 (Spring 1971), 87-98. (Jap)

4994. ———. *Notes on Hospitals*. 3rd ed. London: Longmans, 1867.

4995. O'Connor, R. "American Hospitals: The First 200 Years."
       Hosp, 50(1) (1 Jan 1976), 62-72.

4996. Olch, Peter D., and Floyd M. Nyhus. "Joseph Lister and the
       Old Edinburgh Infirmary." *Hosp Mgmt*, 94 (Jul 1962), 62-65.

4997. Packard, Francis R. *Some Accounts of the Pennsylvania Hospi-
       tal from 1751-1938*. Philadelphia: Engle Press, 1938.

4998. ———. *Some Accounts of the Pennsylvania Hospital: From Its
       First Rise to the Beginning of the Year 1938*. Philadelphia:
       Pennsylvania Hospital, 1938.

4999. Parsons, F.G. *The History of St. Thomas' Hospital*. 3 vols.
       London: Methuen, 1932.

5000. "Pennsylvania Hospital: The Pioneer Hospital of the United
       States." *National Hospital Record*, 5 (1901-1902), 3.

5001. Ransome, J.E. "The Beginnings of Hospitals in the United
       States." *Bull Hist Med*, 13 (1943), 514.

5002. "The Registration of Nursing Homes." *Hospital* (London), 43
       (16 Nov 1907), 192; (23 Nov 1907), 222-223; (30 Nov 1907),
       249; (7 Dec 1907), 275; (14 Dec 1907), 301.

5003. Rosenberg, Charles E. "And Heal the Sick: The Hospital and
       the Patient in the 19th Century America." *J Soc Hist*,
       10(4) (Jun 1977), 428-447.

5004. Scovil, E.R. "The Private Hospital as Owned and Managed by
       Nurses." *Am J Nurs*, 3 (Aug 1903), 892-899.

5005. Seidler, E. "The Hospital Yesterday, Today, and Tomorrow.
       Modern Care of Patients in Its Historical Development."
       Hippokrates, 39 (15 Dec 1968), 893-898. (Ger)

5006. Sturtevant, G.L. "Personal Recollections of Hospital Life
       Before the Days of Training Schools." *Tr Nurs*, 57 (Nov
       1916), 255-260; (Dec 1916), 321-327; 58 (Feb 1917), 67-70;
       (Mar 1917), 127-131. Originally published in *Tr Nurs*
       (1895-1896).

5007. Titus, Shirley C. "The Present Position of Nursing in the
       United States." *Nosokomeion*, 2, 288.

5008. Todd, J., and G.E. Gask. "The Origin of Hospitals." *Science,
       Medicine and History*. Edited by F.A. Underwood. 2 vols.
       Oxford: Oxford University Press, 1953.

5009.   Trexler, Bernice J. "Hospital Patients in Florence." *Bull Hist Med*, 48 (1974), 41-58.

5010.   Twining, Louisa. *Workhouses and Pauperism and Women's Work in the Administration of the Poor Law.* London: Methuen and Co., 1853.

5011.   Winstanley, M.M. "Starting a Nursing Home." *Cath Nurs* (London), 2 (Mar 1934), 4; (Apr 1934), 8.

5012.   Wylie, W.G. *Hospitals, Their History, Organization, and Construction.* New York: Appleton, 1877.

20. NURSES AND NURSING IN LITERATURE

NOVELS

5013. Anderson, Peggy. *Nurse: The True Story of Mary Benjamin.*
New York: St. Martin's Press, 1978.

5014. Arnold, Elliot. *Proving Ground; A Novel.* New York: Charles
Scribner's Sons, 1973. 309 pp.

5015. Bosworth, Allan R. *The Crows of Edwina Hill, A Novel.* New
York: Harper and Brothers, 1961.

5016. Brinkley, William. *The Ninety and Nine.* Garden City:
Doubleday, 1966. 393 pp.

5017. Chase, Mary Ellen. *The Plum Tree.* New York: Macmillan Co.,
1949. 98 pp.

5018. Dickens, Charles. *The Life and Adventures of Martin Chuzzlewit.* New York: Dutton Everyman's Library.

5019. Ellis, A.E. *The Rack.* Boston: Little, Brown & Co., 1958.
414 pp.

5020. Faulkner, William. *Soldiers Pay.* New York: Liveright, 1970.
319 pp.

5021. Gilbert, Anthony. *The Looking Glass Murder.* New York:
Random House, 1967. 215 pp.

5022. Grubb, Davis. *The Voices of Glory.* New York: Charles
Scribner's Sons, 1962. 469 pp.

5023. Hailey, Arthur. *The Final Diagnosis.* Garden City: Doubleday,
1969. 348 pp.

5024. Hartog, Jan de. *The Hospital.* New York: Atheneum, 1964.

5025. Hemingway, Ernest A. *A Farewell to Arms.* New York: Charles
Scribner's Sons, 1929. 355 pp.

5026. Hulme, K. *The Nun's Story.* Boston: Little, Brown & Co.,
1956.

5027.   Kaniuk, Yoram Himmo. *King of Jerusalem.* Translated from the
        Hebrew by Yosef Schacter. New York: Atheneum, 1969.
        246 pp.

5028.   Kesey, Ken. *One Flew Over the Cuckoo's Nest; a Novel.* New
        York: Viking Press, 1962. 311 pp.

5029.   King, Paul. *Hermana Sam.* New York: Coward, McCann & Geoghe-
        gan, 1977. 227 pp.

5030.   Kundera, Milan. *The Farewell Party.* Translated from the
        Czech by Peter Kusse. New York: Alfred A. Knopf, 1976.
        209 pp.

5031.   Rayner, Claire. *Bedford Row.* New York: G.P. Putnam's Sons,
        1977. 278 pp.

5032.   Rinehart, Mary Roberts. *Mrs. Pinkerton: Adventures of a Nurse
        Detective.* New York: Holt, Rinehart and Winston, 1959.
        403 pp.

5033.   Number deleted.

5034.   Slaughter, Frank G. *East Side General.* Garden City: Double-
        day, 1952. 311 pp.

5035.   ————. *Women in White.* Garden City: Doubleday, 1974.
        396 pp.

5036.   Stewart, Fred Mustard. *Lady Darlington; a Novel.* New York:
        Arbor House, 1971. 312 pp.

5037.   Sumner, Cid Ricketts. *Quality, A Novel.* Indianapolis:
        Bobbs-Merrill, 1946. 286 pp.

5038.   Terrot, Charles. *Passionate Pilgrim.* New York: Harper and
        Brothers, 1949. 213 pp. Also published as *Miss Nightin-
        gale's Ladies.* London: Collins, 1948. 255 pp.

5039.   Thompson, Morton. *Not as a Stranger.* New York: Charles
        Scribner's Sons, 1954. 948 pp.

5040.   Woodard, Bronté. *Meet Me at the Melba, A Novel.* New York:
        Delacorte Press, 1977. 268 pp.

PLAYS

5041.   Albright, Hardie. *All the Living.* Based on the book *I Knew
        3000 Lunatics* by V.R. Small. New York: French, 1938.

5042.   Ball, Jack, and Edwin Scribner. *Have Patience, Doctor.* New
        York: French, 1933.

5043. Barry, Mae Howley. *The Nautical Approach.* New York: Dramaticka, 1955.

5044. Berkley, Reginald Cheyne. *The Lady with a Lamp.* New York: French, 1920; also in *Famous Plays of Today.* London: Gollancz, 1930; *Plays of a Half Decade.* London: Gollancz, 1933.

5045. Beuwett, Dorothy. *Quiet Night.* London: French, 1953.

5046. Carlson, Bernice W. "For Soldiers Everywhere." *The Right Play for You.* Nashville, TN: Abingdon, 1960.

5047. Carruthers, J. *Physician in Charge.* New York: Friendship Press, 1954.

5048. Carter, Arthur Philip. *Operation Mad Ball.* New York: French, 1960.

5049. Cavalieri, G. *We Regret to Inform You. Per/Se Award Plays.* New York: The Smith, 1969.

5050. Cronin, Archibald Joseph. *Jupiter Laughs.* Boston: Little, Brown & Co., 1940.

5051. Jeans, Ronald. "Young Wive's Tale." *Plays of the Year*, edited by J.C. Trevin. vol. 3. London: Paul Elek, 1950. pp. 105-210.

5052. Kerr, Sophie. *Home Nursing Review.* London: French, 1951.

5053. Kingsley, Sidney. *Men in White.* New York: Covici, 1933.

5054. Kisser, Fan. "Clara Barton: Angel of the Battlefield." *They Helped Make America.* New York: Houghton Mifflin, 1958.

5055. Lardner, Ring. "Zone of Quiet." *Best Television of 1950* by Kaufman. vol. I. San Jose, CA: Merlin Press, 1950. pp. 75-105.

5056. Lipnick, Ester. "Angel of Mercy." *Fifty Plays for Junior Actors.* Edited by S.E. Kamermon. Boston: Plays Inc., 1966.

5057. Love, Stewart. "Miss Nightingale from Embley Park." *Girls' Plays for Reading and Recording.* Boston: Plays, Inc., 1966.

5058. Nichols, Peter. *The National Health.* London: Faber and Faber, 1970.

5059. Phillips, Marguerite Kreger. *Hospital Zone.* London: French, 1964.

5060. Reach, James. *Doctors and Nurses.* London: French, 1964.

5061.   ————. *Women in White*. New York: French, 1953.

5062.   Richmond, Samuel S. "The Crisis." *Career Plays for Young
        People* by S.S. Richmond. Boston: Plays, Inc., 1949.

5063.   Roberts, Carl E.B., and S. Cecil. *Nurse Cavell*. London:
        Lane, 1933.

5064.   Roberts, Walter C. *Red Harvest*. New York: French, 1937.

5065.   Ryerson, Florence, and Colin Campbell Clements. "Materia
        Medica." *Modern Short Plays* by Felix Sper. New York:
        Globe Book, 1952.

5066.   Sondheim, Stephen. *Anyone Can Whistle, A Musical Fable*.
        Book by Arthur Laurents, music and lyrics by Stephen Sond-
        heim. New York: Random House, 1965.

5067.   Stevens, Henry. *A Secret Voice*. Chicago: Dramatic, 1965.
        Partially based on Cecil Woodham-Smith's biography
        Florence Nightingale. See No. 1670.

5068.   Vvedensky, A. "Christmas at the Ivanovs'." *Russia's Lost
        Literature of the Absurd--A Literary Discovery* by Daniel
        Kharms and Alexander Vvedensky. Ithaca, NY: Cornell Uni-
        versity Press, 1971.

5069.   Watts, Alan S. *As Moths Unto the Lamp*. Boston: Evans,
        distributed by Bakers Plays, 1961.

5070.   Williams, Hugh, and Margaret Williams. "The Happy Man."
        Plays of the Year, 1957-58. Edited by J.C. Trewin, Vol. 17.
        New York: Frederick Ungar, 1958. pp. 341-429.

5071.   Wittlinger, K. "The Night Nurse." *The Best Short Plays,
        1968-1972*. 5 vols. New York: Chilton Book Co., 1968-1972.

5072.   Wood, Margaret. *Out-patients*. London: French, 1960.

SHORT STORIES

5073.   Agnon, S.Y. "The Doctor's Divorce." *Twenty-one Stories*.
        New York: Schocken Books, 1970.

5074.   ————. "Forevermore." *Modern Hebrew Literature*. New York:
        Behrman House, 1975.

5075.   Aiken, Conrad Potter. "Bring! Bring!" *Short Stories*. New
        York: Duell, Sloan. See also *The Collected Short Stories
        of Conrad Aiken*. World Pub., 1960, edited by Sonia Barry.
        A Treasury of Nurse Stories. New York: Fell, 1962.

5076. ————. "Night Before Prohibition." *Short Stories.* New York: Duell, Sloan, 1950. See also *The Collected Short Stories of Conrad Aiken.* Cleveland: World Publishing Co., 1960.

5077. Alcott, Louisa May. "Blue and the Grey." *Hospital Sketches and Camp and Fireside Stories.* Boston: Roberts Brothers, 1869.

5078. ————. "Hospital Sketches." *Hospital Sketches and Camp and Fireside Stories.* Boston: Roberts Brothers, 1869.

5079. ————. "My Contraband." *Hospital Sketches and Camp and Fireside Stories.* Boston: Roberts Brothers, 1869.

5080. ————. "Off Duty." *Treasury of Nurse Stories.* Compiled by Sonia Barry. New York: Fell, 1962.

5081. Anderson, Ethel. "Question of Habit." *Coast to Coast, Australian Stories, 1957-1958.* Compiled by D. Stirens. Sidney: Angus, 1958.

5082. Bacon, Josephine Dodge (Daskana). "The Legacy." *Strange Cases of Dr. Stanchon.* New York: Appleton, 1913.

5083. Bailey, Temple. "So This is Christmas." *So This Is Christmas and Other Stories.* Philadelphia: The Penn Publishing Co., 1931.

5084. Barrangon, Maurice. "Little Student Nurse." *Time of Starting Out.* Compiled by H. Ferris. London: F. Watts, 1962.

5085. Barry, Sonia. "The Silken Glove." *Treasury of Nurse Stories.* New York: Fell, 1962.

5086. Bates, Herbert Ernest. "Time Expired." *Conrad Julian and Other Stories.* Boston: Little, Brown & Co., 1952.

5087. Beattie, Ann. "Magical Scenes." *Distortions.* Garden City: Doubleday, 1976.

5088. Benson, Sally. "Lady with a Lamp." *55 Short Stories from the New Yorker.* New York: Simon & Schuster, 1949.

5089. Berkus, Clara W. "Courier Nurse." *Every Girl's Nurse Stories* by A.L. Furman. Edited by A.L. Furman. Mt. Vernon, NY: Lantern Press, 1963. See also *Teen-age Nurse Stories* edited by A.L. Furman. Lantern Press, 1959.

5090. Bloch, Robert. "The Dynamics of an Asteroid." Mystery Writers of America. *Crimes Across the Sea.* New York: Harper and Row, 1964.

5091. Blundell, Mary E. (Sweetman). "Mrs. Angel." *Simple Annuals.* London: Longmans, 1906.

5092.   Breinberg, Petronella. "It was Rose Hall." *The Haunted and
         the Haunters.* Compiled by K. Lines. New York: Farrar,
         Strauss and Giroux, 1975.

5093.   Brooks, George S. "Poor Sick Boy." *Woman's Home Companion*
         A Diamond of Years. Garden City: Doubleday, 1961.

5094.   Brown, Alice. "Horn-o' the Moon." *Tiverton Tales.* Boston:
         Houghton Mifflin, 1895.

5095.   Brown, Thomas Kite. "Drink of Water." *Prize Stories, 1958.*
         Garden City: Doubleday, 1958.

5096.   Buechler, J. "The Second Best Girl." *Prize Stories 1967:*
         The O. Henry Awards. Garden City: Doubleday, 1967.

5097.   Calderwood, Carmelita Cameron. "Prelude to a Past."
         Prairie Schooner as reprinted in *Prairie Schooner Caravan.*
         Lincoln: University of Nebraska Press, 1943.

5098.   Carhart, Alfreda Post. "Luciych of the Brave Heart" in
         Masoud the Bedouin. New York: Missionary Education Move-
         ment, 1915.

5099.   Carter, Charles Franklin. "La Beata." *Stories of the Old*
         Missions of California. San Francisco: P. Elder Co., 1917.

5100.   Cecil, Henry. "No Expectations." *Portrait of a Judge and*
         Other Stories. New York: Harper and Row, 1965.

5101.   Christie, Agatha. "Blue Geranium." *13 for Luck.* New York:
         Dodd, Mead, 1961. See also *13 Clues for Miss Marple.* New
         York: Dodd, Mead, 1966.

5102.   Coleman, William Laurence. "Nick and Letty, Their Love
         Stories." *Ship's Company.* Boston: Little, Brown & Co.,
         1955.

5103.   Cortazar, Julio. "Nurse Cora." *All Fires the Fire, and*
         Other Stories. Translation by Suzanne Jill Levine. New
         York: Pantheon Books, 1973.

5104.   Curwood, James Oliver. "L'ange." *Back to God's Country and*
         Other Stories. New York: Grosset and Dunlap, 1920.

5105.   Cuthrell, Faith (Baldwin). *Medical Center.* 6 stories:
         "Charge Nurse." "Clinic Aide." "Diagnostician." "Dieti-
         tian." "Intern." "Special Nurses." New York: Blakiston,
         1940.

5106.   Davies, Rhys. "I Will Keep Her Company." *The Chosen One and*
         Other Stories. New York: Dodd, Mead, 1967.

5107.   Davis, Richard H. "Red Cross Girl." *Novels and Stories.*
         New York: Charles Scribner's Sons, 1916. See also *Red*
         Cross Girl. New York: Charles Scribner's Sons, 1912.

5108. DeFord, Miriam Allen. "Mortmain." *The Theme is Murder.* New York: Abelard-Schuman, 1967.

5109. Drake, Robert. "Don't They Look Natural?" *The Single Heart.* Nashville, TN: Aurora Publishers, 1971.

5110. ———. "The Stark Naked Baptist." *The Single Heart.* Nashville, TN: Aurora Publishers, 1971.

5111. ———. "The Trained Nurse." *The Single Heart.* Nashville, TN: Aurora Publishers, 1971.

5112. Fitzgerald, Francis Scott Key. "Alcoholic Case." *Stories of F. Scott Fitzgerald.* New York: Charles Scribner's Sons, 1951.

5113. Flythe, Starkey. "Point of Conversation." *Prize Stories, 1972: The O. Henry Awards.* Garden City: Doubleday, 1972.

5114. Garrett, George. "The Witness." *King of the Mountain.* New York: Charles Scribner's Sons, 1957. See also *A Treasury of Nurse Stories,* compiled by Sonia Barry. New York: Fell, 1962.

5115. Gill, Brendan. "And Holy Ghost." *Ways of Loving.* New York: Harcourt Brace, Jovanovich, 1974.

5116. Gissing, George Robert. "Beggar's Nurse." *Human Odds and Ends.* London: Lawrence and Bullen, 1898.

5117. Glasgow, Ellen Anderson Gholson. "Shadowy Third." *Shadowy Third and Other Stories.* Garden City: Doubleday, 1923. See also *Beware After Dark.* Edited by T.E. Harre. New York: Emerson Books, 1945; *Panorama of Modern Literature.* Garden City: Doubleday, 1934; *Favorite Doctor Stories.* Compiled by A.K. Adams. New York: Dodd, Mead, 1963; *The Collected Stories of Ellen Glasgow.* Baton Rouge, LA: Louisiana State University Press, 1963.

5118. Gold, Michael. "Death of a Negro." *120 Million.* New York: International Publishers, 1929.

5119. Gordimer, Nadine. "Some Monday for Sure." *Selected Stories.* New York: Viking Press, 1976.

5120. Gordon, Arthur. "Old Ironpuss." *Saturday Evening Post Stories.* New York: Random House, 1953. See also *Treasury of Nurse Stories.* Compiled by Sonia Berry. New York: Fell, 1962.

5121. Goyen, William. "The Enchanted Nurse." *The Collected Stories of William Goyen.* Garden City: Doubleday, 1975.

5122. Hagedorn, H. "Edith Cavell." *Heroes, Heroes, Heroes.* Edited by P.R. Fenner. London: Franklin Watts, 1956.

5123.   Hale, Nancy. "Miss August." *Empress's Ring.* New York:
        Charles Scribner's Sons, 1955. See also *Treasury of Nurse
        Stories* compiled by Sonia Barry. New York: Fell, 1962.

5124.   ————. "Who Lived and Died Believing." *Best American Short
        Stories of 1943.* New York: Houghton Mifflin, 1944. See
        also *Treasury of Doctor Stories* compiled by N.D. and H.
        Werner. New York: Fell, 1964; *Between the Dark and Day-
        light.* New York: Charles Scribner's Sons, 1943; *O. Henry
        Memorial Award Prize Stories of 1943.* Garden City: Double-
        day, 1944; *Fifty Best American Short Stories, 1915-1965.*
        New York: Houghton Mifflin, 1965.

5125.   Hamp, Pierre. "Nounou." *People.* New York: Harcourt,
        Brace and World, 1921.

5126.   Harvey, William Fryer. "Account Rendered"; "Arm of Mrs.
        Egan"; "Atmospherics"; "Chemist and Druggist"; "Euphemia
        Intchmaid"; "Flying Out of Mrs. Barnard Hollis"; "The
        Lake"; "No Body"; "Old Masters"; and "Ripe for Develop-
        ment," all in *Arm of Mrs. Egan and Other Strange Stories.*
        New York: E.P. Dutton, 1952.

5127.-
5135.   Numbers deleted.

5136.   Hawthorne, Nathaniel. "Edward Fane's Rosebud." *The Complete
        Short Stories of Nathaniel Hawthorne.* New York: Hanover
        House, 1959. See also *Twice Told Tales.* Centenary edition
        of the works of Nathaniel Hawthorne. Columbus, OH: Ohio
        State University Press, 1974.

5137.   Heggen, Thomas. "The Birthmark." *Best Short Stories of
        World War II.* Edited by C.A. Fenton. New York: Viking
        Press, 1957.

5138.   Henderson, Natalie A. "Cream Puff Girl." *Every Girl's Nurse
        Stories.* Edited by A.L. Furman. Mt. Vernon, NY: Lantern
        Press, 1963. See also *Teen-age Nurse Stories*, edited by
        A.L. Furman. Mt. Vernon, NY: Lantern Press, 1959.

5139.   Herbst, Steve. "Old Soul." *Orbit II.* New York: G.P.
        Putnam's Sons, 1973.

5140.   Hirsch, E.L. "An Aged Man is But a Paltry Thing." *New
        Voices: 4 American Writers Today.* New York: Hendricks
        House, 1960.

5141.   Holtby, Winifred. "Nurse to the Archbishop." *Truth is Not
        Sober.* New York: Macmillan Co., 1934.

5142.   Hopper, James Marie. "When It Happens." *Best Short Stories
        of 1927.* Boston: Houghton Mifflin, 1928.

5143.   Jay, B. "Callie." *Alabama Prize Stories, 1970.* Huntsville,
        AL: Strode, 1970.

5144. Keller, David Henry. "Psychophonic Nurse." *Tales from Underwood*. New York: Pellegrini & Cudahy, 1952.

5145. Kipling, Rudyard. "Legs of Sister Ursula." *Selected Prose and Poetry*. Garden City: Garden City Publishing Co., n.d.

5146. Kotzwinkle, William. "Stroke of Good Luck." *Elephant Bangs Train*. New York: Pantheon Books, 1971.

5147. Kundera, Milan. "Symposium." *Laughable Loves*. Translated by Suzanne Rappaport. New York: St. Martins Press, 1974.

5148. Lardner, Ring W. "Zone of Quiet." *Reading Modern Fiction*. Edited by W.C. Lynskey. New York: Charles Scribner's Sons, 1952. See also *Doctors' Choice* edited by P.M. Blaustein and A.P. Blaustein. New York: Funk and Wagnall, 1957; *Best Short Stories of Ring Lardner*. New York: Charles Scribner's Sons, 1957; *Haircut and Other Stories*. New York: Charles Scribner's Sons, 1961; *The Ring Lardner Reader*. New York: Charles Scribner's Sons, 1963; *Modern American and British Short Stories* edited by L. Brown. New York: Harcourt Brace and World, 1929; *Modern Short Stories* edited by L. Brown. New York: Harcourt Brace and World, 1937; *Cream of the Jug* edited by G.M. Overton. New York: Harper and Brothers, 1927; *Treasury of Doctor Stories* compiled by N.D. Fabricant and H. Werner. New York: Fell, 1946. *Roundup*. New York: Charles Scribner's Sons, 1929; *Collected Short Stories*. New York: Modern Library, n.d.; *Love Nest and Other Stories*. New York: Charles Scribner's Sons, 1926; *Ring Lardner's Best Stories*. Garden City: Garden City Books, 1938.

5149. Ledford, Eliza. "Hold High the Lamp." *Time of Starting Out*. Compiled by H. Ferris. London: Franklin Watts, 1962.

5150. Levine, Ted M. "Elaine's Hope." *Writers for Tomorrow*. Edited by B. Hathaway and J. Sessions. 2nd Series. Ithaca, NY: Cornell University Press, 1952. *Treasury of Nurse Stories*. Compiled by Sonia Barry. New York: Fell, 1962.

5151. Locke, William John. "Echo of the Past." *Stories Near and Far*. New York: Dodd, Mead, 1927.

5152. ⸻. "Women of the War." *Far-Away Stories*. New York: Lane, 1919.

5153. Lorimer, Graeme (Sarah Moss Lorimer). "Mighty Man Was He." *First Love, Farewell*. Boston: Little, Brown & Co., 1940.

5154. Lowry, Robert. "The Sight of Blood." *Park of Dreamers*. New York: Fleet Publishers, 1962.

5155. McCune, Patricia. "The Angry Nurse." *Every Girl's Nurse Stories*. Edited by A.L. Furman. Mt. Vernon, NY: Lantern Press, 1963. See also *Teen-age Nurse Stories*. Edited by A.L. Furman. Mt. Vernon, NY: Lantern Press, 1959.

5156.   ———. "Operation Homecoming." *Every Girl's Nurse Stories.*
         Edited by A.L. Furman. Mt. Vernon, NY: Lantern Press,
         1963. See also *Teen-age Nurse Stories.* Edited by A.L.
         Furman. Mt. Vernon, NY: Lantern Press, 1959.

5157.   Matthews, Brander. "In the Watches of the Night." *Outlines
         of Local Color.* New York: Harper and Brothers, 1897.

5158.   Maupassant, Guy de. "The Derie." *Ball-of-Tallow and Short
         Stories.* New York: Pearson, 1910. See also *Complete Short
         Stories.* New York: Blue Ribbon Books, 1941; *The Horla and
         Other Stories.* New York: Alfred A. Knopf, 1925; *Portable
         Maupassant.* New York: Viking Press, 1947; *Short Stories.*
         New York: E.P. Dutton, 1934; *Complete Short Stories.* New
         York: Hanover House, 1955.

5159.   Mayne, Ethel Colburn. "Campaign." *Inner Circle.* New York:
         Harcourt, Brace and World, 1925.

5160.   Merriman, H. Scott. "Sister." *Treasury of Nurse Stories.*
         Compiled by Sonia Barry. New York: Fell, 1962.

5161.   Milton, H. "A Priceless Strand." *New Voices, '64.* New
         York: Macmillan Co., 1964.

5162.   Munro, Alice. "Images." *Dance of the Happy Shades and Other
         Stories.* New York: McGraw-Hill Book Co., 1973.

5163.   Narayan, R.K. "A Breath of Lucifer." *Horse and Two Goats.*
         New York: Viking Press, 1970.

5164.   O'Connor, Frank. "A Great Man." *A Set of Variations.* New
         York: Alfred A. Knopf, 1969.

5165.   O'Donovan, J. "Tinkling Cymbal." *Shadows on the Wall.* New
         York: William Morrow, 1960.

5166.   O'Hara, John. "The Manager." *Hat on the Bed.* New York:
         Random House, 1963. See also *The O'Hara Generation.* New
         York: Random House, 1969.

5167.   Parker, Dorothy (Rothschild). "Horsie." *Short Story Craft.*
         Edited by L.B. Gilkes. New York: Macmillan Co., 1949. See
         also Harpers Bazaar: *It's a Woman's World.* New York:
         McGraw-Hill Book Co., 1944; *Lady's Pleasure.* Penn, 1946;
         After Such Pleasure. New York: Viking, 1933; *Collected
         Stories.* Reprint. New York: Random House, Modern Library,
         n.d.; *Dorothy Parker.* New York: Viking Press, 1939; *Here
         Lies.* New York: Viking Press, 1939; *About Women*, edited by
         H. Reed. Cleveland: World Publishing, 1943; *World's Best
         Doctor Stories*, edited by N.D. Fabricant and H. Werner.
         New York: Garden City Books, 1951; *The Portable Dorothy
         Parker.* New York: Viking Press, 1973.

5168.   Pincherle, Alberto. "The Nurse." *Roman Tales.* New York:
         Farrar, Straus, 1957.

5169. Piper, Arme. "A Moustache from the Past." *Winter's Tales 8.*
       Toronto: A.D. Maclean, 1962.

5170. Proctor, Roy. "Years in Hamburgerland." *Green River Review,*
       1967-1973. Compiled by A. Wilson. University Center,
       MI: Green River Press, 1975.

5171. Reinbold, James S. "Mrs. Staal." *The Secret Life of Our*
       Times, New Fiction from Esquire. Edited by G. Lish.
       Garden City: Doubleday, 1973.

5172. Rice, Call Young. "Out of Darkness." *Winners and Losers.*
       New York: Century, 1925.

5173. Richmond, Grace Louise (Smith). "Off Duty." *Best Stories*
       of Heroism I Know. Compiled by J.C. Minot. Mede, 1934.

5174. Rinehart, Mary (Roberts). "Error in Treatment." *The*
       Romantics. New York: Farrar, 1929.

5175. ———. "Sanctuary." *The Good Housekeeping Treasury.* New
       York: Simon & Schuster, 1960.

5176. ———. "The Secret." *Treasury of Great Mysteries.* Edited
       by H. Haycroft and J. Beecroft. New York: Simon & Schuster,
       1957.

5177. ———. "Twenty-two." *Community Workers of the New York*
       Guild for the Jewish Blind. New York: G.P. Putnam's Sons,
       1924. See also *Love Stories.* New York: Doran, 1919.

5178. Ross, Lenore C. "Angel of Coyote Hills." "Forced Into
       Murder." *Every Girl's Nurse Stories.* Edited by A.L.
       Furman. Mt. Vernon, NY: Lantern Press, 1963. See also
       Teen-age Nurse Stories. Edited by A.L. Furman. Mt. Vernon,
       NY: Lantern Press, 1959.

5179. Number deleted.

5180. Rubens, Robert. "Two Weeks Beyond Shoreditch." *Winter's*
       Tales. 9. New York: St. Martins Press, 1963.

5181. Schein, Bernice. "Bobby." *Datebook Under Twenty.* New
       York: Association Press, 1963.

5182. Schmidt, Iram. "Extra-Duty." *Teenage Party Time Stories.*
       Edited by A.L. Furman. Mt. Vernon, NY: Lantern Press, 1966.

5183. Scott, Hugh Stowell. "Sister." *Great English Short Stories.*
       Edited by L.S. Benjamin and R. Hargreaves. New York:
       Liveright, 1928. See also *World's Best Doctor Stories.*
       Edited by N.D. Fabricant and H. Werner. Garden City:
       Garden City Books, 1951.

5184. Seifert, Elizabeth. "Quiet Night." *Favorite Doctor Stories.*
       Compiled by A.K. Adams. New York: Dodd, Mead, 1963.

5185.   Sitwell, Sir Osbert. "The Woman Who Hated Flowers."
        Treasury of Nurse Stories. Compiled by Sonia Barry.
        New York: Fell, 1962.

5186.   Sobaler, Leonid Sergevich. "His Sweetheart." *Night of the
        Summer Solstice and Other Stories of the Russian War*.
        Edited by M. Van Doren. New York: Holt, Rinehart and
        Winston, 1943.

5187.   Sommers, M.O. "Haven't We Been Nice To You." *American
        Vanguard, 1956*. Cambridge Publishing Co., 1956.

5188.   Spark, Muriel. "The Curtain Blown by the Breeze." *Voices at
        Play*. Philadelphia: J.B. Lippincott, 1962. See also
        Collected Stories I. New York: Alfred A. Knopf, 1968.

5189.   Strickland, Martha. "Willow, Willow, Willow." *Every Girl's
        Nurse Stories*. Edited by A.L. Furman. Mt. Vernon, NY:
        Lantern Press, 1963. See also *Teen-age Nurse Stories*.
        Edited by A.L. Furman. Mt. Vernon, NY: Lantern Press,
        1959.

5190.   Thomas, Audrey Callahan. "Salon des Refusés." *Ten Green
        Bottles*. Indianapolis: Bobbs-Merrill, 1967.

5191.   Thomason, John William. "Born on an Iceberg." *O. Henry
        Memorial Prize Stories of 1930*. Garden City: Doubleday,
        1931. See also *And a Few Marches*. New York: Charles
        Scribner's Sons, 1943; *Salt Winds and Gobi Desert*. New York:
        Charles Scribner's Sons, 1934.

5192.   Timperley, Rosemary. "The Private Torture Chamber." *The
        Fourth Ghost Book*. Edited by J. Turner. Barrie &
        Rockliff, distributed by DuFour, 1965.

5193.   Touhy, Frank. "A Special Relationship." *Winter's Tales. 12*.
        New York: St. Martins Press, 1966. See also *Fingers in the
        Door and Other Stories*. New York: Charles Scribner's Sons,
        1960.

5194.   Turnbull, Agnes (Sligh). "Dear Little Fool." *Saturday
        Evening Post Stories, 1949*. New York: Random House, 1950.
        See also *Love Will Come*. Compiled by A. Stowe. New York:
        Random House, 1959.

5195.   Ullman, James Ramsey. "Between You and I." *Island of the
        Blue Macaws and Sixteen Other Stories*. Philadelphia: J.B.
        Lippincott, 1953.

5196.   Wharton, Edith. "Writing a War Story." *The Collected Stories
        of Edith Wharton Vol. 2*. New York: Charles Scribner's Sons,
        1968.

5197.   Williams, Ben Ames. "The Nurse." *Treasury of Doctor Stories*.
        Compiled by N.D. Fabricant and H. Werner. New York: Fell,

1946. See also *O. Henry Memorial Prize Stories of 1926.*
Garden City: Doubleday, 1927.

5198. Williams, William Carlos. "The Cold World." "The Paid
Nurse." *The Farmer's Daughter.* New York: New Directions,
1961.

5199. Number deleted.

5200. Wilson, Angus. "Mummy to the Rescue." *Such Darling Dodos
and Other Stories.* New York: William Morrow, 1950. See
also *Stories American and British.* Edited by J.B. Ludwig
and W.R. Pourier. New York: Houghton Mifflin, 1953; *A
Chamber of Horrors Unlocked.* Compiled by J. Hadfield.
Boston: Little, Brown & Co., 1965; *Death Dance.* New York:
Viking Press, 1969.

5201. Wilson, William Edward. "The Answer." *My Favorite Stories.*
Edited by M. Daly. New York: Dodd, Mead, 1948. See also
Novel and Story. Edited by E. Sedgwick and H.A. Domin-
covich. Boston: Little, Brown & Co., 1939.

OTHER

5202. Becker, M.L. "Readers Guide: The Nurse in Fiction."
Saturday Review of Literature, No. 21 (1931).

5203. "Nurse in Fiction." *Nation*, 84 (14 Mar 1907), 239-240.

Stroup, Leora B. 3157
Struthers, Lina Rogers 3153
Stuart, Christina 753
Stuart, F.S. 2264
Studdiford, W.E. 3742
Studer-Von Goumoens, Elisabeth 4285
Stuerzbecher, M. 2732, 2733
Sturtevant, G.L. 5006
Subba, Reddy D.V. 4072
Subhadra, V. 3103, 4073
Sudhoff, K. 331
Suhrie, Eleanor 151, 1174, 3394
Suleiman, Louise Wailus 3395
Sullivan, Howard A. 1638
Sullivan, Judith A. 2823
Sultz, Harry A. 2822, 2823
Sumner, A.B. 3104
Sumner, Cid Ricketts 5037
Sumner, Mary R. 3105
Sundaram, S. 4074
Susman, M.P. 1721
Sutherland, Dorothy J. 2265
Sutlittle, Irene 3459
Suwaia, Z. 4198
Suzuki, S. 3396
Svetliakor, A.G. 4368
Swaffield, L. 3946
Swain, Gladys Perers 1959
Swan, John M. 2266
Swann, L. Alline 1266
Swanson, M. 754
Swanson, R. 3397
Sweatt, Anne 2821
Swort, Arlowayne 4831
Syer, A. 3778
Szasz, Thomas 2940

Tabor, Margaret E. 945
Taft, W.H. 4611
Takahashi, M. 4132
Takahashi, T. 4133
Takami, A. 755
Talbott, John H. 1639
Talcott, Agnes G. 3106
Tanner, Margaret C. 241
Tanno, I. 467
Tarnowska, Maria 4199
Tarrant, W.G. 1640
Taylor, Alice 2485
Taylor, E. 781, 955
Taylor, Effie J. 876, 1933, 1934
Taylor, Henry L. 3398
Taylor, Susie King 1974, 4659, 4660

Tayona, S. 2941
Temple, Sara L. 3107
Tenon, J. 3911
Terney, B. 4010
Terrot, Charles 5038
Terrot, S.A. 1976.1, 2389
Terry, Charles E. 2734, 2735
Thatcher, Virginia S. 2778
Thiede, H. 2713
Thoburn, J.M. 4500
Thomas, Adah H. 508
Thomas à Kempis 756
Thomas, Audrey Callahan 5190
Thomas, D.L. 1165, 1641
Thomas, G.M. 4149
Thomas, G. Morton 4727
Thomas, Henry 1165, 1641
Thomas, Herbert 2736-2738
Thomas, Margaret 243, 1805
Thomas, Margaret W. 2739, 4330
Thomason, John William 5191
Thompson, A. 2390
Thompson, A.M.C. 38
Thompson, Alice M. 39
Thompson, C.J. 2459
Thompson, Campbell R. 293
Thompson, Dora E. 2267
Thompson, Julia 4833
Thompson, Morton 5039
Thompson, W.G. 3460
Thompson, William Gilman 4750
Thoms, A.B. 3400, 4661
Thoms, Adah H. 508, 4662
Thoms, Herbert 2737-2739
Thomson, Elnora E. 515, 4834
Thomson, M. 3401, 4175
Thomstad, Beatrice 4751
Thornton, A. 2741
Thorp, Margaret (Farrand) 1961
Thorup, L. 244
Thorvaldsson, Sigridur 4037
Thurelsen, R. 636
Thurston, Herbert 294
Thurston, Violetta 2391
Thwing, Mary Dunning 2852
Tiffany, F. 684
Timperley, Rosemary 5192
Tinckler, L.F. 2392
Tinkham, Catherine 3108
Tippetts, L.M. 1986
Tirpak, H. 2740
Titus, H. 4912
Titus, Shirley 3461, 4612, 5007
Tjader, Marguerite 1073
Todd, Arthur J. 4913